Buildings for the Performing Arts

Buildings for the Performing Arts

A design and development guide

Ian Appleton

Architectural Press
An imprint of Butterworth-Heinemann
Linacre House, Jordan Hill, Oxford OX2 8DP
A division of Reed Educational and Professional Publishing Ltd

ℛ A member of the Reed Elsevier plc group

OXFORD JOHANNESBURG BOSTON
MELBOURNE NEW DELHI SINGAPORE

First published 1996
Reprinted 1997

British Library Cataloguing in Publication Data
A catalogue record for this book is available from the British
Library

Library of Congress Cataloguing in Publication Data
A catalogue record for this book is available from the Library
of Congress

ISBN 0 7506 1276 2

Typeset by Keyword Typesetting Services Ltd,
Wallington, Surrey
Printed in Great Britain
by The Bath Press, Bath

Contents

Preface viii

Part One   The Context   1
1   Introduction   3
2   Types of production   7
3   Audiences   13
4   Types of client   17
5   Building types   21

Part Two   Approach to Design and Development   67
6   Design and development   69
7   The client   71
8   Consultants   77
9   Stages in design and development   79

Part Three   Specific Studies   89
10   Audiences, companies and staff   91
11   Site considerations   95
12   Initial brief: auditorium and platform/stage   101
13   Initial brief: support facilities   157
14   Building design   199
15   Time-scale   211
16   Financial appraisal   213

Appendix 1   References and sources of information   219
Appendix 2   Main consultants and clients' advisors   221

Index   225

Preface

An aspect of the quality of urban and rural life is the provision of places where people can gather in formal and informal settings. Buildings for the performing arts, at the different scales from metropolitan to local, contribute to a pattern of provision with places for people to gather and appreciate performances of music, dance, drama and so on. This Design and Development Guide is concerned with the realization and design of the different building types covering facilities for a range of performing arts.

Architectural design consists of establishing a multiplicity of information, the resolution of apparently conflicting issues and the application of appropriate technologies to satisfy particular social aims. Most situations are complex and buildings for the performing arts are no exception. Indeed the geometry of the auditorium and performance area, the extent of services, the technical necessities, and the public expectations make these particular building types even more complex than the majority. The main purpose of this Guide is to provide those involved in a building project – client, users, and members of the design team (the architect and specialist consultants) – with a framework and checklist to help them communicate more effectively to produce an appropriate solution to a particular problem.

For every building type there is a wide range of variables: a building may be large or small, simple or complex; the client may be a public body, institution, trust, commercial organization or group of volunteers; those involved as clients may be experienced or inexperienced in the process of achieving a new or adapted building; the design team can vary in size and skills, and may or may not have experience with the particular building type; each design team will have their individual method of working. It is difficult to cover the various combinations in detail to provide guidelines for all clients, users and design teams. There is an inevitable concentration in this Guide towards certain situations. In spite of this, it could be used for not only the simplest but also the most complex of projects.

A distinction is made between the processes of design and briefing, and the information on design standards required within those processes. The design and development processes can be described as a progression of defined, but maybe overlapping, stages, whereas the same information can be used within different stages and at different times, and cannot be 'weighted' towards, or selected exclusively within, a particular stage. As examples, the calculation of sightlines in an auditorium features in the initial stages to establish seating numbers as well as during the detailed design stage of the auditorium: the standards for dressing-room layouts do not change through the evolution of the design.

Also there is no single approach to the process of design and development. The content of this guide should not be seen, or used, as a rigid set of instructions but rather as a broad framework which can be adapted to suit individual requirements.

A building for the performing arts is designed and developed at a period within the evolution of the particular art form and technological advancement. There is a wide and expanding set of building types as a consequence of an increasing number of performers wishing to perform. The client, as the usual initiator of a project, should not become locked into a solution by immediate reference to a particular building type such as a concert hall, as a detailed examination of the local conditions may suggest another type. In this respect this guide places an emphasis on feasibility: that is, for the client, with appropriate advice, to evaluate demand, resources and support to ensure viability before progressing with the project.

Guidance is directed towards the main participants in the process of design and development. It is not always possible to distinguish between that which is specifically for the client and that which is the responsibility of others. Whenever possible an indication is given of who is most likely to be responsible for a particular aspect but it is something to be determined by those involved in each project.

The world of the performing arts is full of strong views held by experienced and articulate professionals including managers, technicians and performers, as well as directors, conductors, choreographers, composers, writers, designers and so on: while buildings for the performing arts are required to satisfy the expectations of a knowledgeable public, architectural critics, theatre critics, urbanists, planners, historians, theorists and those for whom the building is just part of their everyday backdrop. Committing descriptions to paper, even in the simple form of checklists and alternatives, will not satisfy all views and will, no doubt, encourage disagreements. Such publications as this tend to encourage generalizations which should not to be confused with the reality of building design and are not a substitute for the skills and dedication required for the resolution of inevitable problems.

This Guide is divided into three parts: Part One The Context provides background information about the organization of the performing arts, some of the prevailing issues, the client types and the various building types covered by this guide.

Part Two Approach to Design and Development identifies the roles of the client, advisors and consultants; the stages to be achieved including client's proposal, feasibility, the processes of briefing, design and building, and, eventually, hand-over and opening night, with a consideration of the building when in use.

In Part Three Specific Studies are identified and discussed as part of the feasibility of the proposal: these cover assessment of demand, site requirements, initial brief, building design, time scale, and financial viability.

Acknowledgements

The publication of comprehensive information covering briefing and design for all building types commenced in the *Architects' Journal* under the guidance of Leslie Fairweather. Material on buildings for the performing arts was provided by Peter Moro, Roderick Ham and myself. One consequence has been the publication of *Theatre Planning*, edited by Roderick Ham, and a second is this publication, which acknowledges a wider range of building types and accommodates the process of design and development. Over the years various people have contributed directly, indirectly and sometimes inadvertently to this publication; they include theatre consultants, architects, engineers, technicians, theatre and concert hall managers, designers, performers, cultural economists, teachers of the performing arts and the librarians at The Arts Council of England and the Scottish Arts Council. Roy McQueen (Scottish Chamber Orchestra), Roger Spence (Assemby Direct), Moira McKenzie (Usher Hall), Barry Wright (Regular Music) and Julian Sleath (Scottish Opera) provided specific information and references. Dr Roger Savage of Edinburgh University oversaw the definitions of performing arts and any historical references and provided infectious enthusiasm for all forms of performance, while Sally Stote of the Arts Council kindly checked a version of the text. Brian Martin of the Arts Management Training Initiative Scotland provided contacts, references and interest. Marjorie Appleton contributed much assistance and patience.

Acknowledgement of photographs include: Fig 5.1a, *Architects Journal*; Fig 5.1b, Gillanders and Mark; Fig 5.2a, *Architectural Review*; Fig 5.2b, *Architectural Review*; Fig 5.3a, Helsinki Opera House; Fig 5.3b, Helsinki Opera House; Fig 5.4a, *Architectural Review*; Fig 5.4b, *Architectural Review*; Fig 5.5a, Donald Mill; Fig 5.5b, *Architects Journal*; Fig 5.6a, RHWL; Fig 5.6b, RHWL; Fig 5.6c, *Architects Journal*; Fig 5.7a, Stephanie Coutourier; Fig 5.7b, Stephanie Coutourier; Fig 5.8a, HOK; Fig 5.8b, HOK; Fig 5.9a, Wembley Arena; Fig 5.10a, Architectural Press; Fig 5.11a, Max Dupain; Fig 5.11b, Max Dupain; Fig 5.12a, Nicholas Groves-Raines; Fig 5.12b, Nicholas Groves-Raines; Fig 5.13a, Richard Bryant; Fig 5.13b, Richard Bryant; Fig 5.14a, *Architects Journal*; Fig 5.14b, *Architects Journal*; Fig 5.15a, Cloud 9 Photography; Fig 5.15b

Appleton Partnership; Fig 5.16a, *Architects Journal*; Fig 5.16b, *Architects Journal*; Fig 5.17a, Tampere Town Hall; Fig 5.17b, Tampere Town Hall; Fig 5.18a, Tim Renton; Fig 5.18b, Tim Renton; Fig 5.19a, Jo Reid and John Peck; Fig 5.19b, Levitt Bernstein; Fig 5.20a, Richard Hamblett; Fig 5.21a, RHWL; Fig 5.21b, RHWL; Fig 5.22a, Hampshire County Council; Fig 5.22b, Hampshire County Council; Fig 5.23a, Denis Coutts; Fig 5.23b, Denis Coutts; Fig 5.24a, Len Burt; Fig 5.25a, *Architects Journal*; Fig 5.25b, *Architects Journal*; Fig 5.26a, *Architects Journal*; Fig 5.26b, *Architects Journal*; Fig 5.27a, Milton Keynes Development Corporation; Fig 5.27b, Milton Keynes Development Corporation; Fig 5.27d, Kenwood House; Fig 5.28f, Mark Humphries; Fig 5.28g, Mark Humphries; Fig 5.30a, *Architects Journal*; Fig 5.31a, Robert Truman; Fig 5.32a, Gianfranco Fianello; Fig 5,32b, Gianfranco Fianello; Fig 5.33, Arup Associates; Fig 12.9a, Nobby Clarke; Fig 12.11a, Frank Wood, Fig 12.11b, *Architects Journal*; Fig 12.12a, *Architects Journal*; Fig 12.12b, *Architects Journal*; Fig 12.12c, *Architects Journal*; Fig 12.14a, RMJM; Fig 12.17t, *Architects Journal*; Fig 12.36a, Percy Thomas Partnership; Fig 12.36b, *Architects Journal*; Fig 12.36c, *Architects Journal*; Fig 12.36d, *Architects Journal*; Fig 12.36e, *Architects Journal*; Fig 12.36f, *Architectural Review*; Fig 12.36g, Richard Davies; Fig 12.36h, Kors and Ine van Bennekom; Fig 12.36i, Paul White; Fig 12.36j, *Architects Journal*; Fig 12.36k, *Architects Journal*; Fig 12.36l, James R. Grieves; Fig 12.36m, *Architects Journal*; Fig 12.36n, Peter Walsar, Fig 12.36o, Arup Associates; Fig 12.36p, Hurd Rolland; Fig 12.36q, Peter Rourke; Fig 12.36r, HHPA; Fig 12.37b, Percy Thomas Partnership; Fig 12.37c, *Architects Journal*; Fig 12.40e, *Architects Journal*; Fig 12.40f, *Architects Journal*; Fig 12.48ai, Mark Fisher; Fig 12.48aii, Mark Fisher; Fig 12.51a, Paul White; Fig 12.51b, A. S. Green; Fig 13.1a, Alan McCrone; Fig 13.1b, *Architects Journal*; Fig 13.1c, Appleton Partnership; Fig 13.1d, *Architects Journal*; Fig 13.1e, Martii Jaatinen; Fig 13.1f, *Architects Journal*; Fig 13.4a, *Architects Journal*.

Ian Appleton

Part One
The Context

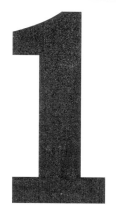

1 Introduction

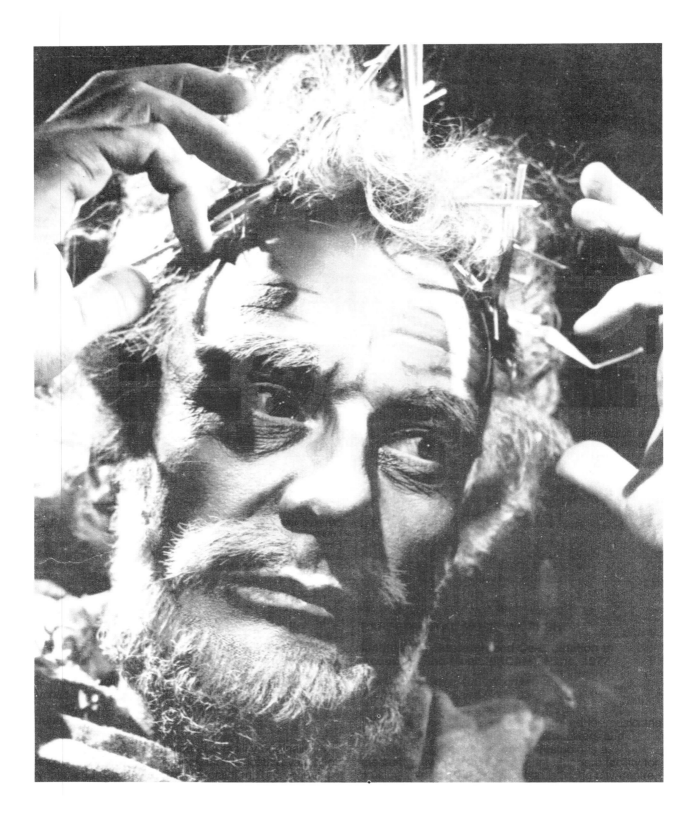

The performing arts cover forms of music (orchestral, choral, pop/rock and jazz), opera, musicals, dance and drama. This Guide concentrates on these. It is acknowledged that the performing arts also cover music-theatre, musical comedies, music-hall, variety, vaudeville, puppet shows, revues, mime, cabaret, folk music, live art, and street performers, as well as experimental theatre, military tattoos and circuses. Essentially though the performing arts are concerned with a space for a live performance experienced by an audience within a set period of time. The space is defined by specific technical and spatial demands and requires a conducive atmosphere for both audience and performer.

The format, an audience focused on the platform or stage, has not changed as an experience since performers first wished to perform and audiences wished to hear and see a performance. Technology has developed, expectations adjusted and experiences have widened, while social aspects, including erosion of social divisions within auditoria and improved status of performers, have reflected changes in the wider society. The expectation is for professional music, dance, drama and other types of performing arts to be available to all in congenial auditoria, and also for facilities to be generally available in the community for amateur groups to perform as a leisure activity.

The performing arts are born of the creative processes of writing plays, composing music, choreographing dance, directing productions and designing settings: realization is found through conductors, musicians, singers, dancers, actors and other performers. All are developing and new music, opera, musicals, dance, drama and other forms of performing art continue to be created. They require the opportunity to be staged within traditional or new methods of presentation, while established works, as well as being staged in traditional and time-honoured ways, are also subject to re-interpretation or presentation in different formats. Experiment in the performing arts may bring new forms of auditorium: electronic music compositions have challenged the requirements of the concert hall whose traditional forms are based on non-amplified acoustic instruments. Similarly promenade drama presentations do not require fixed seating and stage positions, the characteristic of traditional theatre auditoria, while street theatre with only nominal technical back-up contrasts with the increasing sophistication of stage machinery and sound and lighting technology for ever larger theatrical productions.

The pattern of provision includes buildings, either for a resident company or for receiving touring companies, owned and managed by local government, commercial enterprises, private trusts and voluntary bodies. The ratio of public and private provision varies according to country – from complete public provision to predominantly commercial enterprises with a variety of combinations in between, while public funding of the performing arts is, as an example, relatively low in the USA and relatively high in Germany. The principle,

however, of public funding to sustain and support the performing arts is a characteristic of most countries in the developed world, as orchestras, choral groups, opera houses, theatres, etc. rarely balance their books with expenditure exceeding income. They require subsidies as grants from central government agencies and local government as well as commercial sponsorship, and monies from lotteries, foundations and individuals. A consequence has been the close examination of the cultural, social and economic roles of new and existing provision, as well as the adoption of budgeting and marketing techniques and the expansion of income-earning activities to include, for example, conferences to reduce the deficit. Political arguments range from no public intervention to full public control with the actual policy establishing a balance between both, according to the political climate and cultural traditions of a country. The ratio of public to private contribution can change over time with the tension between the conflicting approaches ever present. Justification of support for both capital and revenue funding have included one or more of the following reasons:

- *cultural*: to safeguard an aspect of cultural heritage; continuity of art forms, display of performing skills and sustaining national, local or ethnic traditions; to retain and improve an existing stock of facilities and established companies for the performing arts, or to provide new facilities to ensure cultural opportunities.
- *economic*: direct employment of staff and performers; benefits to secondary businesses such as poster and programme printing and material supply; a widening of the tourist and conference market which, in turn, brings money into the town or city; an attraction to encourage relocation, and location of organizations, institutions, industry and commerce in an area with subsequent employment benefits.
- *educational*: to cultivate an appreciation of the art forms through the exposure of audiences to examples; to form part of an educational programme for schoolchildren, students and those in adult education.
- *prestige*: international, national, regional, city or town comparison; re-inforcement of regional identity emphasizing dispersal from metropolitan focus.
- *quality of life*: performing arts as acceptable complementary activities to work and domestic obligations as a positive use of leisure time which enriches life culturally and also socially.
- *regeneration*: part of a wider programme to re-vitalize an existing city or town centre or to assist in the formation of a new community, to attract industry, commerce, institutions, housing, and so on.
- *cultural democracy*: to stimulate and foster participation in the performing arts by all sections of a community, defined locally, as a creative activity.

General policy for the performing arts tends not to be subject to a national or regional plan in the same way as, say, the organization of health care generates a network of facilities. Provision within the performing arts often emerges from local pressure groups in response to local circumstances. However central government agencies and local government have tended to have their own master plan against which a proposal may be evaluated. This is especially the case if public funds – as grants and revenue subsidies – are involved, where evaluation is the basis of accountability. The roles of the local pressure group and particular individuals should be emphasized as a frequent moving force to initiate and sustain interest in new provision or building adaptation.

Public policy over the geography of provision tends to be focused on giving all sections of the population the opportunity to have access to the performing arts. General policy attempts to avoid *ad hoc* provision to achieve a more coherent plan. The two main areas of concern are the fostering of the highest quality in professional performances and the participation of the public in the performing arts as spectators and amateur performers within local communities. For a given budget, there can be a dilemma over the distribution of funds towards either a concentration on a single major project such as an opera house or a dispersal among community-based projects. This type of dilemma occurs in all sections of public life and debate: invest in the eradication of the common cold experienced by virtually all or a kidney machine for the few, concentrate resources in tertiary education at the expense of primary, and so on. All are concerned with scarce resources and factional interests in the public arena. A distinction for the performing arts lies in their historical and social associations, as well as the values expressed within them: so the content, including the often provocative nature of the performing arts, invades the debate. Actual policy however may be mainly determined by inherited values and facilities: the type of concert hall, theatre, community facility, and so on that are already available; the crisis brought about when a building for a performing art is about to be demolished, an orchestra finds itself on the verge of bankruptcy, and so on.

The history of buildings for the performing arts in the last half century is full of good intentions, and examples can be cited where the project has fallen on fallow ground or held in extended abeyance, relying only on faith rather than the understanding of the economic and social reality and the politics of provision.

2

2 Types of production

The initial consideration in the design and development of a building for performing arts is the choice of production (or productions) to be accommodated. Production type determines size and type of auditorium and the support facilities. Each of the performing arts has its own history, traditions and conventions.

Classical music

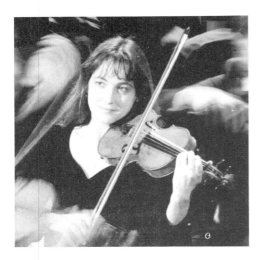

There are various types and scales of classical music which are defined by the size of orchestra (number of instrumentalists) and/or choir (number of singers):

- symphony orchestra with an average of 90 players but may be up to 120, plus sometimes a choir of 100 or more, with conductor and possibly vocal and instrumental soloists.
- chamber orchestra with up to 40–50 players, with conductor, sometimes soloists, and/or small choir.
- small ensemble, with recitals including instrumentalists and soloists.

With orchestral and choral concerts of classical music, the format for live performances has not changed in principle since the formalization of the concert in the early nineteenth century: the conductor standing centrally and in front of the orchestra, usually on a rostrum, with adjacent soloists and choir behind the orchestra. The number of performers may change within an evening's programme of music, but the basic focus of the orchestra, choir and soloists on the conductor remains; though in piano concerts, the piano and player are in front of the conductor on the platform. Some modern orchestral compositions can challenge this traditional format with, for example, the soloists dispersed among the members of the orchestra (sometimes moving about during the performance) and even within the audience seating.

The quality of the sound as received by the listeners – the audience – is paramount and the acoustic requirements for the appreciation of the music is a fundamental condition. However the development of classical music has also experienced variation in the acoustical environment. Until the nineteenth century, music was composed in response to its environment, with, as an example, the liturgical recitation in the basilican church using the effect of the long reverberation time as an integral part of the music. The present-day programming of music requires the understanding historically of the relationship between the composer and the acoustics of the space for which the music was originally written. As well as liturgical music, other periods have distinct characteristics with the rapid music of Mozart and his immediate followers contrasting with the late romantic and choral music and modern classical music. The design of auditoria therefore needs to be suitable for many kinds of classical music, composed in a wide variety of circumstances. Consideration should be given also to the needs of the small ensemble or solo pianist and singer where the acoustic requirements suggest a separate (and more intimate) recital room.

Opera

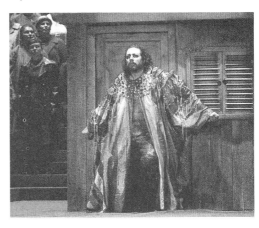

There are various scales of opera production: *large-scale opera* with casts over 200 including principals and chorus and an orchestra of up to 120 players; *standard opera* which consists of medium-scale productions with casts up to 100 including principals and chorus and an orchestra of up to 50 players; *chamber opera* which consists of small-scale productions with casts up to 15 including principals and chorus and an orchestra of up to 20 players; opera as *spectacle* which has cast and orchestra as for large-scale opera but the extent of the stage area, production extravagance and audience numbers are larger.

Opera combines music and drama, each of which modifies the other, and it is an entertainment of ceremony and ritual. Dialogue is mostly in verse and sung to orchestral accompaniment. The primary classification is music with the lyrics as an important element, with the components of conductor, orchestra, principal singers (tenor, baritone, contralto, soprano and so on), chorus of singers and, possibly, dancers.

The scenic setting simulates a particular location and heightens the theatrical context.

For the audience, the quality of music is paramount and, as with classical music, acoustics is a fundamental issue, as are good sightlines. The experience also includes the evocation of atmosphere on the stage and the visual composition of performers and scenic setting.

The traditional format for opera performances has not changed greatly since the initial public opera houses: the proscenium stage with the orchestra in a pit between audience and stage. This form has allowed the conductor in front of the orchestra to control not only the musicians but also the singers on the stage. Opera is illusionary which is not wholly realistic and is necessarily a conventional form of art.

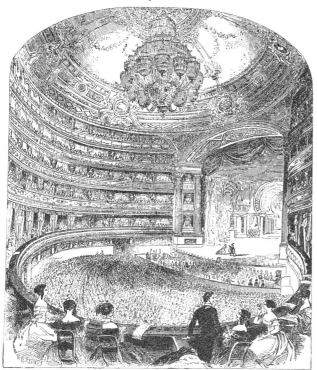

Royal Opera House, Covent Garden, London

The rise of opera began in the sixteenth century. In the hands of Claudio Monteverdi, opera became a vehicle of increased dramatic expression. The first public opera house was opened in Venice in the seventeenth century and took opera a stage further forward from being merely the pastime of princes. The subsequent development of the Italian opera house with elaborate ornamentation, plush furnishings and tiers of boxes about a horseshoe form, provided suitable acoustic conditions for the music of Mozart and subsequent generations of composers. Two further influences were the growing tradition for the audience to see attendance as a social occasion, and the application of the laws of perspective to the stage setting. The large stage and the need to change scenery rapidly within a performance also saw the

introduction of the flytower over the stage and large side and rear stages.

The acoustic and presentation requirements for opera have meant that the traditional format has remained as the predominant solution.

However Wagner did revolutionize the scheme of opera: music, poetry and scenic effect were to have equal importance; the auditorium to be single raked and fan shaped to achieve social democracy; the reverberation time lengthened; the orchestra pit increased in size and was set further under the fore-stage. These aims are seen at his own opera house at Bayreuth, Germany. The basic format though – the proscenium stage, orchestra pit and audience with the conductor as the visual pivot – stayed the same. But the two traditions remain: the Italian opera house with its short reverberation time suitable for Mozartian operas, and Wagnerian opera with different acoustic conditions and greater blending of the orchestra with the singer. The modern opera house is often required to combine these if it is to offer a programme of the major historical productions plus contemporary pieces, usually in repertoire.

Technology has not dramatically changed the traditional format. However, electronic devices allow larger numbers to attend a single performance (with video screens projecting action on the stage and by using amplification), while less costly and physically smaller productions with a small orchestra using amplification (as developed by the Stockholm Folk Opera) makes touring easier and enables larger numbers to experience opera in often modest and rural facilities. With both these examples the intention is to make opera more accessible to the public: the mass audience at one venue and the increasing ease of touring to dispersed populations.

Dance

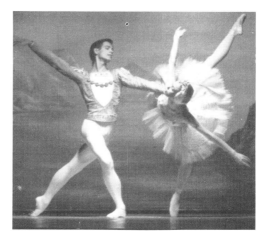

Dance is essentially a form of performance in which a company of dancers perform (usually without words), with expressive physical movements, to music which can be live, recorded or electronic. Dance is conveniently divided into ballet and modern dance.

Ballet is an amalgam of time-honoured conventions, with contemporary innovations, which began in Italy, matured in France in the beginning of the seventeenth century as a separate art form (previously as a combination of opera and ballet) and achieved classic status by the mid-nineteenth century. Twentieth-century development centred in Russia under the impresario, Diaghilev. Thereafter ballet companies in the metropolitan cities in USA, Europe and English-speaking countries have continued its traditions, presenting programmes of classical ballets and new works within the ballet conventions.

Ballet productions can consist of a cast of up to 100 including the soloists and *corps de ballet*, and an orchestra of up to 50 players. The components include conductor, orchestra, soloists (male and female) and *corps de ballet* within a scenic setting. The format is as for opera: the proscenium stage with orchestra in a pit between audience and stage. The conductor is in a pivotal position. For the audience the quality of the music and visual composition as well as the interpretation of the work within the ballet conventions are essential.

Modern dance is concerned with the expression through the physical movement of the performers in a realistic or abstract context, accompanied by live or recorded music (classical, jazz, pop/rock), electronic music and no music. While classical ballet is defined by specific formal movements, conventions and routines, modern dance has extended and supplemented these traditions and explored expression through movement in response to a wide range of themes, musical forms and ethnic dances. The second half of the twentieth century has seen the expansion of dance in America, Europe and other English-speaking countries with the strong influence of companies led by Martha Graham and Merce Cunningham in the USA who can be identified as the pioneers.

Two formats may be considered for the presentation of modern dance: the traditional relationship, as for ballet, with the orchestra pit between stage and audience; no orchestra pit if the performance relies on taped music, or musicians on or off stage. The lack of orchestra and modest setting associated with modern dance productions can be economical and make them easier to take on tour than traditional ballet productions.

Musicals

Musicals follow a similar format to the description under opera, with soloists, chorus, dancers, orchestra and conductor: the stage/orchestra pit/audience relationship remains the same as for opera, with the same pivotal role of the conductor. Extensive stage scenery and often spectacular staging effects rely on the ease of change that a flytower and large side and rear stages offer.

Amplification of the music is accepted, and, with the use of video coverage of the conductor so that he is seen on screen by the performers, has questioned the

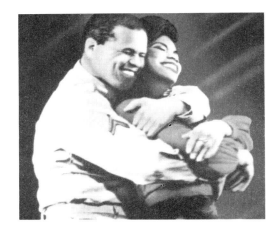

position of the orchestra in its traditional location between stage and audience. The orchestra can be located away from the stage area in a specially designed room. The music is received by the audience through the amplification system.

The musical is essentially a twentieth-century performing art which developed from nineteenth-century Parisian and Viennese operetta and the light operas of Gilbert and Sullivan of the late nineteenth century. The tradition and conventions were developed by the American musical in the 1920s, with a particular boost in the 1940s. Since the 1950s development seems to have occurred either side of the Atlantic. The musical has become recognized as part of theatre heritage and certain musicals are now hailed as classics.

Jazz

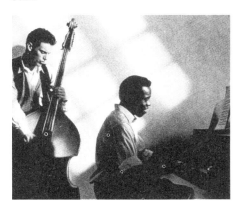

Jazz, born in New Orleans from African-American roots, has absorbed gospel, dance band, folk, gypsy and other music and has developed in content and musicianship worldwide. Styles vary and evolve but the combination of ensemble and solo playing, strong rhythm, improvisation and showmanship in presentation remain.

Jazz has risen to the formal location of the concert hall from the informal, often basement, atmosphere of the club. Jazz performances have borrowed the format of the concert hall and recital room for the appreciation of the music. The club scale is concerned with the intimacy of the experience for audience and performer and is usually connected with the activities of eating and drinking. Provision exclusively for jazz music is rare and it is the club location which predominates.

The number of players vary from solo, trio, groups up to 10, and orchestras up to 30 with soloists as instrumentalists and singers. Amplification is an accepted feature of the music and indeed for orchestral works can be an integral part of the performance.

Pop/rock music

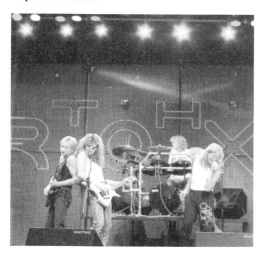

For concerts of popular music, the orchestra is usually on the stage behind the singers and dancers in the tradition of the dance band and hall. The focus is on the principal singer or group of singers supplemented by dancers and other singers. The orchestra can be up to 50 musicians. Amplification of the music is normal.

The rock concert tends to be only for a group of instrumentalists and/or singers. Not only is amplification a normal ingredient of the music but also the electronic guitar is an essential instrument in the development of the music. Rock music has borrowed from jazz, folk and popular music, and is constantly evolving: once classified, the music is immediately re-defined. It has developed a variety of distinctive approaches including theatrical staging and lighting effects which can be on large and spectacular scales.

Both popular music and rock music are closely linked to the recording industry with concerts consisting of touring singers and groups whose popularity is defined by the record sales. Such concerts play to large and very large (mass) audiences.

The mass audience can range from 10 000 to 30 000 and considerably more, usually as one-off events with temporary staging and facilities. Sports stadia, gardens of stately homes and open spaces have been adapted to accommodate such concerts for outdoor events, as have large indoor enclosures, such as the arena. Large video screens and amplification aid the visual and aural presentation. Rock music is also played on a much smaller scale in clubs, usually with the club owner as promoter, who books groups to perform in relatively modest venues.

Scale apart, the format remains simple with a raised stage and the audience facing the stage. A fore-stage may extend into the audience for the principal singer.

Drama

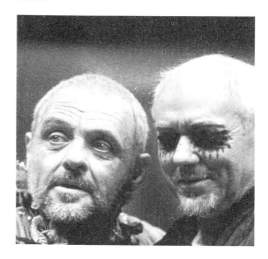

There are various scales of drama production: *medium* or normal scale which consists of casts of up to 20, *large* scale such as Shakespearean histories with many extras, and *small* scale with casts restricted to under 10 (this scale refers to the small touring company playing in studio and school theatres.) For medium and large scales an orchestra may be required of up to 10 players.

Drama productions (also referred to as plays) are essentially concerned with the spoken word, but also to a great extent with facial expressions and body language. They are presented by a company of actors within a scenic setting to a script by a playwright and under the interpretation of a director. The performance aims include comprehension of the text, interpretation through dramatic effect and the communication with the audience by the acting and setting. The acoustic aim is to ensure that every member of the audience can hear clearly the spoken word: the visual aim is for the audience to see the facial expressions and physical gestures of the actors. Actors require that they can command the audience while the stage space and scenery neither dwarf nor crowd them.

Prior to the mid-nineteenth century, one particular format for drama tended to dominate its particular period and country: Euripides wrote his plays for the amphitheatres in Hellenistic Greece, as an example. The late nineteenth and twentieth centuries, however, have seen a full vocabulary of past experience and forms available to the auditorium and stage designer, with the formats classified broadly under the proscenium stage and open stage.

The *proscenium stage* may be seen as the mainstream format, as the direct descendant of the Baroque horseshoe opera house. The format places the audience so that they are facing the acting area on one side only: the audience sees the acting area through an architectural opening. The acting area may project a nominal distance into the auditorium as a fore-stage or apron. The audience and actors are, in effect, in separate rooms. The proscenium opening creates a limited but unified fixed frame for the pictorial composition of the performance. Scenery can be developed as a major design element.

The *open stage* formats are those arrangements where the audience in part, or wholly, surround the acting area, and descend from Greek, Roman, Restoration and Elizabethan theatres, with links also to classical oriental theatre. They place the audience in the same space as the performance, in possibly larger numbers and at less cost, and consequently places the audience closer to the performance. Open stage formats heighten the three-dimensional and live nature of a performance. They require particular approaches from directors and actors, in order to accommodate the diffused orientation of the performance and the particular difficulties of exits and entrances onto the stage – including from the audience. With open stage formats, scenery does not necessarily play such a significant role as tends to be the case with the proscenium stage. The legitimacy of the advocacy of an open stage format lies in part with historical precedent (Shakespeare wrote for a thrust open stage as seen at the Globe Theatre) but also with concern for the heightened sensation of the art of a drama performance.

Selection of format seems to be underlined by two related issues:

- There are two broad categories of play type: the naturalistic and the epic. The former is concerned with simulating a slice of reality, whereas the epic category does not accept the illusion of realism and acknowledges the characters as actors, settings as symbols and the stage equipment (for example, the stage lighting) as part of the performance. The naturalistic play is more sympathetically presented within the proscenium format while with the open stage it is less easy to accommodate the illusionary content of naturalism and so it is the preferred home of the epic approach.
- Plays may have been strictly written to a particular format or may be assumed to require accommodation within the predominant format of the time of writing. Artistic policy may respond to the original context following a measure of historical authenticity and thus require a reproduction of that format, or play selection may be limited to match the available format.

3

3 Audiences

The experience of attending a performance by members of an audience is not restricted to the time spent in the auditorium. Five distinct sequential phases can be identified: each requires to be satisfied and all affect marketing, location and accessibility, and the standard of building, management and performance.

1. Planning and anticipation – audience members must:

- have knowledge of and made a selection of performance: awareness by advertising, reviews, word of mouth;
- organize friends and relations;
- have time available for attendance, including travel;
- assess cost of attendance, including ticket, refreshments, travel;
- have an accessible method of purchasing tickets.

2. Travel to facility – audience members need to decide upon:

- travel time and method (walking, car, bus, coach, train), which will be affected by
- ease of parking or convenience of public transport.

3. Experience of facility – impressions will be formed of:

- sequence of activities to and from seating: quality of entrance, foyer, cloakroom, toilets, auditorium;
- quality of the performance: ability to see and hear; content of play, show or concert; ability of performers, and directors/choreographer/conductor;
- associated activities such as eating, drinking and visits to art gallery, exhibitions and shops;
- staff response to public: box office, access to seats, directions.

4. Travel from facility – in addition to travelling before a performance, post-performance factors include:

- travel time and method;
- convenience of public transport (if appropriate) with services running after a performance a critical issue.

5. Recollection – after the event audience members will:

- evaluate the quality of the experience. This phase may commence the cycle again for another visit to the facility.

Studies of the social characteristics of audiences attracted to existing facilities for the performing arts have shown broadly the attributes of the traditional participant in musical and theatrical activities. Characteristics though vary according to type and quality of production with classical music, pop/rock, opera, musicals, dance and drama attracting almost distinct audiences. Travel times vary also and relate to production quality and type: for example, those who attend opera performances tend to travel further than those for drama, while the Royal National Theatre company on tour will attract audiences from a larger area than the local dramatic society can.

Therefore a simple calculation based on a catchment area (defined by the number of people living within a certain distance of a proposed building) does not indicate the correct potential for participation. The potential requires the identification of those who have the characteristics of the traditional audience with distance being defined by the travel time to and from the proposed building. However this provides only the *potential* market: the *actual* market is subject to the particular programme, quality of facility, costs, awareness through publicity, tradition of participation in musical events and theatre-going in the area and the effect of competing leisure attractions for the same market. In addition there is the *embryonic* market, made up of the non-traditional participants. Studies should be carried out to establish the reasons why people do not attend performances to identify those barriers. These may include cost, distance and time, but may also relate to the experience, including the quality of the building design.

There are 3 further groups of users who may require consideration:

- public use of non-performance spaces such as restaurant, coffee bar and bar as informal activities;
- groups and organizations using the auditorium for non-performance activities such as conferences, lectures and commercial presentations;
- meeting rooms for hire by groups and organizations within the building complex for activities not necessarily related to attendance at a performance: seminars, gatherings, social occasions.

Each of these relates to availability within the general programme of events and are examples of management policies to maximize the use of facilities primarily provided for the function of the performance.

Changes in audience numbers

The counter-attraction of other leisure activities, in particular cinema and television, saw the decline in attendance at the performing arts, and exacerbated by the rising costs of productions and theatre buildings were perceived as becoming obsolete. Recent decades have arrested and indeed reversed this decline. This trend has been the result of various factors which have included:

- Changes in supply: the improved quality of the facilities, with increased audience comfort as an example. Ancillary accommodation, such as bars and restaurants, has become more attractive for the public. Facilities for performers and technicians have improved substantially. New and noticeably improved buildings, less civic in character, have generated interest and stimulated attendance.

- Improvement of the product – the live performance – in content and presentation.
- Marketing has become more positive and exposure for the performing arts has widened in the media in general.
- Active support from the public sector for music, dance, and drama, endorsed by a political concern to sustain cultural activities. Subsidies in the form of government grants have removed both deficits and the pressure to be profitable. A result has been the allowance of a level of risk in form and content which has made experiment possible. This has encouraged in particular new writing, musical composition and developments in dance, as well as live art and new collaborative work.
- The level of tourism has grown due to increased affluence in the population and improved, and less costly, travel arrangements. A result has been for live performances to become an identifiable attraction for the tourist visiting a city. The West End theatres in London, for example, rely on and are sensitive to, the tourist market. The music/drama festival has proliferated, and many cities and towns benefit from annual general and specialist festivals, with visitors from within a country and abroad as cultural tourists.
- Higher educational attainment, more disposable income and increased mobility – all attributes of the traditional public for the performing arts – among the population as a whole have contributed to an increased demand. Also specific management policies have reduced perceived barriers, encouraging non-traditional members of an audience to become involved as viewers of, or even participants in, the performing arts.
- The decline of the use of the city centre has been halted. The decline was the result of the increased spread of low density suburban areas, the relocation of rental outlets and offices to out-of-town sites, parking difficulties, and, in some cities, an adverse reputation, with a consequential reduction in transport systems serving the centre. Each contributed to the decline in numbers of people with ease of access of a city centre facility. Housing, shopping and work have been encouraged back, while transport networks have improved access and car parking facilities.
- An increase in real leisure time remains debatable. Any real increase has not released blocks of time suitable for the attendance at a performance which usually takes 3–4 hours. However increased time does affect the non-performance use of facilities, the participation in community music and drama as an active recreation, and, with an increasing elderly population for example, groups in society with periods of time during the day available for active and passive involvement in the performing arts.
- The perception of programmes as being part of a wider role: organization of travel facilities, provision of all-day activities in the facility, organization of supporter's clubs, special programmes to attract young people, co-operation with local education authorities with visits to schools through a Theatre-in-Education programme.

While audience numbers and those participating actively in music and drama increase, the performing arts remains a minority activity with variations in popularity among the production types. Probably the pop concert, rock concert and musicals attract the largest numbers within a population, while experimental drama will rely on a particularly small following however ardent their interest.

4

4 Types of client

There are various types of client for buildings for the performing arts covering public bodies, commercial organizations, private institutions and voluntary organizations. This chapter indicates the broad groups of potential clients and their potential contribution.

Local government

Local government can be concerned with three main building types for the performing arts, each having a distinct public policy. These cover the following building types:

- Facilities with a resident professional company for music, ballet, dance or drama. The building may be seen as a focus for regional activity with the company touring around the region. The capital expenditure and company are supported by grants and subsidies from local taxes and central government. Subsidies to companies tend to be on an annual basis.
- Facilities to host touring companies. Buildings to meet the requirements of the subsidized national touring companies, commercial companies and local amateur companies performing opera, musicals and dance. These regional touring buildings are a link with the metropolitan centre. With buildings receiving touring companies, there may be little distinction between the local government and commercial facilities. The local government hires out the facility with a charge which covers overheads, permanent staff, publicity and profit.
- Facilities for community use. Community facilities vary considerably. They do, however, serve local requirements including performances by amateur companies as well as by touring medium- and small-scale professional companies.

Educational institutions

This category includes:

- Places of higher education specializing in the teaching of, and training for, music and drama performances, including stage management, design and administration as well as development of music and drama skills.
- Departments in Universities and Colleges concerned with the study of music and drama including performance.
- State and private schools concerned with the appreciation of music and drama including development of skills. A school may be the location of a Theatre-in-Education programme.

Facilities for the performing arts may be exclusively attached to a teaching programme and the location for student or schoolchild performance, or made available for public performances as well.

Facilities may be sponsored by a place of higher education providing concert hall, recital room or theatre as for public and student access and not attached to a teaching department. Such an approach is a link with the local community.

University theatres have tended to be experimental in design and have made a significant contribution to their local community. Local educational authorities have been encouraging the use of schools for community use especially during times when schools are closed.

Commercial sector

The commercial contribution is to sell live performances for profit. The financial aim influences the selection of production type, audience capacities, ancillary accommodation and location. Various arrangements can exist:

- A building may be for a company's own use. This category of owner–occupier includes buildings which host touring companies, which are permanent homes of professional companies, and metropolitan theatres (such as West End theatres in London and Broadway theatres in New York) which present new productions where long runs make it possible to stage elaborate productions which would be uneconomic elsewhere.
- A building may be provided as a speculative project with an unknown occupier or for occupation by a known occupier, by sale or lease, which could be another commercial organization, local government or private trust.
- A building might be provided as part of a large development with the brief for a performing arts facility provided by the local government. In effect, the commercial organization, as developer, pays for the new facility – to be occupied by others – in return for permission to build the more lucrative sections of the overall development.
- The development may replace an existing building for the performing arts within a larger commercial re-development which increases the density of the site.

A further role of the commercial sector is as promoter of music, dance and drama productions. A promoter arranges performers/company, venues and programme.

Commercial organizations can be small (perhaps owning a single facility), medium sized (owning a few facilities) and large (with an extensive set of buildings not just for the performing arts but a multiplicity of leisure provision).

The commercial sector used to be the exclusive provider. Competition from cinema and television reduced audience numbers and the costs of production increased, which made the performing arts financially unattractive. A consequence was a reduction in the contribution of the commercial sector which, in Britain tended to concentrate its efforts in the West End of London, a few regional cities and popular resorts. Professional touring companies remained but reduced the extent of their activities concentrating on proven successes for their main productions. The number of buildings receiving touring companies diminished with the remaining few often purchased by local government or subject to a conservation policy which halted their demolition.

However, recent decades have seen an increase in the commercial touring company although the type of production has changed: drama with celebrity stars, proven musicals initiated in the metropolitan centre, pop/rock concerts responding to record sales popularity and entertainments.

Private trust

A trust is an independent organization which tends to be a registered charity and a non-profit making limited company. The client is usually a board of trustees with funds obtained from a wide range of sources including central and local government, industry and commerce, and through professional fund raising activity. Funds from the public sector are an essential component of the finances.

Voluntary sector

Some facilities for the performing arts are run privately by voluntary organizations like a music or drama amateur company, a religious organization or a society such as the Young Men's Christian Association (YMCA) who might wish to provide a facility for their own use, either with general public access to performances or with access restricted to members. The provision may be exclusively for the performing arts or might supplement principal activities such as within a church.

Capital funds may come from private sources, fund-raising activities, or grants from trust bodies, a national body or public funds. Amateur companies are usually not subsidized as professional companies are but may receive a grant from local government as a local voluntary organization. The amateur drama, music and choral tradition is an important characteristic of local, social and cultural life.

Provision includes:

- hiring of theatre or concert hall;
- purpose-built facilities;

- hiring of local village hall, church hall, community centre or school hall/facility.

Community organization

Such an organization serves a community, defined territorially. The client comprises representatives of the community the facility serves. A characteristic of such an organization is their direct control over the resources, management and facility. Their aim is to involve all sections of the community in the performing arts, as performers and audience, with the facility also available for small-scale professional touring groups. A distinction is made between predominately professional venues for the performing arts and the facilities involving communities which are essentially amateur and educational.

Funds are available from the public sector and fund raising: the organization may be registered as a charity.

The 1970s saw a dramatic expansion in community-based art centres. These are non-institutional in character, consisting of a resource-based centre as provision and multi-purpose by nature. Participation by various groups in the community is in not just the performing arts but in arts in general and also in social activities: all encouraged by an active management. There has been a tendency for such centres to be conversions of suitable existing buildings.

Approaches towards community theatre range from the simple provision of a theatre or auditorium for amateur use, to situations where the mere participation of members of the community is the aim and overrides any consideration of quality. Participation is the main objective, including creating as well as spectating. The *animator*, associated with community arts centres, stimulates and fosters the participation by all sections of the community in the performing arts as spectators and performers.

Other client bodies

Others may regard performances as supplementary activities to a principal activity such as those within a museum, art gallery or church with, for example, music recitals.

5

5 Building types

Buildings for the performing arts are grouped together in this book to discuss their design and development, since they share common features and, as institutions, many of the same concerns. There are also important distinctions, with each of the performing arts having its own specific requirements. The common feature of all buildings is the core activity of the live performance and the reciprocal experience between audience and performer. To cater for the wide range of requirements for the different performing arts, various building types have emerged such as concert hall, opera house, theatre and so on. The majority are purpose-designed around a predominant activity, while others may be part of a multi-purpose space or a secondary activity to a non-performance primary activity.

The categories of building types can follow the conventional names such as the concert hall, opera house or theatre. However within these categories there are variations and a wide interpretation. A more realistic definition of a category should consider the following factors:

- Location: defined by catchment area, numbers in the population and level of accessibility:
  - metropolitan centre,
  - regional centre,
  - town centre,
  - neighbourhood centre,
  - resort: urban, rural, seaside,
  - specialist centre,
  - one-off event.
- Owner and/or occupier:
  - local government,
  - educational institution,
  - commercial organization,
  - private trust,
  - voluntary organization,
  - community organization.
- Type of production:
  - predominant type of production: classical music, opera dance, musicals, jazz, pop/rock music, drama,
  - combination of compatible productions and/or other activities, such as sports, in a multi-purpose auditorium.
- Auditorium form:
  - proscenium stage format,
  - open platform/stage format: single direction, partially or fully surrounding the performance area by the audience,
  - combination of formats.
- Seating capacity, standard and scale of auditorium:
  - under 250,
  - 250–500,
  - 500–1000,
  - 1000–1500,
  - 1500–2000,
  - 2000 +,
  - mass audience events.
- Role of facility:
  - housing resident professional company,
  - hosting touring professional companies or groups,
  - for community use,
  - for teaching purposes,
  - for festival use.
- Production selection:
  - new works,
  - established works,
  - experimental.
- Pattern of use
  - repertoire (several productions are presented intermittently),
  - repertory (productions run for a limited period),
  - seasonal,
  - one-off event.
- Audience type and numbers:
  - open to all,
  - restricted to a particular section of the public, e.g. children,
  - targeted towards a particular section of the public,
  - tourists.
- Financial policy:
  - profit making,
  - non-profit making with or without subsidies.
- Building policy:
  - permanent or temporary,
  - indoor or outdoor,
  - formal or informal,
  - degree of adaptation,
  - standard of provision, including space allocation, finishes and fittings, environmental factors such as ventilation, acoustics, sound isolation to the auditorium.
- Associated activities:
  - complementary functions in auditorium, e.g. conference,
  - production facilities on site if resident producing company,
  - public facilities such as bars and restaurant,
  - other arts facilities,
  - other activities.
- Building complex
  - more than one auditorium and support facilities,
  - larger complex, such as an educational institution.

Building types by location

In urban areas, there is a pattern of provision within a locational hierarchy which places national institutions at the top of a pyramid with regional centres at the second level, town centres at the third level and district and neighbourhood centres at the fourth and fifth levels. Each level is determined by catchment, as the number of people within a given travel distance of a facility.

oooo	Metropolitan centre
ooooooo	Regional centre
ooooooooo	Town centre
ooooooooooo	District centre
ooooooooooooo	Neighbourhood centre

An implication is that the cultural dispersal starts from the top of the pyramid. This is not the case. Cultural innovation and techniques emerge at various points within the pyramid and disperse in all directions.

The larger and more specialized the building type, the higher its location in the pyramid: the large opera house occurs in the metropolitan centre, while the small multi-purpose hall is found in the neighbourhood centre. In addition there are specialist centres, including rural and seaside resorts, festival centres and historic building and/or setting. Each of these categories relies on visitors from nearby centres of population and the tourist market.

Metropolitan centre

Metropolitan centres are traditionally the main focus of cultural activity within a country, with a concentration of companies and facilities for the performing arts, their organization, creative activity and education of performers, management and production staff. Such centres benefit from the major concentration of population and national focus of transportation networks. There are several categories as follows:

Opera house

National subsidized professional resident company in repertory or repertoire and visiting comparable companies of international standard providing large-scale opera productions. Such a facility may be exclusively for opera or combined with ballet.

Ballet/dance theatre

National subsidized professional resident company as described under opera house, but exclusively for ballet and dance.

Concert hall

Classical orchestral and choral music, jazz and pop/rock music, with the leading subsidized professional orchestras and groups. Either housing a resident orchestra for their exclusive or seasonal use, or a touring facility hired by promotional organizations including the orchestras and groups.

Recital room

Medium- and small-scale classical orchestral and choral music, jazz and pop/rock music also with readings such as poetry. Either housing a resident orchestra for a season or, more often, hosting touring companies and groups.

Experimental music workshop

Facility for the development of new forms of music with a prevailing concentration on electronics and amplification.

Commercial theatre

Drama and musical productions usually initiated by the management or promoting organization with long runs over several months. Such theatres usually present new plays and musicals and originate the new productions. They may also be initiated by the subsidized sector and transferred to the commercial theatre.

Arena

Facilities for the presentation of very large-scale pop/rock concerts and other spectacles covering opera, music and musicals, hired by commercial organizations who initiate and promote groups and companies as one-off events or part of a tour.

Drama theatre

National subsidized professional resident drama company in repertory, or repertoire and visiting companies of national and international standard, producing new and established works.

Small- and medium-scale drama theatre

Small theatres presenting new plays and experimental productions, with or without subsidy to supplement revenue, relying on low overheads and benefiting from a large catchment area from which audiences are attracted.

Other categories

- Universities and Colleges including Schools of Music and Drama, providing theatres and concert halls for their own and public use.
- Open-air auditoria for seasonal concerts and drama productions.
- Informal external spaces for street theatre, music and entertainments.
- Theatres with restrictions on company (e.g. Youth Theatre) and audience (e.g. club theatres with restricted membership).
- One-off events including stadium concerts and festivals.

Regional centre

Regional centres are the major cities which are the focus of their hinterland, providing a range of buildings for the performing arts, and including the following categories:

Concert hall

Classical orchestral and choral music, jazz and pop/rock music, with regional subsidized professional company either resident or hiring the facility for a season and receiving touring orchestras and groups.

Recital room

Medium- and small-scale classical orchestral and choral music, jazz and pop/rock music. Either housing a resident orchestra for a season or, more often, hosting touring companies and groups.

Touring theatre

Facility host to professional touring opera, dance, musicals and large-scale productions, including the national companies on tour. Run by local government and/or commercial organizations and hired by promoting organizations usually on a weekly basis. Such a facility may also be the base for regional professional subsidized opera and ballet companies.

Touring music and drama

Where demand may not justify a separate concert hall and touring theatre, then the activities described under each of the above categories may be combined in a single auditorium.

Drama theatre

Resident professional drama company receiving subsidy, with productions in repertory or repertoire covering new and established works. Run by local government or private trust.

Arena

Facilities for the presentation of very large-scale pop/rock concerts and other spectacles covering opera, music and musicals, hired by commercial organizations who initiate and promote groups and companies as one-off events or part of a tour.

Small- and medium-scale drama theatre

Facility as host to the smaller touring professional drama companies and/or resident company. The concentration is on new plays and new forms of presentation.

Other categories

- Universities and Colleges, including Schools of Music and Drama providing theatres and concerts halls for their own and public use.
- Open-air auditoria for seasonal concerts and drama productions.
- Informal external spaces for street theatre, music and entertainments.
- One-off events including stadium concerts, and festivals.

Town centre

Community theatre

Medium-scale facility hosting touring companies covering drama, opera, ballet, musicals, etc., with a multi-functional auditorium, for both professional and amateur companies.

Arts workshop or centre

Drama and music facilities as focus of creative and social life in a community, along with other arts acting also as a resource centre. The emphasis is on participation as spectator and performer.

Amateur theatre

Facilities for the predominant use by amateur music or drama groups provided by a voluntary organization or local government.

District centre

Community school

Drama and music facilities for use by both school and community within the local school.

Multi-purpose hall

Hall provided by local government accommodating a wide range of activities not just music and drama.

Neighbourhood centre

Multi-purpose hall

Local hall, provided by a voluntary organization, local government, housing association, church or primary school, accommodating a wide range of activities not just music and drama.

Resort

Urban, rural and seaside locations where the market for the presentation of performing arts includes the tourist and holiday-maker as the predominant categories. The local community benefit from the provision. The pattern of use is seasonal, usually in the summer. The attraction is enjoyed by those travelling who stop over in a resort or make a specific visit to enjoy various productions.

Historic building

Music or drama productions which gain from the historic setting internally or externally.

Rural area

Multi-purpose hall

Local hall, provided by community church, primary school or local government, accommodating a wide range of activities not just for music and drama. Facility host to small-scale professional touring music and drama companies.

Mobile theatres

Professional touring music and drama company providing and erecting their own mobile building in remote areas not served by appropriate permanent facilities

Building categories

The following series of photographs, plans and descriptions illustrate the variety of building types identified in Chapter 5.

CONCERT HALL

Royal Glasgow Concert Hall, 1990

Seating capacity: 2461
Architects: Sir Leslie Martin with RMJM

The building is located in Glasgow city centre, at the junction of two of the principal shopping streets. The design integrates the concert hall into the shopping pattern offering the ground floor frontage as a continuation of the shopping streets.

The main use is for classical orchestral and choral music concerts, but is also used for rock, pop and jazz concerts and conferences. The building is essentially for touring companies and is the principal civic venue for concerts in the city.

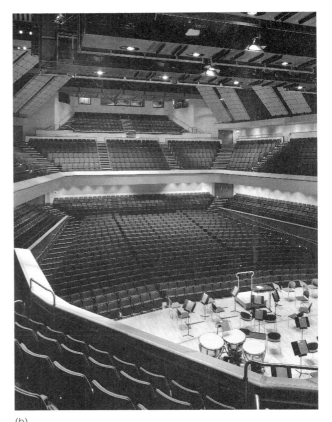

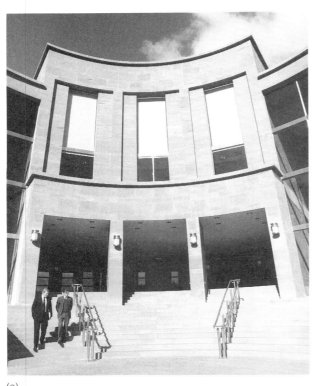

(a)

(b)

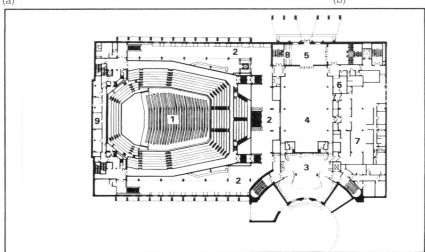

(c)

Fig. 5.1 *Royal Glasgow Concert Hall. (a) Pedestrian entrance to the south. The steps rise over a shopping arcade at ground level. (b) Rectangular auditorium with seating semi-surrounding the platform, combining traditional format with modern flexibility. (c) Level 5 plan: 1 auditorium, 2 foyer, 3 restaurant, 4 conference, 5 ante-room, 6 cloakroom, 7 kitchen, 8 bar, 9 offices.*

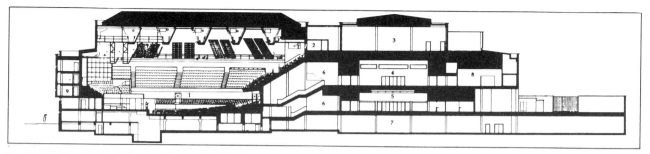

Fig. 5.1 continued *Royal Glasgow Concert Hall. (d) Long section: 1 auditorium, 2 control rooms, 3 plant rooms, 4 conference, 5 reception/ exhibitions, 6 foyers, 7 shops, 8 kitchens, 9 changing rooms*

The ceiling consists of adjustable acoustic panels and technical bridges linked to technical platforms at a high level on either side of the auditorium. Internal flexibility of use is achieved by different performance lighting and sound systems as well as adjustment of the platform shape and size.

The building is in the ownership of Glasgow City Council, and was built for the Year of Culture 1990, replacing a previous hall which had burnt down.

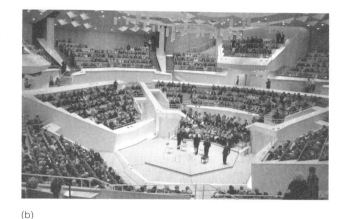

(b)

RECITAL ROOM

Chamber Music Hall, Berlin, 1987

Seating capacity: 1022
Architects: Hans Scharoun and Edgar Wisniewski

This is a purpose-built chamber music hall in the city centre as part of a grouping of cultural buildings. The building, owned by the Berlin City Council, is exclusively for chamber music, for the Berlin Philharmonic Orchestra and other visiting orchestras.

(a)

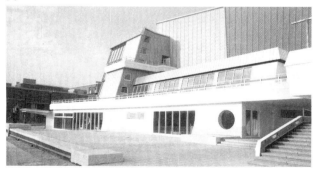

Fig. 5.2 *Chamber Music Hall, Berlin. (a) General view of the southside, looking at the public entrance. Virtually an isolated building linked to the adjacent concert hall. (b) Interior of the auditorium, showing the encirclement of the platform by the audience. The balcony fronts assist reflecting sound. (c) Auditorium level showing enclosing nature of the seating and the vertical circulation (staircases and lifts) from the foyer below.*

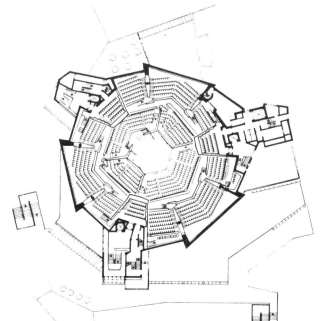

(c)

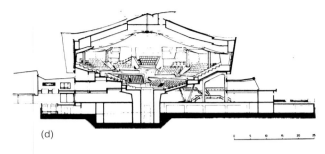

Fig. 5.2 continued *Chamber Music Hall, Berlin. (d) Long section through auditorium*

OPERA HOUSE

Opera House, Helsinki, Finland, 1993

Seating capacity: 1385
Architects: Hyuamaki-Karhunen-Parkkinen

The building is located in central Helsinki, along a lake, to which other buildings for the performing arts relate. The principal view from the site is towards the lake with the main road, car parking and entrances at the rear. The building is placed in a landscaped setting, placing the main frontage along the water edge. The service road and unloading areas are below ground level at the rear, thereby reducing the apparent bulk of the building.

The form is further sub-divided into smaller-scale elements, with bays allowing the surrounding landscape to be integrated into the design.

The main use is for opera productions with the building housing the Finland National Opera Company, who initiate and develop their own productions within the opera house.

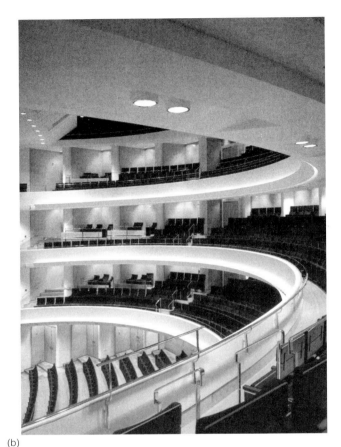

(b)

The purpose-built provision is owned by the national company. The move was prompted by the inadequacy of their previous facilities.

(a)

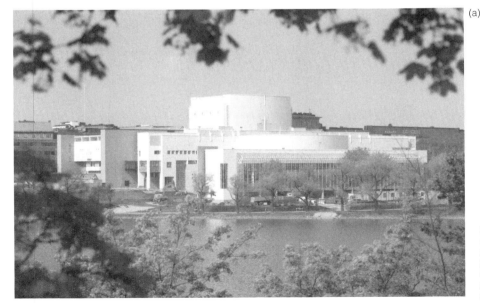

Fig. 5.3 *Opera House, Helsinki. (a) General view from the south, showing its relationship to the lake. The main public entrance is from the rear. (b) Horse-shoe auditorium and proscenium stage. Three shallow balconies.*

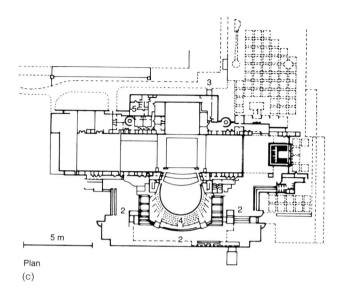

5 m

Plan

(c)

Section

(d)

5 m

Fig. 5.3 continued *Opera House, Helsinki. (c) Main foyer level: 1 main entrance, 2 foyer, 3 stage door, 4 auditorium, 5 dressing room. (d) Long section: 1 foyer, 2 auditorium, 3 orchestra pit, 4 orchestra rehearsal room, 5 stage, 6 flytower, 7 rear stage, 8 staff restaurant, 9 offices, 10 dressing rooms, 11 unloading bay and services road, 12 storage*

DANCE THEATRE

Netherlands Dance Theatre, The Hague, Netherlands 1987

Seating capacity: 1001
Architects: OMA

The building is located near the city centre in a part of The Hague which is not particularly attractive and it therefore acts as a focus and stimulus for further development. It is one of few purpose-built theatres for dance.

The dancers are able to rehearse in the building.
The building is in the ownership of a limited company rented to the Netherlands Dance Company and is for the resident and touring dance companies, rehearsal and teaching.

(a)

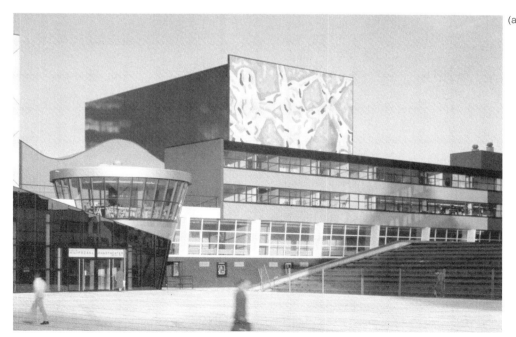

Fig. 5.4 *Netherlands Dance Theatre, The Hague. (a) General view of the building. Each functional section of the building is expressed by form and materials.*

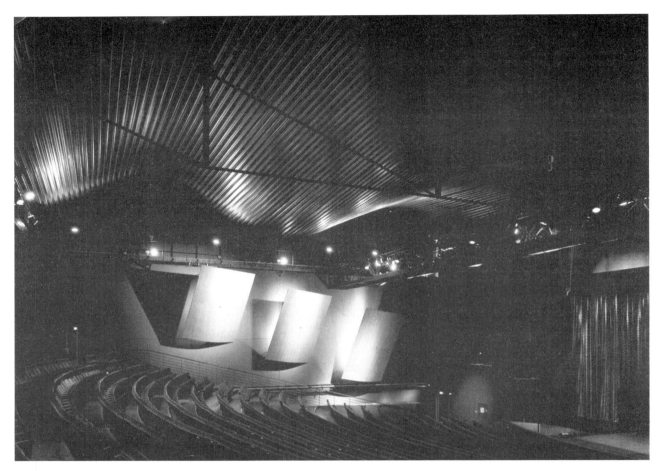

(b)

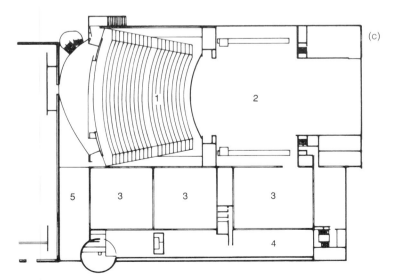

(c)

Fig. 5.4 continued *Netherlands Dance Theatre, The Hague. (b) Simple auditorium with modest fan, and proscenium stage. Visual interest achieved by undulation of walls and ceiling, and auditorium lighting. (c) Upper level plan: 1 auditorium, 2 stage, 3 rehearsal studio, 4 green room, 5 foyer.*

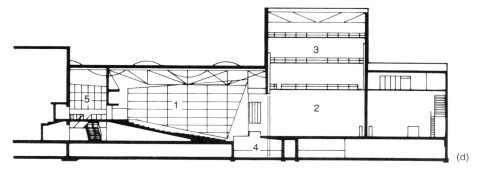

Fig. 5.4 continued *Netherlands Dance Theatre, The Hague. (d) Long section: 1 auditorium, 2 stage, 3 flytower, 4 orchestra pit, 5 foyer*

DRAMA THEATRE

Royal National Theatre, London, 1977

Seating capacities: 1160 (Olivier Theatre), 890 (Littleton Theatre), 400 (Cottesloe Theatre)
Architects: Denys Lasdun and Partners

This major national facility houses the three auditoria for the resident Royal National Theatre Company and includes all production and administration provision.

The building is located along the south bank of the Thames and is adjacent to other cultural facilities, with a main railway station and underground station nearby. The building is owned by a trust.

(a)

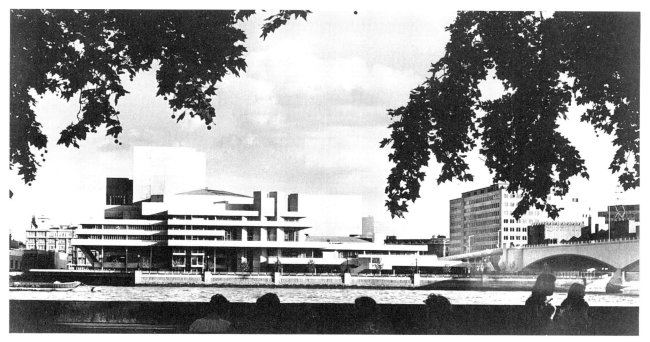

Fig. 5.5 *Royal National Theatre, London. (a) General view of the building from the riverside entrances and terraces.*

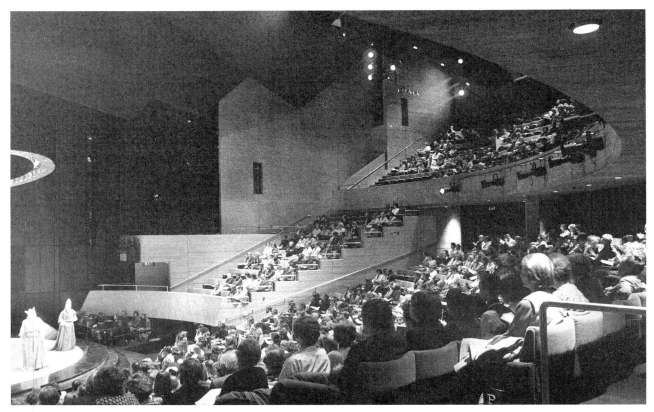

(b)

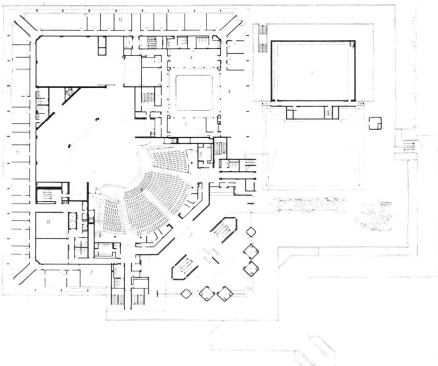

(c)

Fig. 5.5 continued *Royal National Theatre, London. (b) View of the largest of the three auditoria, the Olivier Theatre: a 90° fan seating layout on two levels. The balcony drops at the sides to link with the lower level. The curving rows of the seating embrace the stage. (c) Plan at Olivier Theatre stalls level: 1 Olivier Theatre, 2 foyer, 3 Lyttelton Theatre flytower, 4 costume workroom, 5 wig workroom, 6 offices, 7 conference room, 8 rehearsal room.*

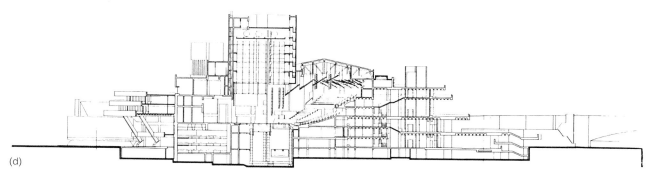

(d)

Fig. 5.5 continued Royal National Theatre, London. (d) Long section through Olivier Theatre

COMMERCIAL THEATRE

Old Vic, London, 1818/1871/1984

Seating capacity: 1077
Architects for the restoration: Renton Howard Wood
Levin

Commercial theatres are concentrated in metropolitan centres with occasional theatres in other cities, located usually in the commercial district of the central area.

This is an example of a restored theatre in London, originally designed by Frank Matcham. The commercial sector tend to use, and adapt, existing theatres, usually sensitive to location and ease of access from a large catchment area.

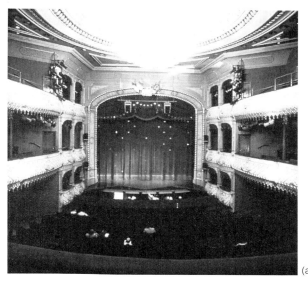

(a)

(b)

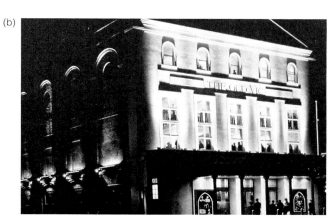

Fig. 5.6 *Old Vic, London. (a) External view of the Old Vic at night, after restoration. (b) Internal view of the auditorium looking towards the stage with the restored proscenium opening.*

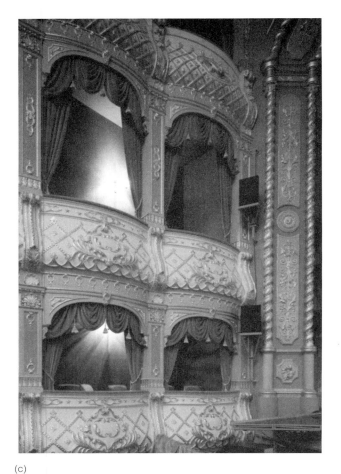

(c)

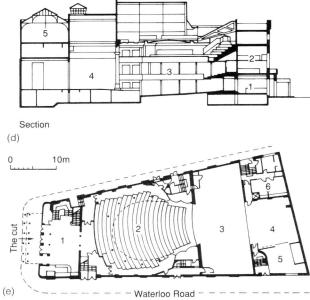

Section

(d)

0   10m

Plan

(e)

Fig. 5.6 continued *Old Vic, London. (c) Detailed view of boxes. (d) Plan: 1 foyer, 2 auditorium, 3 stage, 4 rear stage, 5 scene dock, 6 dressing rooms. (e) Section: 1 foyer, 2 bar, 3 auditorium, 4 stage, 5 rehearsal area*

POP AND ROCK CONCERTS

Zenith 2, Montpellier 1986

Seating capacity: 6400 maximum
Architects: Philippe Chaix and Jean-Paul Morel

One of a proposed series of Zenith buildings throughout Europe offering a 80 m × 80 m clear space for rock and pop concerts. A lightweight pre-fabricated structure of metal and PVC sheeting responding to the demands of youth culture, costs and technical requirements.

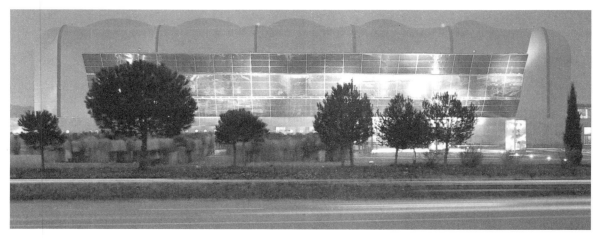

Fig. 5.7 *Zenith 2, Montpellier. (a) General external view showing entrance canopy and the undulating plastic skin of the structure.*

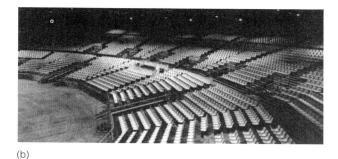

(b)

The roof covering is in square modular sections stretched across the structure: air-conditioning is provided by 16 extractor fans in the roof surface and by a sprinkler network onto the cover stretched over the whole structure.

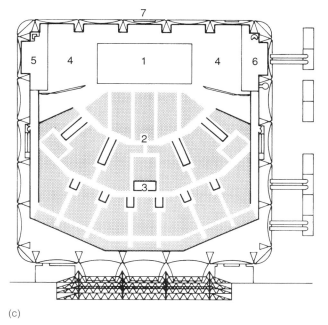

(c)

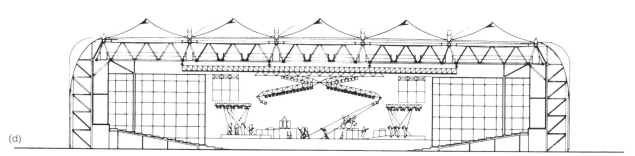

(d)

Fig. 5.7 continued *Zenith 2, Montpellier. (b) View of seating areas. (c) Plan of auditorium and stage: 1 stage, 2 auditorium, 3 sound control, 4 slide stage, 5 dressing room, 6 technical room, 7 technical access. (d) Cross-section through the auditorium looking towards the stage, showing the metal structure bearing theatrical equipment and incorporating the technical bridges at a height of 13 m.*

ARENA

Birmingham Arena 1991

Seating capacity: 1300 maximum
Architects: HOK Sports Facilities Group

This large facility is multi-use, combining rock and pop concerts by touring groups with sporting events and conferences.

The Arena in Birmingham is located in close to the International Convention Centre using land which was formerly derelict industrial sites. The Arena includes separate indoor sports facilities. It is built over a railway track.

The building is owned by Birmingham City Council.

(a)

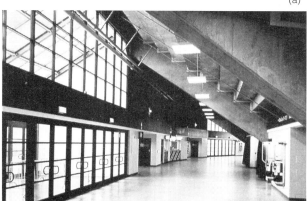

Fig. 5.8 *Birmingham Arena. (a) Internal view of concourse.*

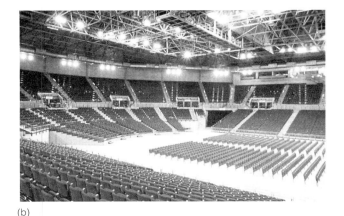

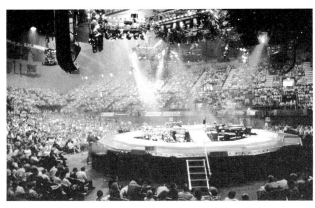

(b)

(a)

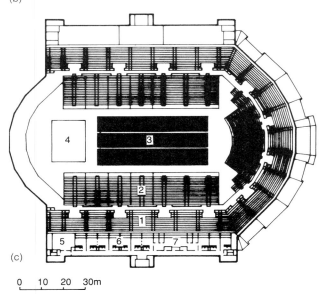

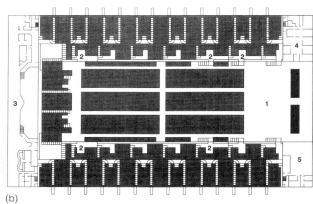

(c)

0   10   20   30m

Fig. 5.8 continued *Birmingham Arena. (b) Internal view of the arena: fixed seating to the gallery with telescopic seating and loose seating within the area surrounded by the gallery. All seats have clear views of the performance areas. (c) Plan of auditorium and stage: 1 fixed seating, 2 retractable seating, 3 temporary seating, 4 stage, 5 catering, 6 VIP rooms, 7 press room*

(b)

Fig. 5.9 *Wembley Arena, London. (a) Rectangular auditorium with permanent seating on all sides. Various formats can be configured to achieve a range of events including pop/rock concerts. Such concerts can be fully seated or part standing/part seated. This view of the interior shows an island stage with the audience in the centre section focused on the performance. (b) Seating and first floor plan: 1 stage, 2 wheelchair position, 3 restaurant, 4 offices, 5 social club*

ARENA

Wembley Arena, London, 1934 (original building) 1990 (adaptation)

Seating capacity: 12,000 maximum capacity
Architects: Sir Owen Williams (original building); Gibberd, Hedes, Minns (adaptation to form current arena)

The building is an adaptation of a facility originally designed as a swimming pool. It now hosts a variety of events, and is run by a commercial firm. The venue is intensely used for mass events (as well as indoor sporting activities such as ice hockey) and is a major metropolitan facility.

EXPERIMENTAL MUSIC WORKSHOP

Institute for Research and Co-ordination in Acoustics and Music (IRCAM), Paris, 1977

Seating capacity: 400 maximum
Architects: Piano and Rogers

IRCAM is a set of studios below ground for musicians and researchers with administration towers and building above ground. The main studio is a mechanically variable acoustic interior as a facility for musical experiment. The location is in the city centre, adjacent to the Centre Pompidou.

The facilities are essentially for experimental music and research with support facilities and archives.

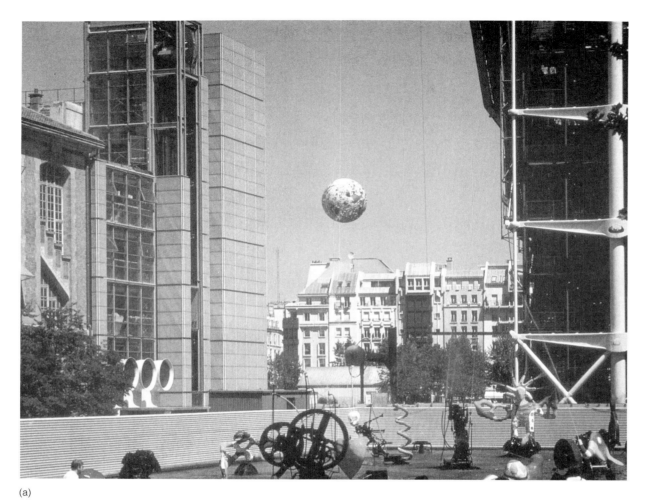

(a)

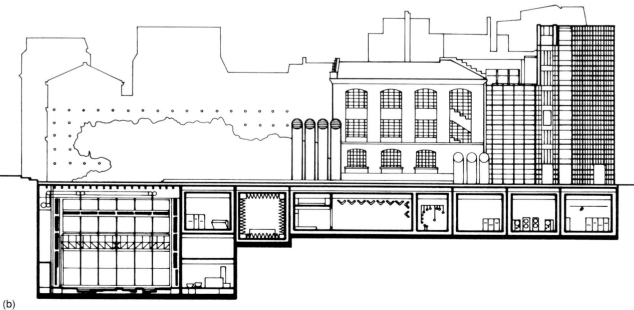

(b)

Fig. 5.10 *IRCAM, Paris. (a) General view of the facilities above ground level: the studios are located below the open space. (b) Long section showing subterranean sound centre and overground facilities*

SMALL AND MEDIUM DRAMA THEATRE

Sydney Theatre Company, Walsh Bay, Sydney 1984.

Seating capacity: 350
Architects: Vivian Frazer

Facilities for a resident drama company stretched along an existing wharf and converted warehouse, including offices, workshops, rehearsal spaces as well as the theatre and support provision, located near the city centre. The design combines careful remodelling while retaining and emphasizing the original structure.

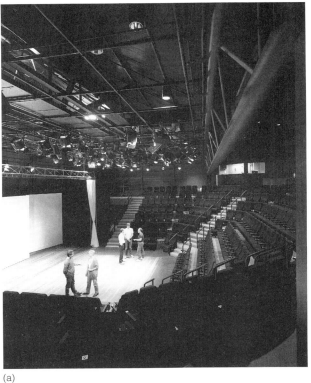

(a)

(b)

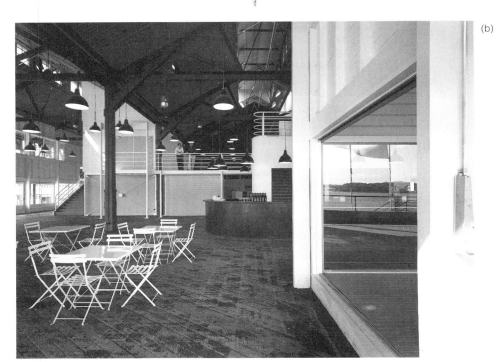

Fig. 5.11 *Sydney Theatre Company. (a) View of the auditorium: flexible seating allows different configurations. (b) View of foyer, which is located at the end of the existing wharf building. From an upper level, the public spaces overlook Walsh Bay and give long views across Sydney harbour.*

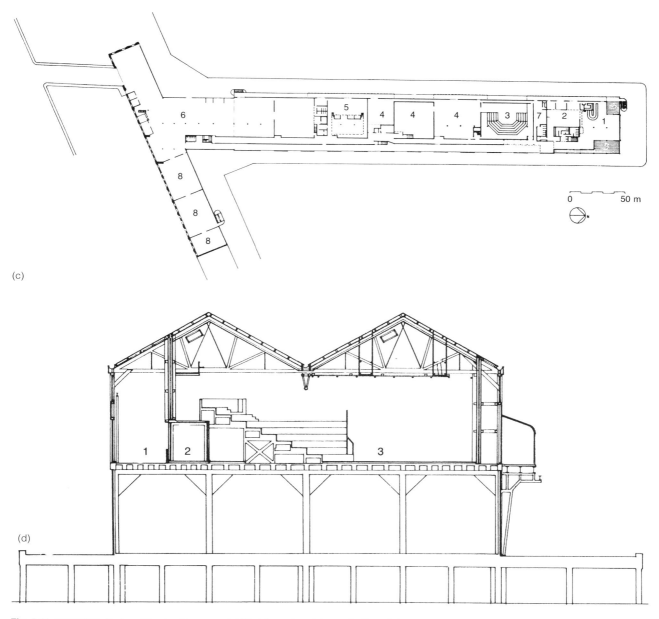

0   50 m

Fig. 5.11 continued *Sydney Theatre Company. (c) First floor plan: 1 foyer, 2 office, 3 theatre, 4 rehearsal room, 5 wardrobe, 6 workshop, 7 dressing room, 8 store. (d) Cross-section through auditorium, which is on the first floor: 1 entry gallery, 2 fire tunnel (necessary to provide a protected exit back to the main land), 3 auditorium*

SMALL AND MEDIUM DRAMA THEATRE

Traverse Theatre, Edinburgh 1992

Seating capacities: 280 (large auditorium), 100 (small auditorium)
Architects: Nicholas Groves-Raines

The shell was provided by the officer developer and the interiors were fitted by the owners – a trust – to form two flexible auditoria and support facilities.

The policy is to put on new plays and operetta in various formats, and therefore is in the tradition of experimental productions in small- and medium-scale theatres located in a city centre but not within the commercial core.

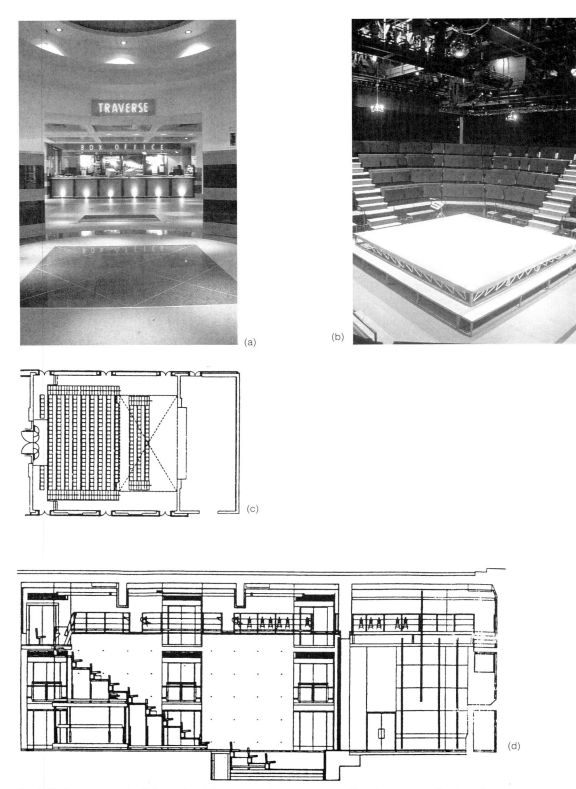

Fig. 5.12 *Traverse Theatre, Edinburgh. (a) The entrance is part of a new office development. The box office is on the ground level and theatres are below in the basement of the block. (b) The main auditorium is a 'black box' solution offering a multi-form space in which the banks of seating can be moved to create different formats. (c) Seating layout of main auditorium, showing end stage format. (d) Section through main auditorium with seating layout for end stage productions*

UNIVERSITY PROVISION

Performing Arts Centre, Cornell University, Ithaca, New York State, 1989

Seating capacity: 456
Architects: James Stirling, Michael Wilford and Associates

A university-owned provision for students and public, run by the Department of Theatre Arts of a major place of higher education, covering opera, drama, dance and film. Rehearsal spaces and scenery and other workshops are included in the complex. The facilities are used for teaching as well as performances.

(a)

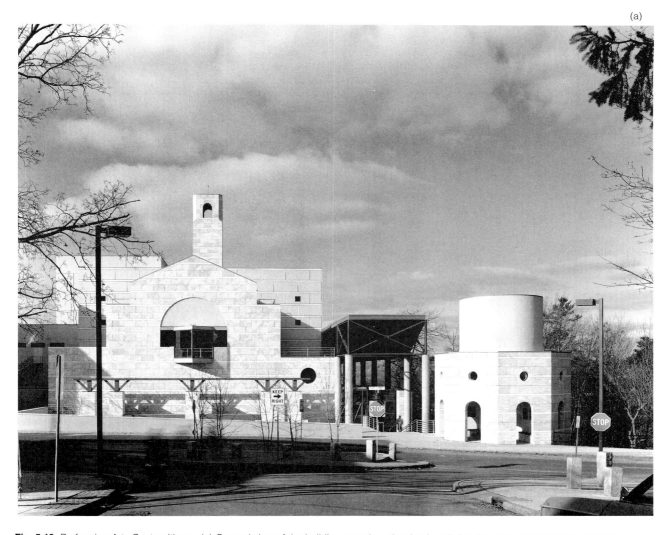

Fig. 5.13 *Performing Arts Centre, Ithaca. (a) General view of the building complex, showing its relationship to the escarpment and linking loggia.*

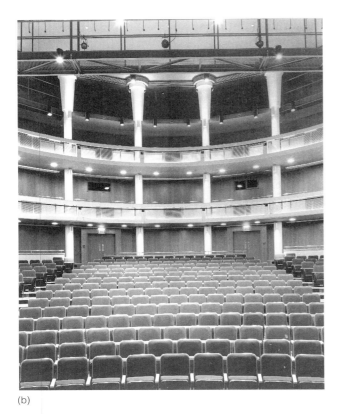

(b)

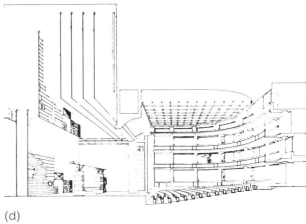

(d)

SCHOOL OF MUSIC AND DRAMA

Royal Scottish Academy of Music and Drama, Glasgow, 1988

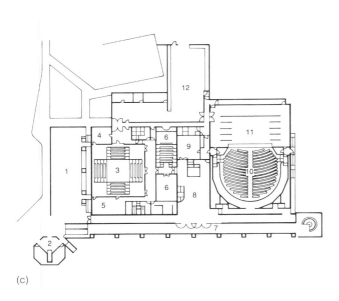

(c)

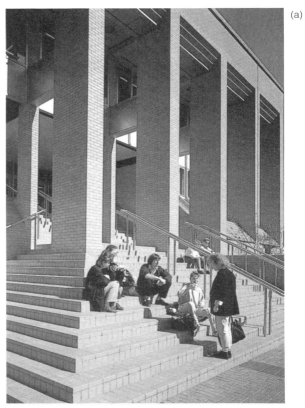

(a)

Fig. 5.13 continued *Performing Arts Centre, Ithaca. (b) View of the horseshoe auditorium interior, showing the two balconies with a single row of seats at each level. (c) Plan at the level of the public entrance: 1 piazza, 2 kiosk, 3 flexible theatre, 4 electrical workshop, 5 lighting laboratories, 6 classroom, 7 loggia, 8 foyer, 9 green room, 10 auditoria, 11 stage, 12 scenery workshop. (d) Perspective section through proscenium theatre*

Fig. 5.14 *Royal Scottish Academy of Music and Drama, Glasgow. (a) General view of the building from the main street, showing the characteristic brick piers which unify the elevations.*

Seating capacities: 344 (theatre), 363 (concert hall), 125 (recital room)
Architects: Sir Leslie Martin, in association with William Nimmo & Partners

A facility primarily for the teaching of music and drama, offering public performances in three auditoria and experimental theatre. A large complex on a city centre site, owned by the Academy, the auditoria include public performances .

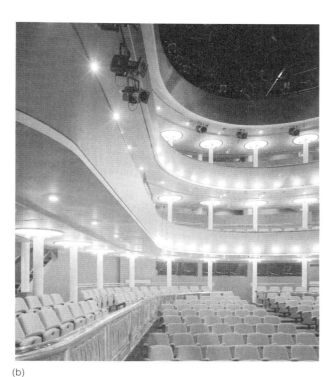

(b)

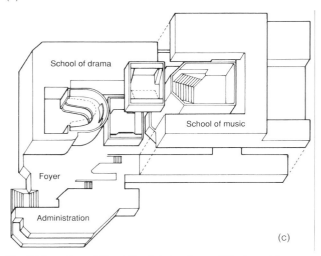

(c)

Fig. 5.14 continued *Royal Scottish Academy of Music and Drama, Glasgow. (b) View of one of the auditoria, the theatre, with its horseshoe form and shallow balconies. (c) Diagrammatic projection showing the main elements of the building*

DRAMA THEATRE

The West Yorkshire Playhouse, Leeds, 1992

Seating capacities: 750 (Quarry Theatre), 350 (Courtyard)
Architects: The Appleton Partnership

The building is located on the edge of the city centre, conveniently served by public transport and adjacent car parking.

The main use is for drama productions by the resident company, with productions by touring companies. The facilities are used for conferences, lectures and workshops. The public facilities are in use through the day as well as the evening and is the base for a Theatre-in-Education programme.

The building is owned by a trust.

(a)

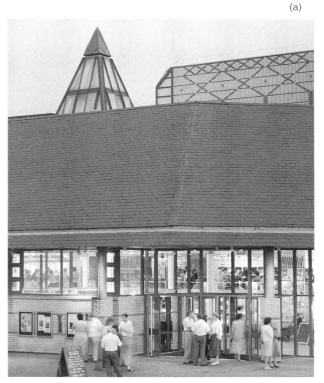

Fig. 5.15 *West Yorkshire Playhouse, Leeds. (a) General external view of the public entrance.*

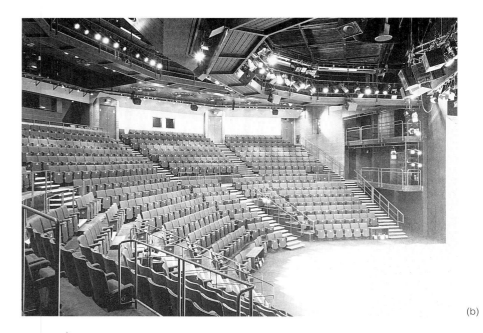

(b)

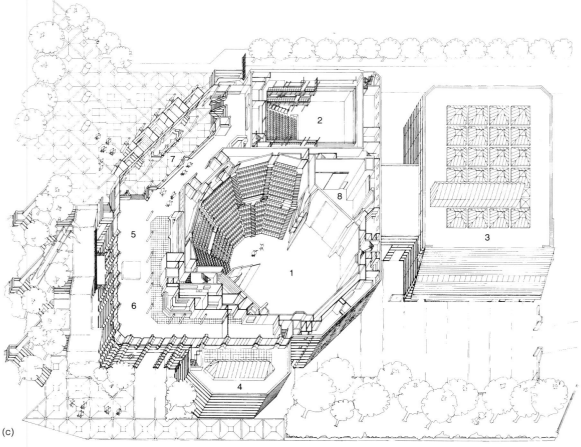

(c)

Fig. 5.15 continued *West Yorkshire Playhouse, Leeds. (b) View of the larger of the two auditoria, the Quarry, showing the 90° fan seating layout on a single level. The audience and stage are within the same space. (c) Projection view of the theatre complex showing the two auditoria, the public spaces and workshop block at the rear of the stages. 1 Quarry Theatre, 2 Courtyard Theatre, 3 workshops, 4 rehearsal room, 5 bar, 6 restaurant, 7 entrance foyer*

TOURING MUSIC AND DRAMA

Theatre Royal, Newcastle 1837/1901/1988

Seating capacity: 1294 (maximum)
Architects for the restoration: Renton, Howard, Wood, Levin

A city-centre building receiving touring companies, covering musicals, opera, dance, drama, pop concerts, and other entertainments, owned and run by the Newcastle City Council. The building has been adapted over time with the recent refurbishment of 1988 seeing the restoration of the auditorium interior and exterior, and the adjustment of the public spaces and back-stage accommodation.

(a)

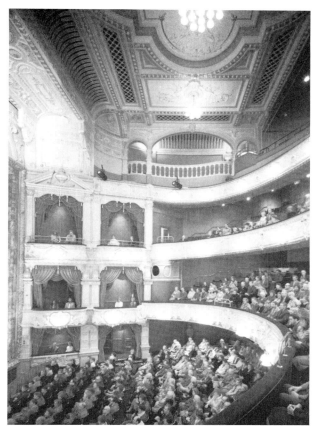

(b)

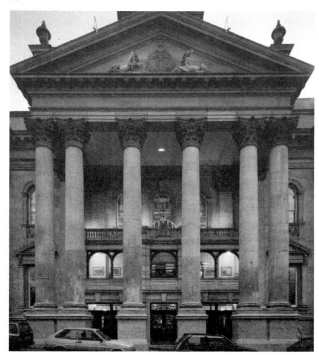

Fig. 5.16 *Theatre Royal, Newcastle. (a) Restored exterior showing the quality of the nineteenth-century inherited theatre buildings. (b) View of auditorium recently restored to match the original drawings by Matcham. The auditorium has three balconies and side boxes, with a proscenium stage. (c) Ground floor plan: 1 auditorium, 2 stage, 3 foyer, 4 buffet, 5 dressing room, 6 workshop, 7 green room, 8 box office. (d) Long section through restored auditorium and support facilities*

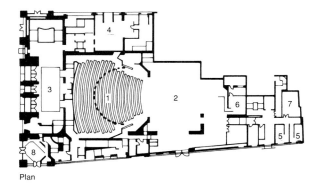

Plan

(c)

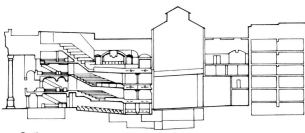

(d)   Section

TOURING MUSIC AND DRAMA

Tampere Hall, Finland 1990

Seating capacity: 1806 (main auditorium), 489 (smaller auditorium), 230 maximum (studio theatre)
Architects: Aartelo and Piironen

The building is located in a spacious park adjacent to the university campus in the city centre. It consists of

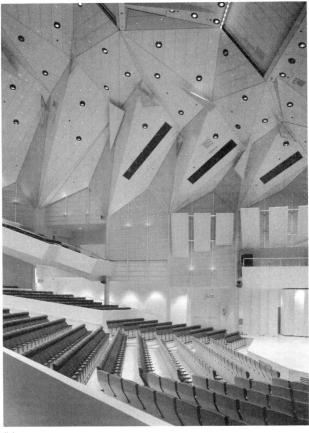

(b)

three auditoria, the concert hall/opera house, lecture theatre/recital room and experimental theatre. The uses combine concert and opera in the main auditorium as well as drama and conferences.

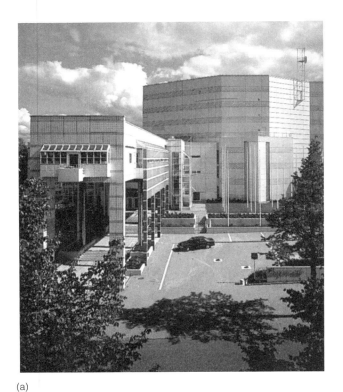

(a)

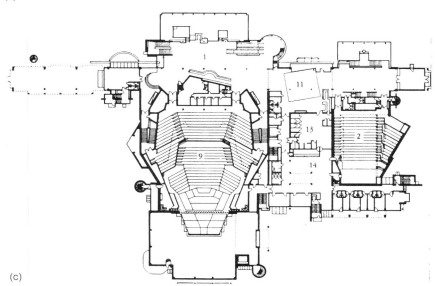

(c)

Fig. 5.17 *Tampere Hall. (a) The building faces a park, with the public entrance at the side. The conservatory includes a coffee bar at ground level and the main foyers look through the conservatory to the view beyond from upper levels. (b) The main auditorium, within a rectangular box and with a single balcony and extended sides to the balcony. The angular ceiling, the main visual feature of the interior, acts as an acoustic umbrella to the auditorium. (c) Plan of the main entrance level: 1 foyer, 2 main auditorium, 3 stage, 4 restaurant, 5 function room, 6 small auditorium.*

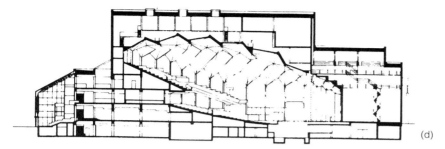

(d)

Fig. 5.17 continued *Tampere Hall. (d) Longitudinal section through main auditorium. An enclosure for an orchestra on the stage can be wheeled into position to provide the acoustic shell*

COMMUNITY THEATRE

Jacksons Lane Community Centre, London, 1989

Seating capacity: 170
Architects: Tim Ronalds Architects

The building is owned and run by the Jackson's Lane Community Centre Association and is a converted Sunday School hall. Initiated by the Community Association, the facilities include provision for drama, music, cabaret, and social activities by local groups, serving the needs of the community in which the building is centrally located. The design combines restoration of an existing building with the introduction of new uses and their technical requirements in a compatible manner. Adaptation of format is achieved manually by moving rostra and seating.

(a)

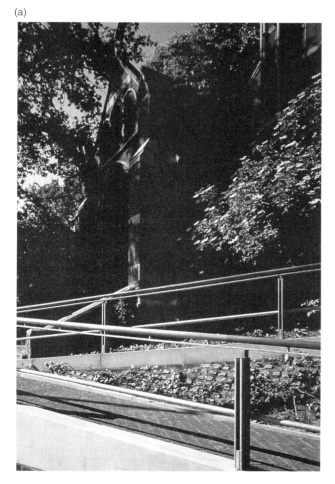

(b)

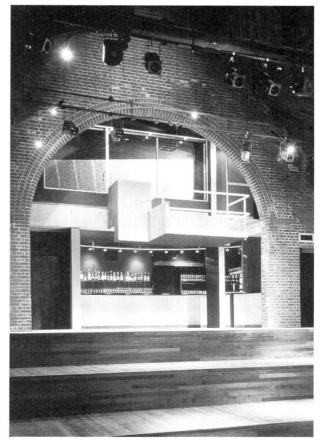

Fig. 5.18 *Jacksons Lane Community Centre, London. (a) General view of the community centre of which the theatre is part. (b) View of interior showing conversion of a hall into a multi-use space.*

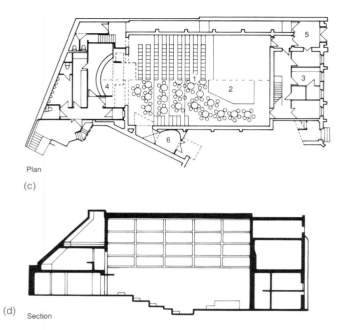

Plan

(c)

(d) Section

Fig. 5.18 continued *Jacksons Lane Community Centre, London. (c) Ground floor plan, showing both layout as theatre, with end stage and nine straight rows of seating, and cabaret, with thrust stage and tables: 1 auditorium, 2 stage, 3 dressing room, 4 bar, 5 stage door, 6 foyer. (d) Long section showing theatre, control room, bar and dressing rooms. The wider tread for tables when the auditorium is used for cabaret is achieved by removal of the intermediate raked floor*

COMMUNITY THEATRE

Wilde Theatre, Bracknell 1984

Seating capacity: 330 maximum plus 70 standing
Architects: Levitt Bernstein Associates

Flexible layout with possible proscenium format (with or without forestage or orchestra pit), open stage (with or without forestage or orchestra pit) or concert hall as well as cabaret, promenade performances, indoor sports, exhibitions and informal jazz.

The building, owned by a trust, serves its local community and provides facilities for touring professional companies and local groups. Its location, adjacent to an eighteenth-century house also benefits from its parkland for outdoor performance of jazz and folk music.

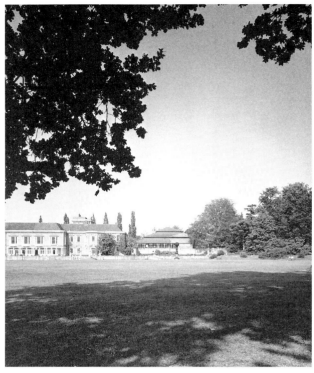

(a)

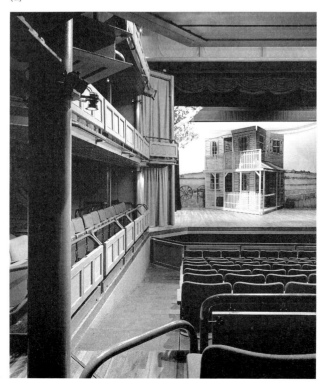

(b)

Fig. 5.19 *Wilde Theatre, Bracknell. (a) View of building from outside. The building is a wing to an existing house. (b) View of auditorium showing the courtyard format with two shallow balconies on three sides and proscenium stage.*

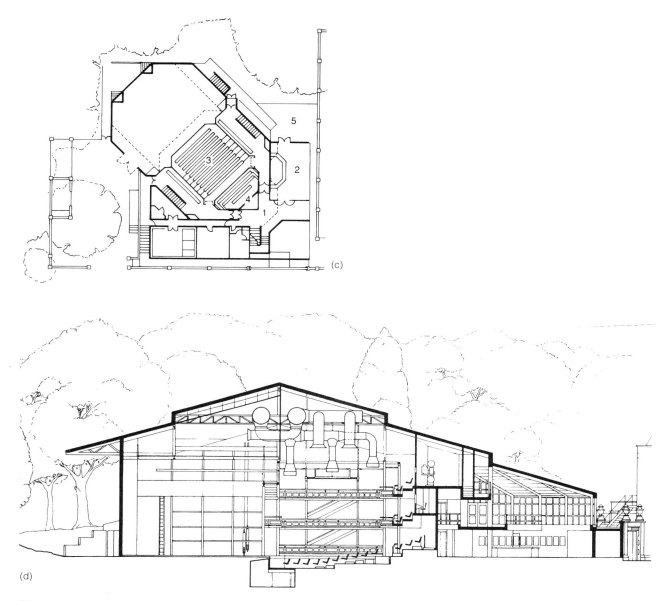

Fig. 5.19 continued *Wilde Theatre, Bracknell. (c) Plan of first floor level showing: 1 foyer, 2 bar, 3 auditorium, 4 control room, 5 terrace. (d) Long section through auditorium with 1 foyer, 2 auditorium, 3 stage, 4 orchestra pit, 5 projection room*

ARTS WORKSHOP

Edinburgh Theatre Workshop 1990 (current phase of development)

Seating capacity: 153
Architects: Richard Hamblett Associates

The building is located in a neighbourhood near to the city centre and is both a focus for local community activities and city-wide events. The design is a conversion of an existing terraced building with additions at the rear. As well as performing arts – drama and dance – the workshop is a location for art classes and is used by, as well as servicing, the local schools, disabled persons and ethnic groups.

The building is owned by the City of Edinburgh District Council and run by an independent trust.

The small auditorium consists of a bleacher unit, easily retracted to provide a flat floor for other workshop activities.

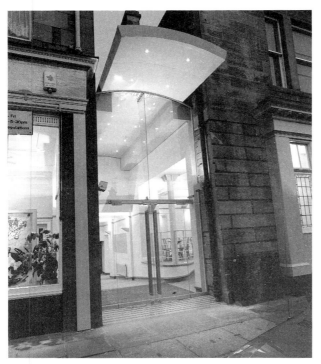

(a)

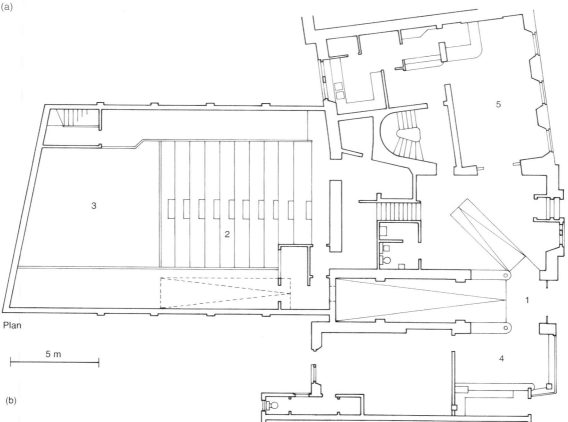

Plan

5 m

(b)

Fig. 5.20 *Edinburgh Theatre Workshop. (a) External view of entrance with access to restaurant and box office, and the auditorium beyond: the design and art class facilities are on the first floor. (b) Ground floor plan: 1 entrance, 2 auditorium, 3 stage, 4 box office, 5 cafe.*

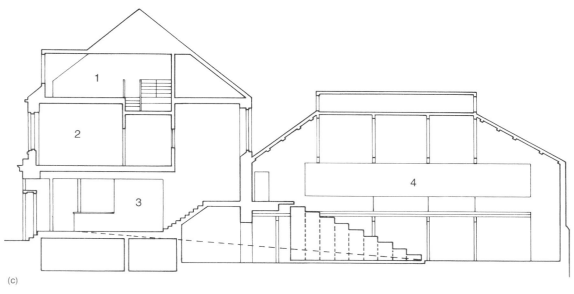

Fig. 5.20 continued *Edinburgh Theatre Workshop. (c) Section. 1 office, 2 workshop, 3 entrance, 4 theatre*

COMBINED MUSIC, DRAMA AND OTHER FUNCTIONS

Derngate, Northampton

Seating capacity: 1472 (concert format) 1172 (proscenium theatre)
Architects: Renton Howard Wood Levin

A multi-form multi-function theatre, receiving touring music and drama companies as well as housing social assemblies and some indoor sports: a solution for the town centre where demand suggests a single flexible auditorium rather than a set of single-purpose buildings. The flexibility relies on a kit of mobile parts able to be combined to form different configurations.

The building is owned and run by the local authority.

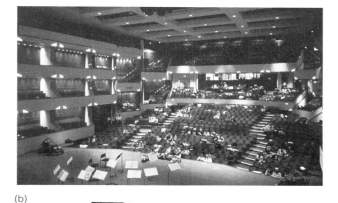

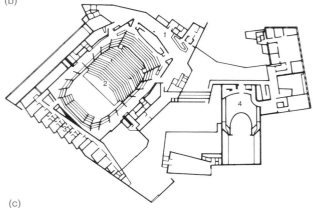

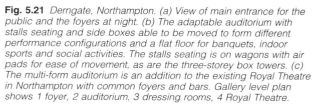

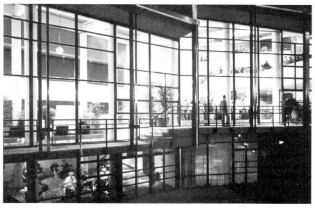

Fig. 5.21 *Derngate, Northampton. (a) View of main entrance for the public and the foyers at night. (b) The adaptable auditorium with stalls seating and side boxes able to be moved to form different performance configurations and a flat floor for banquets, indoor sports and social activities. The stalls seating is on wagons with air pads for ease of movement, as are the three-storey box towers. (c) The multi-form auditorium is an addition to the existing Royal Theatre in Northampton with common foyers and bars. Gallery level plan shows 1 foyer, 2 auditorium, 3 dressing rooms, 4 Royal Theatre.*

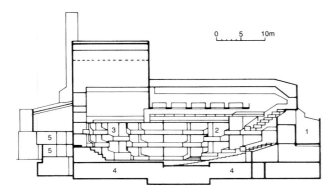

Fig. 5.21 continued *Derngate, Northampton. (d) The longitudinal section through the auditorium showing 1 foyer, 2 auditorium, 3 stage area, 4 seat wagon store, 5 dressing rooms*

COMMUNITY SCHOOL

Barton Hall, Horndean Community School, Hampshire 1993

Seating capacity: 450
Architects: Hampshire County Council, Architects Department

This simple and effective multi-purpose hall is an addition to an existing school, designed to be shared by outside groups from the local small community. The hall is for the programmed use covering school assembly, examinations, dances, aerobics, karate, etc. as well as for drama and concerts. The hall is also used for lectures, displays, banquets, wedding receptions, conferences and as a cinema. Bleacher seating for 300 has been installed so that the floor can be completely cleared. Various staging configurations are possible using the bleachers and by building raked seating and stages off the flat floor. The projection box (as stage control room) and stage lighting suspended from the roof structure are provided for performances. Daylight is closed off by motorized blinds to control glare and provide black

(a)

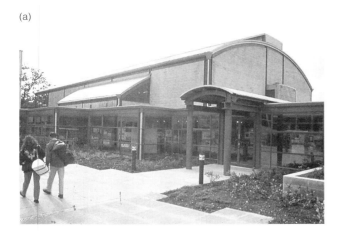

out. The internal atmosphere is easily transformed by variations in the artificial and natural lighting while appropriate acoustic and ventilation standards for the range of activities are achieved.

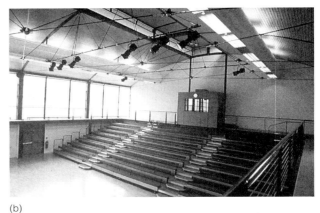

(b)

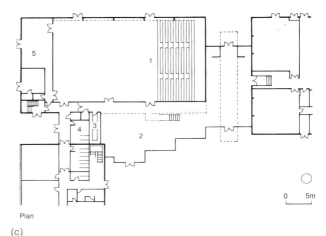

Plan

(c)

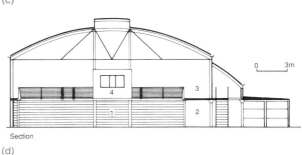

Section

(d)

Fig. 5.22 *Barton Hall, Horndean Community School. (a) External view of the hall showing the barrel-vault roof and zig-zag shape of the foyer areas. (b) Internal view from the stage of the bleacher seating and projection room at balcony level: daylight can be easily blanked out for performances. (c) Ground floor plan showing: 1 bleacher seating, 2 foyer, 3 bar, 4 toilets, 5 store. (d) Traverse section showing: 1 hall, 2 foyer, 3 balcony, 4 projection booth*

MULTI-PURPOSE HALL

Clickhinin Leisure Centre, Shetland Islands

Seating capacity: 1000 maximum
Architects: Faulkener-Brown, Hendy, Watkinson, Stonor

The building is essentially a sports hall (36.5 × 26m) accommodating hockey, badminton, basketball and so on, including spectator tournament sports, with support facilities. Such accommodation is made suitable for concerts as well as exhibitions, dances, dinners and festivals. A modest facility offering a range of activities, the Centre serves a mainly rural community over a large area of the Shetland islands, responding to the inclement weather both in the range of indoor activities and the external architectural detail.

The building is owned and run by the local authority, and receives local amateur groups and touring professional companies.

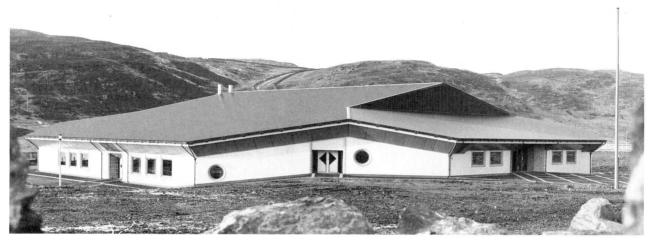

(a)

(b)

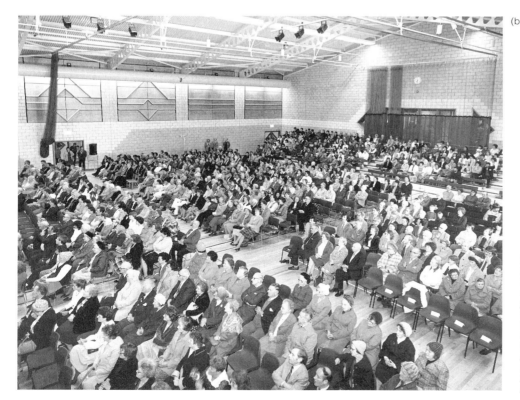

Fig. 5.23 *Clickhinin Leisure Centre, Shetland Islands. (a) The building nestles in a valley by a loch: the large pitched metal roof follows the line of the landscape and hills beyond. (b) The main hall with a large audience suitable for concerts and public meetings. Mobile bleacher units are in place providing raked seating for the rear five rows only.*

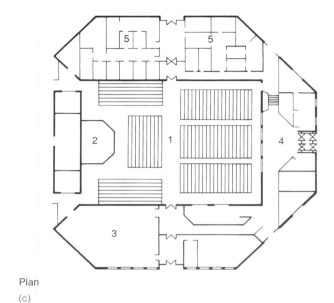

Plan
(c)

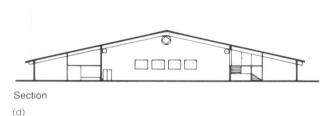

Section
(d)

Fig. 5.23 continued *Clickhinin Leisure Centre, Shetland Islands. (c) Ground floor plan showing a layout for concerts on the central main hall: 1 main hall, 2 stage, 3 green room, 4 public entrance, 5 changing facilities. (d) Traverse section showing the high hall centrally located, surrounded by the lower accommodation*

COMMUNITY THEATRE

Stantonbury Campus Theatre, Milton Keynes

Seating capacity: 452 maximum (208 raked, 52 loose, 192 retractable)
Architects: Milton Keynes Development Corporation

Small theatre located within one of a series of 'villages' which constitute the overall structure of Milton Keynes. The theatre, part of a larger leisure complex, serves the local neighbourhood and also city-wide interests. The majority of the seats are on a single faxed-raked level with the use of additional bleacher seating. The programme of use covers a wide range of uses and users in the community including school and student use, professional touring companies and groups, local amateur companies and groups, opera, dance, musicals and drama, as well as social functions.

The building is owned and run by a trust.

(a)

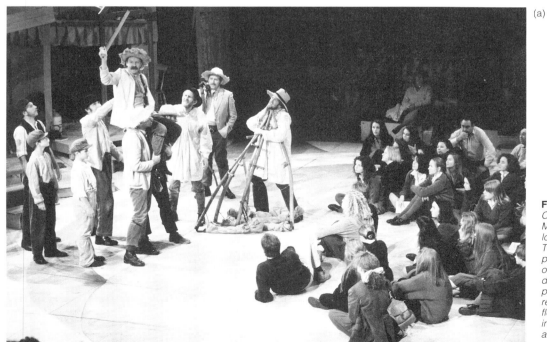

Fig. 5.24 *Stantonbury Campus Theatre, Milton Keynes. (a) The local Stantonbury Theatre Company's promenade production of Lark Rise demonstrating the potential of the rectangular box and its flexibility. The plans indicate different stage and seating arrangements:*

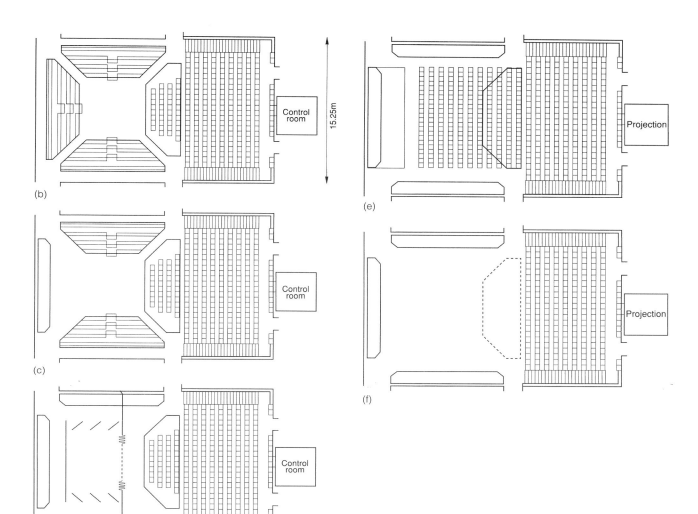

15.25m

Fig. 5.24 continued *Stantonbury Campus Theatre, Milton Keynes.*
(b) Theatre-in-the-round: bleacher seating extended on three sides;
seating capacity: 452. (c) Thrust stage: side bleacher seating
extended; seating capacity: 396. (d) Proscenium stage: bleacher
seating retracted; removable curtains borders, etc. in position;
seating capacity: 264. With the orchestra pit in use, the seating
capacity is reduced to 212. (e) Cinema, lectures, concerts: the
orchestra pit is covered, bleacher seating retracted, loose seats set
on the flat floor, temporary end stage; seating capacity: 451. (f)
Display, exhibitions and social functions: pit covered, bleacher
seating retracted, maximum flat floor area exposed

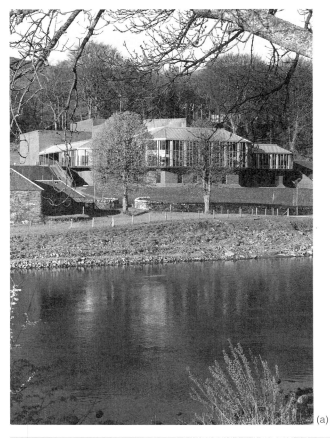

(a)

RURAL RESORT

Pitlochry Festival Theatre, Pitlochry 1981

Seating capacity: 544
Architects: Law and Dunbar Nasmith Partnership

The theatre, owned by a trust, provides a repertoire of drama productions through the summer season in a small town with a large influx of visitors as part of tours through Scotland. The resident, but seasonal, company initiates its own productions and has workshop facilities adjacent. The foyer includes a restaurant and exhibition facilities.

Fig. 5.25 *Pitlochry Festival Theatre. (a) View of the theatre from across the river. The car parking is to the left. (b) View of auditorium. A single level seating layout with cross-gangway and proscenium stage.*

(b)

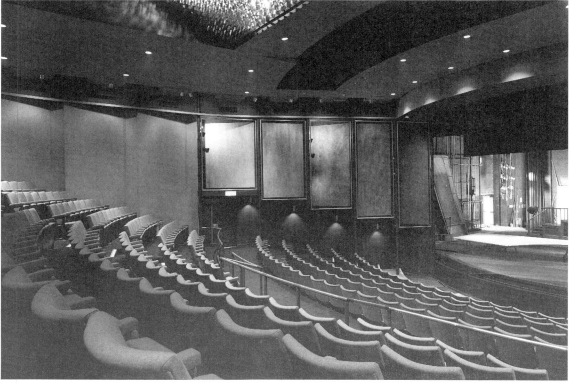

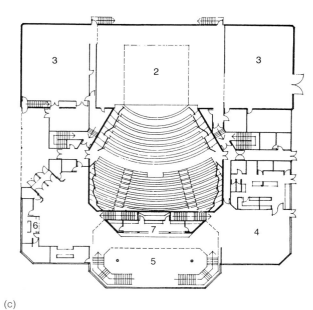

(c)

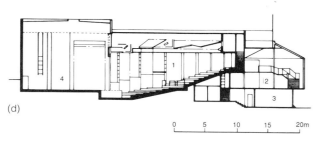

(d)

0 5 10 15 20m

Fig. 5.25 continued *Pitlochry Festival Theatre. (c) Plan of main level: 1 auditorium, 2 stage, 3 scene store, 4 restaurant, 5 foyer, 6 box office, 7 bar. (d) Long section showing: 1 auditorium, 2 foyers, 3 dressing rooms, 4 stages*

SPECIALIST THEATRE

Young Vic, London: Young People's Theatre Complex 1969

Seating capacity: 450
Architects: Howell, Killick, Partridge and Amis

Inexpensive, modest standard of provision: facility to encourage young performers and theatre-goers. Located, at the time, in a derelict area of London but near a main line railway station in the city centre.

Building was an adjunct of the National Theatre Company, especially for youth productions.

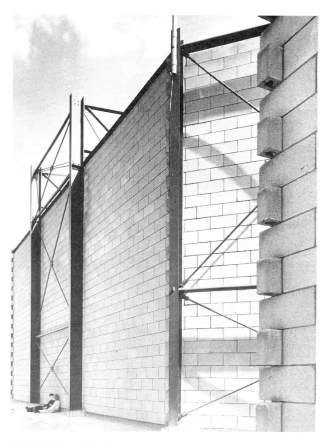

Fig. 5.26 *Young Vic, London. (a) General view of the exterior showing expressed structure and modest materials.*

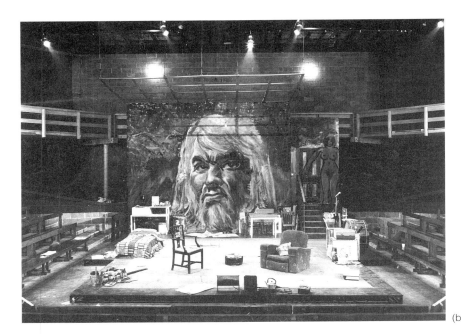

Fig. 5.26 continued *Young Vic, London. (b) View of auditorium: the thrust stage is surrounded by bench seating. (c) Ground floor plan: 1 auditorium, 2 stage, 3 rehearsal room, 4 coffee bar, 5 foyer, 6 dressing rooms, 7 scenery store. (d) Long section*

(b)

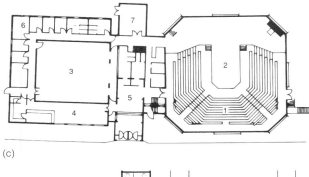

(c)

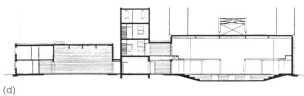

(d)

OPEN-AIR AUDITORIUM

Milton Keynes Bowl, Milton Keynes

Seating/standing capacity: 60,000
Architects: Milton Keynes Development Corporation

A major facility for pop/rock concerts in easy reach of London and Birmingham as well as its own hinterland, run by a commercial organization. The facility is used also for classical concerts, entertainments and community activities.

(a)

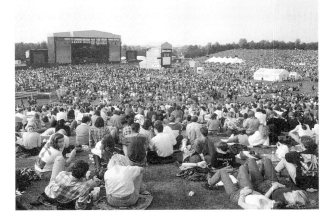

Fig. 5.27 *Milton Keynes Bowl. (a) The large natural bowl focused towards the enclosed stage, with the sound and lighting control positions located centrally within the audience.*

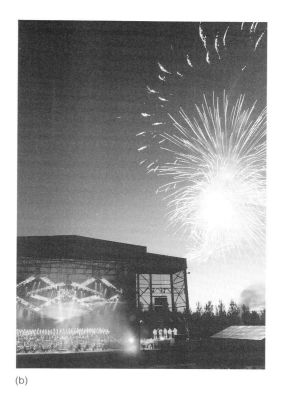

(b)

Concert Bowl, Kenwood House, London 1950

Seating capacity: 2082 (formal), 6000 (informal)

An outdoor auditorium for mainly classical music, set up for summer seasons. The canopy and platform are temporary structures, removed for the winter.

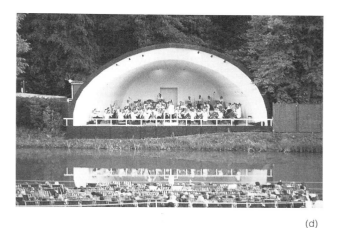

(d)

(c)

Fig. 5.27 continued *Milton Keynes Bowl. (b) View of the stage at dusk during a performance. (c) Layout of the arena: 1 stage, 2 control tower, 3 bars, 4 disabled persons platform, 5 disabled persons toilets, 6 concession facilities, 7 box offices, 8 police area, 9 first aid area, 10 hospitality area, 11 information/public telephones, 12 public toilets, 13 emergency vehicle entrance, 14 auditorium. (d) Concert Bowl, Kenwood House, London. The natural bowl of the landscaped grounds of Kenwood House for the audience, directed towards the concert platform and canopy across a small lake. The water acts as a reflective surface for both the sound of the orchestras and the platform and its setting*

JAZZ CLUB

National Jazz Centre, London, 1982 (not completed)

Seating capacity: 381, plus standing
Architects: Sandy Brown Associates

Conversion of a building to form a national focus for jazz performances. The layout illustrated shows a centre stage and gallery in a relatively formal arrangement. The proposal allowed for tables and chairs, as opposed to rows of seats, while the stage could be located along one side of the auditorium.

Ronnie Scott's Jazz Club, Birmingham, 1991

Seating capacity: 300, plus standing
Architects: Mark Humphries

Conversion to form a city-centre club for jazz performances, with an addition of a cafe/bar. The stage seating, bars and dining areas are within one level, with central seating/dance floor dropped to form stage and tiered seating. The cellar and further dressing rooms are located at a lower level.

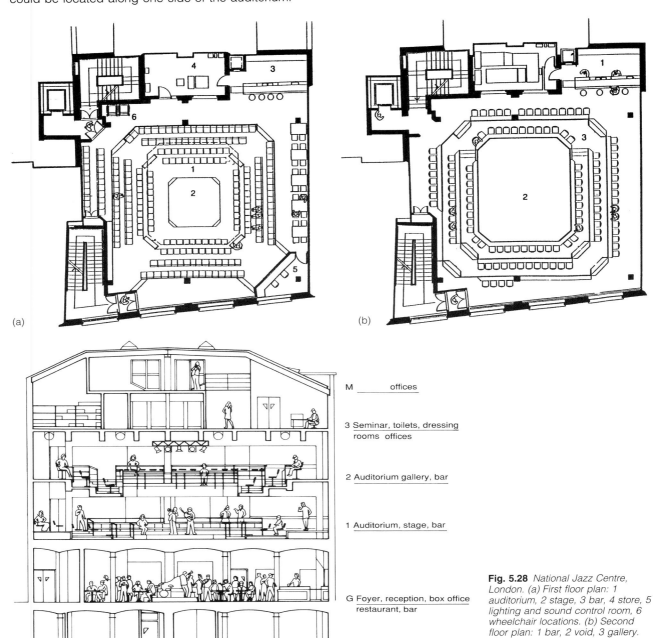

(a)

(b)

(c)

M   offices

3 Seminar, toilets, dressing rooms offices

2 Auditorium gallery, bar

1 Auditorium, stage, bar

G Foyer, reception, box office restaurant, bar

B Practice, rehearsal rooms kitchen, toilets, stores

Fig. 5.28 *National Jazz Centre, London. (a) First floor plan: 1 auditorium, 2 stage, 3 bar, 4 store, 5 lighting and sound control room, 6 wheelchair locations. (b) Second floor plan: 1 bar, 2 void, 3 gallery. (c) General section through the main auditorium and support facilities.*

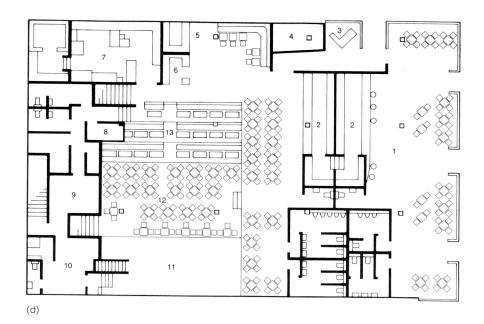

(d)

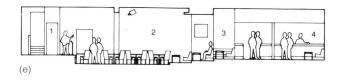

(e)

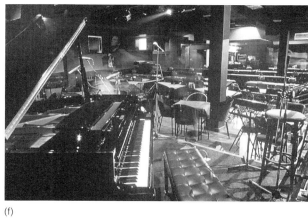

(f)

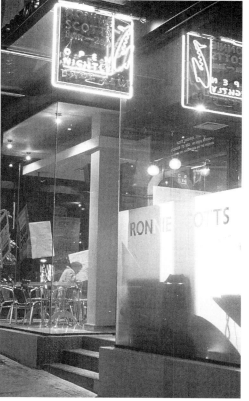

(g)

Fig. 5.28 continued *Ronnie Scott's Jazz Club, Birmingham.*
(d) Ground floor plan: 1 cafe/bar, 2 servery, 3 box office, 4
cloakroom, 5 cocktail bar, 6 waiter station, 7 kitchen, 8 sound
control, 9 rehearsal room, 10 dressing room, 11 stage, 12 dance
floor/seating, 13 tiered seating. (e) General section through jazz
club: 1 stage, 2 dance floor/seating, 3 tiered seating, 4 cocktail
bar. (f) General view of the interior of the jazz club. (g) General
external view

MOBILE THEATRE

Royal National Eisteddfod Mobile Theatre of Wales, 1983

Seating capacity: 540 maximum
Architects: John Dangerfield Associates

A solution to providing performances in areas of low population or demand is to develop a mobile theatre in the tradition of the travelling circus, by erecting a temporary enclosure, seating and staging with the attendant support facilities. This example of a mobile theatre uses natural ventilation through ventilators at the head of the masts: summer use only means no heating is required. The layout is flexible and suitable for music and drama. The kit of parts is moved by trailer: the trailer becomes the dressing rooms and green room attached to the tent when erected. The owner is the Royal National Eisteddfod.

MOBILE THEATRE

New Bubble Theatre Project, London, 1978 (unbuilt)

Seating capacity: 350 maximum
Architects: Pentagram Design

The mobile theatre was designed for a professional drama company, funded by the local authority, to give informal performances in parks and similar locations in the various London neighbourhoods as an introduction to theatre.

The proposed structures consisted of free-standing rigid pneumatic structures, based on a series of tubular ribs. Free standing lighting rigs were to be erected within each of the structures. The auditorium consisted of tables and chairs to retain the informality of the theatre-going experience.

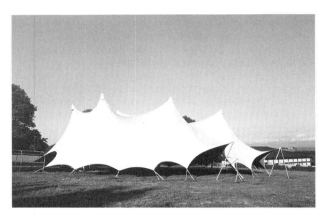

Fig. 5.29 *Royal National Eisteddfod Mobile Theatre of Wales. External view of the erected tent: the membrane consists of a polyester fabric, triple-coated in PVC to the outer surface and a blackout layer and coloured lining to the inner, with aluminium supports*

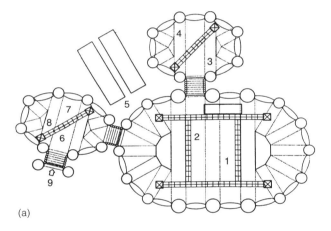

(a)

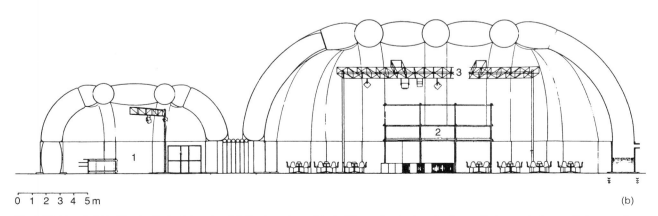

0 1 2 3 4 5m

(b)

Fig. 5.30 *New Bubble Theatre Project, London. (a) The layout consisted of the main structure for the auditorium and stage, with two smaller structures. The plan consisted of: 1 auditorium, 2 stage, 3 dressing room, 4 green room, 5 trailers, 6 display, 7 bar, 8 box office, 9 public entrance. (b) The longitudinal section shows: 1 foyer, 2 auditorium, 3 lighting rigs*

TEMPORARY BUILDING

Garsington Manor, 1993

Seating capacity: 321
Architects: Atelier One

Temporary auditorium set up each summer in the grounds of a historic building, Garsington Manor, a Tudor manor house near Oxford, using the grounds and house as the setting for operetta performances. A carriage hood structure can be opened over the raked seating set up in the Italianate gardens.

The facility is privately owned and the summer season is organized by the owners.

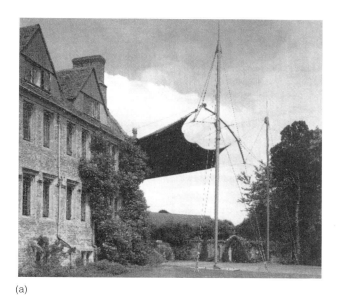

(a)

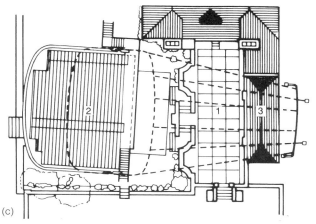

(c)

Fig. 5.31 *Garsington Manor. (a) View of retractable canopy at the side of the existing manor. (b) Isometric of overall structure of the retractable canopy. (c) Main Level: 1 stage, 2 auditorium, 3 existing building.*

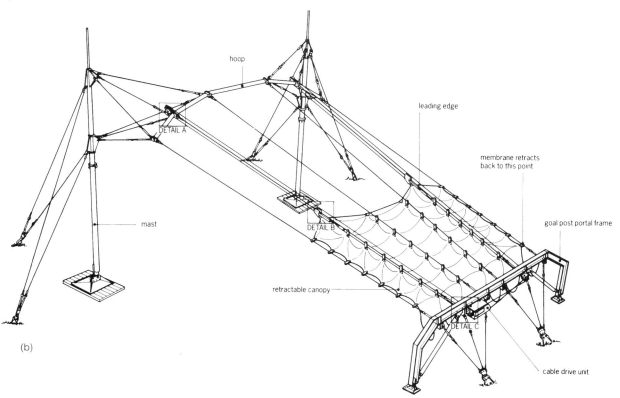

(b)

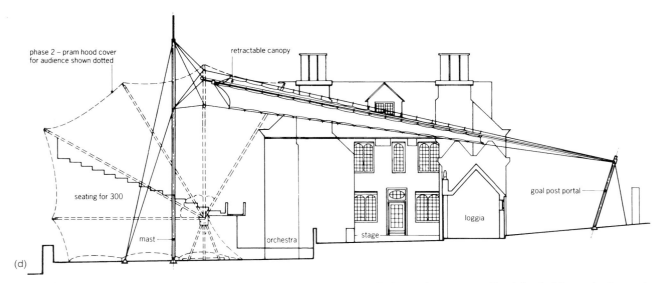

Fig. 5.31 continued *Garsington Manor. (d) Long section showing built-up auditorium and stage area with existing building as background*

USE OF HISTORIC BUILDING

Verona Amphitheatre, Italy

Seating capacity: 16 000

(a)

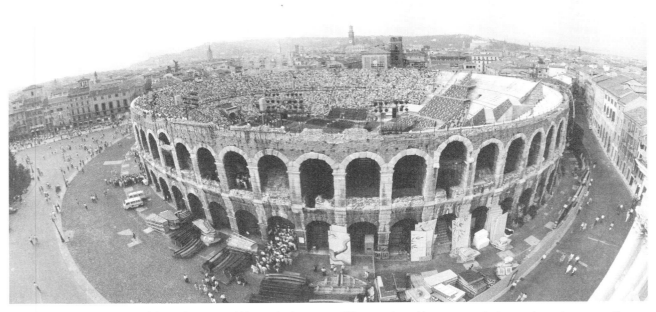

Fig. 5.32 *Verona Ampitheatre. (a) The Roman amphitheatre in the centre of Verona adapted for opera, and other music, performances. The amphitheatre form has been adapted to accommodate opera on a spectacular scale, with the staging using the rear stone raked terraces as part of the setting.*

(b)

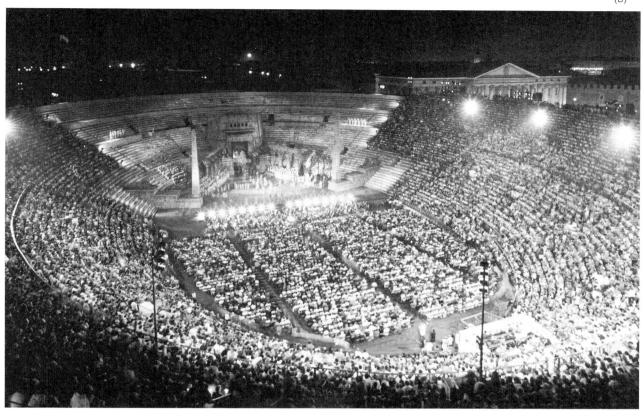

Fig. 5.32 continued *Verona Ampitheatre. (b) View of the inherited auditorium set for an opera*

INFORMAL EXTERNAL SPACES

Broadgate, London 1989

Architects: Arup Associates

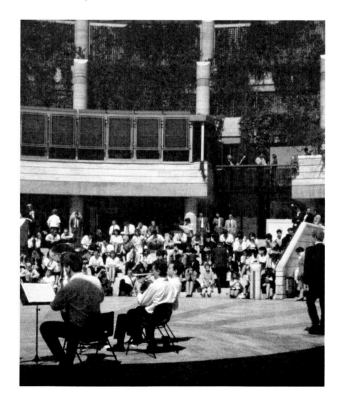

Fig. 5.33 *Broadgate, London. Open space formed by commercial development with provision for outdoor performances – street theatre – as an informal activity attracting users of the open space and from the adjacent developments*

Part Two
Approach to Design and Development

6

6 Design and development

The design and development of a building for the performing arts has become increasingly complex, involving a multiplicity of issues, intentions and interests, and responses to technological advancement. Complexity is due to various factors: the increased number of approaches to design with more feasible ideas, materials, technologies and specialists. There are also more issues to be resolved: controls, regulations and standards; new imperatives such as energy conservation; economic constraints; increased extent of information; an expectation of guaranteed performance-in-use. As the design and development process becomes more involved and prone to delays, time becomes a scarcer commodity and physical developments are expected faster. A consequence has been for the design process to become less easily reliant on experience and intuition. It is acknowledged that a degree of systematic progression ensures those involved in the process are fully informed.

The initial aim may appear to be simple, to provide a concert hall or theatre, but the processes involved to achieve such a building require consideration and resolution of often disparate interests. The requirements of public, performers, technicians, management and production staff, as well as the technical necessities, all need to be integrated into the building design, while an appropriate visual image, both externally and internally, must be achieved.

Ultimately the building becomes a back drop to the intense activity of staging a performance in an appropriate environment to an expectant audience. The performance space – the auditorium and platform or stage – is the predominant volume and focus of the overall layout, with support facilities, functionally linked to either the auditorium or platform/stage for the public, performers, technicians and management, as well as for rehearsal and, in the case of opera, dance, musicals and drama production, for the preparation of scenery, properties and costumes.

This Guide raises the issues to be considered and provides guidance on the decisions which define the intentions and eventual use of the building. There is an emphasis on the relative importance of those issues which require architectural resolution. The critical issues lie with the correct initial definition of the category of building for the performing arts, and its feasibility in terms of demand, resources and time-scale. All buildings for the performing arts are unique and therefore any consideration of standardized approaches and solutions is inappropriate. However the following chapters in this part outline those factors which appear to be constant for each situation and the wide range of categories classified under buildings for the performing arts indicate the choices available for the decisions to be made by the main participants.

The process commences when a client puts forward a proposal for a new or adapted building, setting out the reasons for building and outline requirements. Before detailed design can be progressed, the proposal needs to be tested and assessed as a feasibility study. This includes initial research to establish whether there is a demand in the particular locality, identification of the users to be accommodated, location and site characteristics, management of building, and financial viability, including sources of funds. Once feasibility is established, user requirements can be extracted and assessed in detail in the form of a comprehensive brief, as the written description of the eventual building. The building design can be developed in response to those detailed requirements by the architect and other consultants, and documentation prepared for its eventual construction and client occupation.

Those involved in the design and development process – the main participants – are the client and the users of the proposed building; the architect and other members of the design team as the professional consultants; the client's advisors; authorities such as planning, building regulations, licensing and fire; and funding organizations.

7

7 The client

The client is the person or organization who initiates and develops the building project. The client is also the authorized body who pays for the design, development and implementation at the various stages in the process.

There are various types of client involved in the buildings for the performing arts and they range from individuals to large public, commercial and private organizations. Not only does the type vary but also the objectives, requirements, resources and constraints. Some clients build for their own use, while others provide buildings to be used by others. For some, the basic motive may be concerned with education, culture, prestige, community development or urban regeneration.

The various types of client were categorized and the roles described in Chapter 4. While the types demonstrate a wide range of approach, each one will need to go through a similar design and development process whatever the initial reason for building. Broadly the client's interest in a project is to plan, fund and construct a new or adapted building:

- either for their own use as a resident company or to host touring companies.
- or to be handed over, leased to or sold to another organization as a resident company or to host touring companies

Those who initiate a building for the performing arts tend to be one of the following types:

- Local government initiating a new or improved building which they propose to manage directly or lease to a company or another organization.
- Educational institution requiring a new or improved building for the performing arts for its own exclusive use, for community use as well.
- An established, or newly-formed, independent music, dance or drama company requiring a new, improved or permanent facility for their own use as a resident company.
- Commercial organization building for their own use, for sale or for lease.
- Development organization initiating a building for the performing arts as part of a large development project. Such a development organization may combine public and private sector interests.
- Pressure group – group of individuals, community group or voluntary organization – requiring a building for the performing arts in their city, town or district, or maybe seeking the re-use of an existing building as a venue for a performing art. Such pressure groups may work well within the initial stages, including feasibility, on an *ad hoc* basis. Design and development will need a more formalized client organization.

A distinction is made between the initiating client, development committee and management structure. The *initiating client* refers to the person or group who prepares the initial statement outlining the intentions

leading to a new or adapted building and explores the basic ideas. These become the basis of the initial brief and feasibility study. As requirements become more defined then the final brief, and indeed the intentions, may vary from the initial assumptions. The *development committee* refers to those responsible for the detailed briefing and design development of the building project, including exploration of specific issues: the initiating client may be expanded to accommodate representatives of appropriate interests, or a new committee may be formed. The development committee requires to liaise with the building users to elicit detailed information and also to keep the wider public in touch with developments. With proposals which consist of a partnership between various parties then the development committee should include all the client bodies and associated interests. The *management structure* refers to the staffing arrangements for the new or adapted building when complete and in use.

These may be three separate functions: those who initiate a proposal pass over the intention to the development committee who, when the building is constructed, hand over to a management organization who run the facility. In other situations, especially where there is an established resident company re-locating or expanding, then the three functions can be carried out by the same people.

Further divisions may occur between land ownership, organizations who initiate and develop the construction of a building and management of the building use. For example the land may be owned by local government, the initiating client may be a pressure group, the development carried by an independent trust, and the building leased and managed by a commercial organization. Each landlord may place conditions on the leasees over development and use.

Clients within the *public sector* are controlled by predetermined rules and procedures which affect approvals, funding, accountability and time-scale. Departments can initiate projects, select sites, instruct consultants and monitor the progress, and can also produce the initial brief and preparing documents for outline planning application, loan sanctions and so on. Clients within the *private sector* – commercial, trusts and voluntary organizations – have a relative freedom. If it exists then the private client may rely on its own organization for the briefing to a brief-writer. The client body may be a *partnership* where the design and development may be more complex: the balance, constitution, membership and leadership of the client committee responsible for development will need to be agreed before decisions are made.

Client decisions

The client should define their organization and resources, covering:

- Management structure;
- Client organization;

- Decision-making structure;
- Fund raising;
- Building or site acquisition;
- Public and political support;
- Project management;
- Client's advisors.

Management structure

The management structure of the building when complete and in use, may be classified as one of the following:

- Independent organization, either as a limited company or trust, with a board of directors or trustees. The board defines policy including artistic and financial responsibility. An alternative is for an independent organization to be constituted as a co-operative with all members of say, a company, having equal shares in the assets.
- Public sector, with the local government running a building directly, who can benefit from the central services of the authority such as marketing, consultation expertise and personnel management. Dis-benefits included restrictions often placed on a company by the local government procedures.
- Educational institutions, such as a University, where the management may be part of an existing department (such as Drama), or a separate unit within the institution. Facilities in schools tend to be managed by a number of staff, as their sole function or combined with a teaching responsibility.
- Commercial organization, as an individual, small independent company or part of a large company, with the company being limited and constituted with directors, who manage a building.

Local government may lease a facility to a commercial organization to manage, while retaining building ownership. The proposal would require to be financially viable to encourage commercial interest. The leasing arrangement may require conditions covering type of productions, pattern of use and so on. Local government may also lease to an independent organization, as a trust, to run the building: a benefit is the distance achieved between the political process and the artistic policy. Similarly educational institutions may lease to a commercial organization or a trust.

The staff categories of a building for the performing arts are considered under two broad headings:

- Building with a resident company. The management structure may be divided into functional areas of responsibility:
  - public-related staff: usherettes, sales staff, box-office staff, fire officers, house manager;
  - management: artistic and financial direction, administration, audience development, publicity;
  - performance-related staff: actors, musicians, singers; stage lighting, sound, machinery and management; repair and maintenance staff;

stage door keeper – these may be production related, seasonal contracts or longer term;
  - production-related staff: company, organization, rehearsal and practice, storage and the preparation of scenery, properties and costumes, if applicable.
  - building maintenance: maintenance staff, cleaners.
- Buildings that host touring companies. The functional requirements include administration, artistic policy and the planning and development of an annual or seasonal programme of productions and events. These may be carried out by one person – the director – with or without back-up staff according to the scale of the operation. Permanent staff can also include technicians (which may be restricted to an electrician and repair and maintenance staff), usherettes, firemen, sales staff and box office staff, and also cleaners, maintenance staff and a stage door keeper.

In large facilities offering a multi-use auditorium and stage with frequent changes, staff (whether permanent or temporary) will be required to effect the changes.

The larger the organization, the more hierarchical the structure tends to be, with department sections, heads and staff. Roles within such an organization are usually clearly defined and are focused on staging a performance at least once daily and on preparing for a production. The larger companies refer to the major opera, dance and musical companies with their own facilities, producing scenery, properties and costumes, where staff numbers can exceed 1200 (Royal Opera House, London) including performers. In contrast a small touring company may travel together in a single van, where performers double as technicians, and play in a church hall, managed by a part-time caretaker.

Any marked distinction between different groups within an organization have been eroded over time but depend on the type of organization. High performance stage lighting, sound and machinery has encouraged improved skills among technicians while more professional management and accounting systems have been encouraged in the administration. Performers have improved their social status and the standards of back-stage accommodation have developed in parallel.

The style of management varies according to organization and ranges from the highly structured to the relatively informal as seen with the smaller companies. It is noted however that buildings for the performing arts, especially those housing their own company creating productions, require a combination of managerial approaches: the creative activities of the artistic director, designers and performers as well as directors/choreographers; the financial and auditing functions of the administration; the exactness of the technical staff during a performance; the manufacturing processes required for the production of scenery, properties and costumes including craft skills.

A move to a new building or an adjustment of an existing building inevitably means change within an existing organization by re-deployment or increases in staff as well as alterations to the management structure.

Client organization

A client organization is required to be formally, legally and properly constituted. Where no such organization exists then one will need to be formed. This becomes especially the case once it is necessary to employ consultants and project staff, purchase a site or building and be involved in other expenditure.

Clients within the private sector – commercial organization, private trust or voluntary organization – have the opportunity of becoming a company limited by guarantee. Such a format prohibits the company from having shareholders and distributing profits to its members. This format is regulated by the Companies Act.

Also, for non-profit making organizations, the question of charitable status should be considered. The benefits include tax concessions and eligibility for certain types of grant aid. The Charity Commission in England, for example, provides information on the method of applying for registration.

Clients within the public sector – local government or educational institutions – will be part of organizations already constituted. They may consider the formation of a private trust, independent of the public sector as a limited company with charitable status for the building project during its design and development, and also when up and running.

Decision-making structure

The client should set up an appropriate structure for decision-making and management of the project. Individuals and small organizations can rely on a simple line of contact between participants. The more complex the client body, then the larger the number of interests involved. It is therefore essential that the roles and responsibilities of everyone involved in the project – whether in a management, professional or advisory capacity, and that the channels of communication, especially day-to-day, are clearly defined.

The client needs to determine:

- who will be responsible for the initial statement;
- who will be making the decisions, giving approvals and instructions;
- a method of liaison between the client and the various consultants and advisers;
- the functions of those in the client's organization who will be involved in the project.

In addition the client should consider the:

- initial statement of intent describing the reason for the building project;
- objectives and brief of the proposed project;

- selection and appointment of the professional consultants and advisers, including the definition of their roles, responsibilities and remuneration;
- time-scale of the project and the method of monitoring progress, including the time-table for briefing, feasibility, design and construction;
- method of formally recording decisions;
- sources of funds and arrangements for fund raising, including the possible appointment of professional fund raisers;
- continued public and political support for the project and possible appointment of a public relations officer;
- management of the project including the possible appointment of a project manager.

Fund raising

Fund raising is a characteristic of the majority of projects for buildings for the performing arts. Unless all money for the capital expenditure is forthcoming from the client, as may be the case with an individual benefactor, public sector or commercial organization, then all or part of the amount required will have to be obtained from the public, industry, commerce and foundations.

There are two stages requiring funds, covering the cost of the feasibility study and the building project including design and construction. It is advisable to consider funds for the feasibility study (which covers the cost of the initial brief, market research, development analysis and design implication) as a separate amount from the fund raising for the building project. The amount for the feasibility study is a relatively small amount compared with the ultimate capital expenditure but is a critical investment to ensure the basis of the project is sound. Funds can be obtained from the parent organization, private sector, public, foundations and some arts boards. The major fund-raising campaign should concentrate on the building project with the amount to be raised based on accurate figures and ensured viability of the project. A strategy for fund raising should include methods targeted at specific funding organizations and at the general public. The appeal for funds needs to be planned well in advance with clear, accurate and comprehensive information about the project to be laid before potential fund givers.

Fund raising requires to be co-ordinated and conducted in a systematic manner by a single person as a full-time activity. The client should consider the employment of a specialist in development fund raising, appoint a specialist consultant or seek advice from a specialist consultant. Fund-raising consultants usually do not run an appeal but can advise a client body on methods, including presentation techniques. Only where the extent of funds to be raised is high should a client consider appointing such a consultant to carry out the task. Otherwise the fund raising could be carried out from within the client organization.

Promotional material, as back-up material, needs to be well designed with the potential funders in mind. A graphic designer should be commissioned to produce the material in consultation with the fund raiser and also the public relations officer.

Building or site acquisition

The search for a suitable building or site in an appropriate location at a reasonable cost may take some time. A search is subject to market opportunities as a building or site, after evaluation, may require to be purchased speedily. A building or site may be leased, usually with conditions, from the local government or a commercial organization. Outline planning permission (at least) should be obtained before purchase/lease and the location needs to be checked to ensure access, size, shape and position are suitable. Site requirements are discussed in detail in Chapter 11.

Public and political support

Support throughout the design and development of the building project must be sustained among the users, funders, public, agencies and politicians, as well as local media and interest groups. If money is from public funds then any political argument against such an allocation can continue after a decision in favour of the project. Such support and political sensitivity may necessitate the appointment by the client of a public relations officer, directly or as a consultant, who can keep the public and interested parties informed of progress to ensure a positive involvement. The opportunity can be taken at the completion of the various stages within the design and construction of informing the public of progress and thereby sustaining interest.

Project management

Except for the smallest of building projects, a project director should be identified within the client's organization or a new appointment made to a post with full-time or predominant responsibility for coordinating the building project. The functions of the project director include developing the brief in consultation with building users and professional consultants, negotiating with funding bodies and making grant applications, planning over time the building project and communicating the proposals at the various stages of development to the client body.

Client's advisors

During the briefing and feasibility stages various advisers may be necessary. These will be, mainly, short-term or *ad hoc* appointments to resolve particular issues, such as site or building acquisition, organization structure and constitution, security, public liability and so on. Such advisers can include: legal adviser, estate agent, insurance adviser, accountant, management consultant, surveyor. In addition the client may employ or have within their organization – as may be the case with local government – architectural and cost advisers who may evaluate the advice provided by members of the design team. National and regional arts organizations are available to give advice over the formation of the client's organization, procedure and also proposals. Legal advice should be obtained to ensure the correct formation of a limited company and charitable trust, including the responsibilities of the trustees. For details of advisers and the services they offer, refer to Appendix 2.

8

8 Consultants

The design and development of a building for the performing arts requires knowledge and expertise across a wide range of issues from the establishment of demand through to the exacting technical requirements. This range is not found with other building types such as houses and offices. Appointment of specialists to advise and direct the client become essential to advance the project. Professional consultants can offer:

- experience in areas where the client may be lacking;
- familiarity with solutions which may be workable, appropriate, and cost effective, and those which are not;
- credibility with funders, community and authorities;
- assistance over the questions to be asked and identification of specific issues.

The client should determine which consultants are required during the briefing and feasibility stages, and which are required during design and development.

Before any work on the design of the building can commence the architect at least should be appointed for the feasibility study, with other consultants, specialists and advisers as considered appropriate. The full design team will need to be selected for the design and construction of the building project. Formal agreement should include definition of limits of responsibilities, scope of service, time implication, fee agreement including expenses, etc. A standard form may be used or an exchange of letters.

Professional consultants will be necessary at different stages in the development of the project to assist the client. These include:

- professional brief writer, briefing specialist, or theatre consultant;

- architect;
- surveyor: for obtaining accurate site information or when adapting/converting an existing building;
- quantity surveyor or cost consultant, for cost estimates and cost control;
- acoustic consultant, lighting consultant, stage machinery consultant;
- other specialists such as landscape architects and interior designer; the brief may suggest conference and restaurant design specialist, specialist advisers on access for all disabilities (mobility/hearing/sight).

The client should investigate suitable firms and ascertain services provided, fees, contracts, etc. Consider, amongst other aspects:

- the experience of architects and other consultants in dealing with similar buildings;
- personalities: ensure compatibility between all concerned.

Selection of an architect may be by competition, interview, experience, recommendation or qualitative analysis.

A *theatre consultant* may be employed to provide a full service which could include defining the brief, advice on the organization of the management structure, the provision of detailed technical information. The service may be partial, such as covering technical information on stage machinery, or nominal, such as acting as a second opinion or bringing experience from elsewhere to bear on a project. A theatre consultant is an essential appointment if the client has no experience of the proposed building type.

For details of consultants and the services they offer refer to Appendix 2.

9

9 Stages in design and development

This section is concerned with the various stages in the design and development of a project. Each stage is described within distinct headings, although each may overlap with some of the others as well as being individually identifiable. The aim is to raise the aspects to be considered within each stage and, where appropriate, the options available. Design and development has been broken down into the following headings:

- *Client's proposal*: The initial stage is the client committing objectives, reasons for building and defining the project, including the exploration of ideas, opportunities and support.
- *Feasibility study*: Testing client's proposal to establish its feasibility including a series of studies: demand, resources and constraints, initial brief, building design, time-scale, financial viability.
- *Briefing process*: Establishing user requirements; list of activities, shape and size of spaces and their relationship, and their technical necessities, equipment and furniture.
- *Design process*: The three-dimensional creation of the building design, the detail design, and the production of information for the construction of the building and inviting tenders from building contractors.
- *Building process*: The construction of the building, within a specified period of time, and its commissioning.
- *Hand-over and opening night*: The client taking over the completed new or adapted building: staffing, rehearsing and other activities in preparation of the start of the new season or one-off event.
- *Building in use*: The consideration of the cost-in-use of the building over its lifetime covering maintenance requirements.

An emphasis in this guide is placed on the client's proposal and feasibility study as two discrete stages, placing importance on the correct definition of the type of facility required and the testing of the proposal in a rigorous manner before progressing into the design process and commitment of resources, such as fund raising and building or site acquisition.

Client's proposal

The client initiates a building project by putting together a *proposal* in sufficient detail to provide a broad outline of their requirements. The proposal should be the result of an exploration of ideas for a new or adapted building, which can be tested to determine the actual feasibility.

The aim of this stage is to outline the general requirements and to plan future action, with the client, possibly with professional help, defining the problem and considering the questions who? what? where? when? how? by whom? why build and create a new or adapted facility?

For those existing organizations or companies, the members should be consulted and encouraged to assist with the formulation of objectives. Experience can be sought from local interest groups, comparable organizations and visits to similar facilities elsewhere. To generate and develop ideas and establish priorities, techniques such as brain-storming and value analysis may be applicable. The opportunity should be taken to evaluate the initial statement of objectives and to consider alternative, and wider, views of the role of the proposed facility.

The initiating client should consider the following:

- nature and character of the client body;
- reason for building;
- client's objectives and priorities;
- proposal scope and requirements;
- community and political support;
- development options;
- decision.

Nature and character of the client body

The client body should be described as fully as possible, including evaluation of the current position: function or purpose for existence, and activities; philosophy and history; economic assets and liabilities; sources of funding; management structure. For those with their own facility, its adequacy should be assessed and the current audience characteristics, numbers and pattern of use should be recorded. All types of client should also establish the level of experience in the design and development and running of the proposed building for a performing art.

Reason for building

The client's initial reason for considering a building project can include one (or more) of the following:

- an existing company or organization seeking a more adequate building due to changes in their programme of use, management objectives, building image, funding method or technical and physical standards;
- an existing company or organization seeking a new facility due to re-location;
- the identification of a gap within a regional pattern of provision, requiring a new facility;
- a one-off or annual event, such as an arts festival, requiring a temporary facility;
- the re-use of a vacant building or site, seen as a development opportunity;
- part of a wider strategy of revitalization, tourist/ conference policy, or economic/community/cultural development;

- seeking justification to allocate resources within the local political context or parent organization.

Whatever the initial reason, the client requires to fully explore the reality of development covering demand, resources, finance and time-scale, and the reasons for embarking on a building project need to be assessed. Broadly the initial motivation lies with the identification of a need or with development opportunities.

Client's objectives and priorities

The client requires to define short- and long-term objectives in terms of the following objectives and activities.

Artistic objectives

- *Type and scale of production*: Establish if the production(s) is/are to be music, opera, musicals, dance or drama and if the scale is small, medium or large. The client needs to recognize the primary functions and the priority of use. The client may ask for several types of production to be housed in the same auditorium but there are restrictions on the level of adaptation.
- *Operational category*: Establish if the building is to host touring companies only, house a resident company which initiates its own productions only, or whether a combination is required to host touring companies and house a resident company or companies.
- *Programme selection*: Establish if the programme of productions is:
  - not subject to any restrictions or policy;
  - to concentrate on a particular policy such as presenting established classics, new works, experimental formats or performances following local, national or ethnic traditions.
- *Type of company*: Establish if the performers, as members of a resident company or visiting companies, are:
  - amateur and/or professional.
  - restricted to particular social groups (ethnic, people with disabilities, youth) or restricted to location or parent institution.
  - small-, medium- or large-scale.
    Consider standard of performance: standards range from international centres of excellence to local community participation as a recreational activity. If a resident company then it may already be established and will transfer to the new or adapted building, or, if not established, a new company will be formed. If the building is to host visiting companies then the client should consider the type of companies and their availability.
- *Pattern of use*: Establish if the building is to be open continuously, seasonally (e.g. summer season only), intermittently (occasional use of an auditorium for performance), or for a one-off event. Determine the

hours the facility will be open to the public: if performances occur in the auditorium only in the evening or at other times, if the building is to be open during non-performance times. More than one company may use a single auditorium within a day: children's workshops in the morning, rehearsals in the afternoon, evening performance by resident company, late night show by touring company.

Social objectives

Clarify the *role in the community* of the proposed building and if it is, or they are:

- To serve a metropolitan, regional, town, district, or neighbourhood catchment area, or a resort, specialist centre or institution. The client needs to define the market for which the facility and programme of use is intended.
- Open to all sections of the public, with or without targeting of non-traditional audiences, or restricted to members of a parent organization (e.g. University) or social group (e.g. children).
- To provide an attraction for the tourist, conference and other visitors.
- For community use:
  - to encourage participation in creative leisure activities and appreciation of the performing arts;
  - to provide a social focus and meeting place;
  - to act as an information point and resource centre for a particular performing art or art in general;
  - to provide a base and/or performance space for clubs in the community.
- For educational use:
  - to teach the art and craft of performance;
  - to act as a base for Theatre-in-Education;
  - to provide performances and workshops for schoolchildren and students within an educational programme.
- For festival use: to act as a focus or one of a series of locations for a concentrated period of time, when all performances relate to a specific theme or general display of music and drama by companies defined geographically (local, regional, national, international).

Financial objectives

Establish the primary economic objectives, such as:

- If the aim is to make a profit or to be non-profit making, with or without relying on subsidies and sponsorship.
- To own, hire or lease land and building.
- To include associated commercial activities and franchises: conferences, lectures, meeting spaces for hire, restaurant, bars, shops.
- To maximize use of provision.
- The method of raising capital and revenue funds.

Management objectives

Consider objectives which assist the management of the facility such as:

- the layout to ensure efficient management, minimum maintenance costs, maximum use of the spaces, flexibility and future change;
- ease of control, supervision and security;
- management structure;
- marketing methods and audience development.

Associated activities

Consider the inclusion of the following types of activities:

- complimentary activities in the auditorium such as conferences and lectures;
- supplementary activities such as an art gallery, painting workshop, or as part of an *arts complex* with additional facilities for painting, sculpture and other arts participatory activities, and exhibition spaces and display areas.

Building objectives

Consider the following possibilities:

- whether to erect a new building, to adapt, convert or extend an existing building or make an existing facility more effective by adaptation;
- whether the facility needs to be indoor or outdoor, permanent or temporary;
- level of flexibility required and allowance for future change;
- standards of finishes and internal environments – lighting, heating, air-conditioning and other services;
- if the building is to be developed in phases;
- establishing links with other functions within the catchment area and/or a larger, existing building complex.

Development objectives

Consider the following:

- conservation of an existing building;
- regeneration of a run-down area;
- community focus;
- improvement of an area's image;
- attracting commercial and industrial development.

The client's primary motivation may be one or another of the factors: improving a derelict area, providing a drama company, community emphasis. Whatever the motivation, all factors apply and the feasibility requirements remain. These objectives should be examined to establish medium- and long-term needs and priorities and to evaluate the ability to achieve all these ends.

Proposal scope and requirements

The client must formulate in *general* terms the scope of their proposal including:

- demand for the proposed building and the activities it is required to accommodate, including the type of production (music, opera, musicals, dance, drama), audience capacity and requirements of the users;
- building's life-span and flexibility: possible changes of use over time and phasing of the project;
- character and standards envisaged;
- location characteristics and linkage with other activities within the community;
- cost implications; capital, income, running costs, access to funds;

Overall the client should identify the building category described in Chapter 5, with the classification based on location.

Community and political support

Local community and political support is essential throughout the various stages of the design and development and ultimately for the success of the building. The client should consider, as background information to the proposal, the following:

- Holding discussions with local business, commercial and political interests as well as officials in local government and others active within the community to be served by the proposed building. This may help to establish how they would see the proposal contributing to the local social, cultural and economic life. Similarly if the proposal is restricted to being within a parent organization, the discussion should take place with representative members to establish the contribution to the social, cultural and perhaps educational life of that organization.
- Running workshops to include local interest groups and public within the community or members of the parent organization to exchange ideas and heighten interest in the proposal.

The client may have to justify the need for a building for a performing art as beneficial to the community or parent organization: in Chapter 1 particular forms of justification were categorized as: cultural, economic, educational, quality of life, regeneration, cultural democracy.

The client may have to justify the proposal to the wider community the facility is designed to serve, potential funding organizations and decision-makers (politicians, parent organization) of the return on investment of money and possibly time.

Development options

For an existing organization or company with their own facility then the first option is to consider the use of the existing accommodation more effectively by internal physical change or by adjustment of management policy. Otherwise the building options for all clients include:

- Construction of a new building on a green-field site or the replacement of an existing building. New build provides a purpose-designed facility without the possible compromise of the brief to accommodate the activities within an existing building. There is relative freedom with the design of a new building which allows a number of alternative layouts and the incorporation of a higher level of technology if necessary.
- Conversion of an existing building requiring change of use, internal adaptation and possible extension. An existing building requires careful assessment to establish the fit between the existing building structure and the space volumes required by the brief. Redundant churches or chapels, for example, are more sympathetic volumes as the auditorium for a building for the performing arts. This can be the case for recitals where the existing volume may be compatible with the building interior. Building types with columns at close centres and low ceiling heights may demand prohibitively high conversion costs to produce the large spaces required.

  The character of an existing building may lend itself to a public building while avoiding the impact of the new. An existing building may occupy a desirable location and, due to planning restrictions on its use, have a low selling price. An existing building may be brought into use at a low cost and may allow ease of phased work. This may be more applicable where a pilot scheme is considered necessary to develop an audience for a particular type of production.
- Adaptation of an existing building for the performing arts, including internal modification and additions. Adaptation offers an established facility in a known location to continue, including, possibly, during the construction period.

The land for new build or an existing building may be rented, leased or purchased. Renting and leasing places a continued burden on the revenue as a fixed cost while purchase may mean the erosion of capital at a time when the pressure on capital is the greatest – covering the construction costs.

A possible method of achieving a dedicated building for the performing arts is for a developer of a large scheme to contribute to the capital cost of a building for the performing arts within the complex. Contributions can take the form of a lump sum from the developer, a construction of a new facility or conversion of an existing building, or the provision of a shell, an enclosure, which is fitted out by the client body. This concept of a contribution by a developer is combined with planning permission to develop a larger, usually commercial, scheme. For such a developer, in addition to actually obtaining the permission sought, the inclusion of a building for the performing arts generates a wider interest and brings in people who may also use the commercial facilities such as restaurants, cafes, shops and so on.

Decision

A decision has to be made by a client to proceed to the next stage – the feasibility study. This is a preliminary decision only and relates to the investment of time and funds to commence the formal process of briefing and design in order to investigate in detail the feasibility of the proposed project. As new information becomes available through later stages, it may be necessary to review the decision. The initiating client should prepare a written statement summarizing the factors which condition the proposal.

Feasibility study

Before the building design can be developed in detail, the client's proposal will need to be evaluated both physically and financially to ensure its feasibility. This is seen as a distinct stage in the design and development process. Feasibility is critical as the pivot linking the proposal with the design and its implementation. The importance of the feasibility study lies with the assurance the framework offers for subsequent stages. It becomes increasingly more costly to rectify mistakes as the project progresses. This underlines the main benefit of an investment of time and money to ensure viability of the project. Preparatory work should be carried out in a sound manner: short cuts and the obvious solution should be treated with caution.

The feasibility study relates the reality of *demand* for the client's proposal to the reality of *supply*, and is concerned with the following *local* conditions:

- Assessment of demand and support for the proposed programme of uses, including the selected type(s) of production and ancillary functions, if required, such as restaurant, art gallery and conference facilities.
- Availability of appropriate resident company, touring companies or local community companies as well as management, technical, production and other staff: also the availability of appropriate exhibitions for the art gallery and similar functions, if included in the brief.
- Analysis of sites for a new building or existing buildings for conversion or improvement in terms of availability, location, access, size and shape to accommodate the activities.
- Production of the initial brief; the requirements of the visitors and users of the proposed building, expressed as activities and their relationships, and the spaces required to house them.
- Building design; evaluation of different layouts and the architectural implications of the project including standard of provision and building character.

- Analysis of time-scale; including the programme for the design, development and building work, and possible phasing of the project including effect on programme of use.
- Financial viability; examination of level of capital expenditure, revenue and income including sources of funds, level of subsidy or profit and cash flow.

These issues, outlined above, should be considered together, each having a consequence on the others. A significant link is the *audience or seating capacity* as both an expression of demand and principal component of the income calculation. To answer the specific question posed by the list above, a series of studies will need to be carried out. Possible studies are outlined and discussed in Part Three, and cover:

- Audience, companies and staff;
- Site considerations;
- Initial brief: auditorium and platform/stage;
- Initial brief: support facilities;
- Building design;
- Time-scale;
- Financial appraisal.

In addition the feasibility study should include an evaluation of the community and political support and, in particular, the ability to sustain the efforts to achieve the project: which interests will assist and which may hinder.

The feasibility study can be carried out by:

- the client, assisted by professional advice;
- a number of consultants commissioned to carry out separate studies constituting the feasibility, with the client coordinating the evidence;
- a single (or lead) consultant appointed to carry out the entire feasibility study.

How the feasibility study is actually carried out will be dependent on the context, the scale of the proposal, its complexity and the degree of available information. The larger the proposal then the more politically sensitive the project may be which should encourage a more exacting testing.

Feasibility requires the input and involvement of the client and the eventual users, as well as market research expertise (to establish demand), architect, surveyor, brief-writer/theatre consultant, acoustician and legal adviser. The process requires dialogue between all concerned to explore ideas and to determine what is feasible.

The depth of analysis and design sufficient to prove feasibility varies and depends on, in part, the proposal's compatibility with other examples. The closer the existing example the less analysis and design needed. A unique and especially experimental situation would require more exploration. In all situations it is better to progress into the feasibility as deeply as resources reasonably allow.

Data collection needs to be done in relation to stated objectives and within a restricted time period. A balance is necessary between the penalty of insufficient information against the cost of obtaining it. New information will be added through the briefing and design processes, so the data needs to be stored in such a manner that new information can be added easily.

The documentation for feasibility can vary in length and format, depending on the nature of the proposal. A small proposal could achieve statement, initial brief, building design and costing in a single exercise and document. Large projects may require a series of specific studies presented as interim studies.

A specific study, which may be a critical exercise determining the category of building, is the design of the auditorium and platform/stage, independent of the general layout of the building. Studies can examine seating capacity, relationship between platform/stage and auditorium, acoustics of the auditorium, sightlines for the audience and so on. This examination would involve the architect, acoustician, theatre consultant, as well as the client and also model-makers and/or computer simulation. The necessity to carry out a discrete study of the auditorium and platform/stage becomes more acute in the following situations:

- Where the auditorium is for the appreciation of productions including music, if without amplification. The concert hall auditorium, for example, is particularly sensitive to the acoustic performance.
- Where maximum seating capacity is critical with capacity requiring to be calculated within the constraints that determine the maximum enclosure of the auditorium.
- For experimental forms, where precedent cannot illustrate the format being proposed, and a detailed examination is required to show that the form can satisfy the needs as well as illustrating the proposal.

The client should select an option as the recommendation for development. The selection needs to be recorded and presented, including the reasons for the selection, in an appropriate manner. The key questions that are to be answered remain: proven demand, available resources, funding viability and support to progress until completion.

If the questions are not adequately answered then the proposal cannot be progressed or parts of the proposal require to be re-thought. If the costs are too high then a reduced scheme could be considered or an alternative funding package.

If the decision is to progress then the client should carry out the following:

- The objectives should be restated and made generally available as the common basis of the project for those involved.
- The site or building should be acquired. This is critical, as without acquisition the development will be inhibited; acquisition can be conditional on planning approval.
- Planning approval should be obtained.

- Re-organization of the committee. The client should consider the committee membership and functions of funding, briefing, consultants, public relations and programme.
- Development of a design and building programme.
- Commencement of fund raising.
- Presentation of the scheme, preparation of drawings and models of presentation to fund raisers, press and interested parties.

The results of the feasibility study may be used to raise funds and publicize the project, and will act as the basis for subsequent stages in the design and development.

Briefing process

The brief is a statement of the client's intentions and the requirement of the users of the proposed building, presented as a list of activities, the shape and size of the spaces required to accommodate them, and the relationship to each other. A detailed brief includes for each space the type of enclosure, equipment and furniture, and environmental requirements. In general, the brief for a building for the performing arts requires definition of the user requirements for the following:

- auditorium and platform/stage;
- public spaces and their support areas;
- performance and management spaces;
- production space, if applicable, covering rehearsal spaces, company administration, wardrobe, and scenery and properties workshops.

Proper briefing is important to the success of a building project. Conversely inadequate and incorrect briefing will be reflected adversely in the building when in use.

There are various identifiable stages in the briefing process:

- The written statement outlining a proposal including the reason for building and the client's objectives.
- The initial brief, listing the activities and space requirements and their relationships, expressed as a schedule of accommodation.

These – the proposal and initial brief – are components of the feasibility study.

- The detailed brief, when the initial brief is expanded, will include, for each space, function, size and shape, users, special needs and linkages as well as furniture, fitting, finishes, layouts, enclosure, environmental requirements and structural issues.

The *detailed* brief follows the foundations established in the feasibility study. Such a detailed brief can be prepared for the option which the feasibility identifies.

The brief is derived from consideration of many factors: the primary factor is the identification of user requirements but it is also influenced by budget,

climate, site conditions, legal constraints, change over time and the trade-offs between requirements, costs and viability.

The brief states a set of desired conditions and it is a way of defining, ordering and specifying objectives and user requirements systematically, as well as outlining the methods for achieving them.

The brief tends to be presented as a report and can vary in length, content and form. These depend on the nature of the project. As well as a record of objectives and user requirements, the brief also acts as the instructions given by a client to their appointed architect, establishing the basis for the design of the building. The initial brief can assist the client in selecting the appropriate architect and the other professional consultants, while a detailed brief may be used as a competition document as a further method of selecting an architect. The brief can also form part of a contractual document within a legal agreement between the client and others.

The brief needs to be specific (covering all the requirements of the different categories of users) and flexible (so that the architect can contribute through the creation of the building as a whole). With the conversion of an existing building there can be a greater interaction between the existing form and fabric and the user requirements.

Starting with a preliminary statement prepared by the client (possibly with professional help), the brief is developed and constantly refined through a process of communication, investigation, analysis and evaluation. The process of briefing becomes one of dialogue between all concerned; a process of finding as well as solving problems; of determining and defining objectives, constraints, resources, subjective and objective criteria; of determining and exploring what is appropriate and possible, evaluating proposals and making recommendations. Briefing is often controversial, since, while technical requirements can usually be quantified, this is often not possible with other more abstract criteria. It should therefore be a process of debate and a means of decision-making, encouraging participation by, and feedback from, all the participants.

The brief, therefore, changes and grows continuously as the design proceeds. The design solution evolves from the brief and can, in turn, clarify and expand it through early design work which helps to identify problems, objectives and criteria. When it is realized in the completed project, it also has a role in post-construction evaluation. After a certain point in the design process, which will vary from project to project, major changes to the brief can lead to abortive work and have cost implications for the client or the design team.

There is no single way of approaching briefing, it always forms the foundation of the design process and constitutes an integral part of this process. This defines the intimate relationship between the object of design and the design process that is crucial to the general sense of competence. For these reasons, and because there are usually so many factors and variable involved in the design of even the simplest building, it is important that the brief be objectively, imaginatively and comprehensively developed, whatever the method used.

The users

Central to the briefing process is the identification of the users of the proposed new or adapted building, and their specific requirements. The users refer to those who will actually function in the building: categories of users include the visitors to the public facilities including the audiences, performers (as resident or touring company), management, technicians and production staff. It is important to understand, and be responsive to, the implications of their requirements. The client and the users may be distinct: where a proposed building is for an existing organization or company the users are known; a client may build speculatively where the specific users are not known at the time of the briefing.

Visitors, as members of the public or a parent organization, who will be attending a performance and/ or the foyer, refreshment areas and other attractions, are unknown. Their requirements may be identified by:

- relying on the experience of the management;
- relying on the experience of comparable facilities elsewhere and/or the traditions of similar buildings;
- market research studies to establish visitor preferences;
- workshops and discussions with representative groups from the catchment area;
- general research studies into visitor response to public facilities.

Visitors may be restricted (e.g. from a particular parent organization) or targeted towards a specific group in the community (e.g. children) and obviously the requirements need to be defined in response to the particular situation.

Where the proposed building is to be designed to accommodate an existing organization, then the permanent or regular staff, as the users, can be actively involved in the definition of their requirements, with a study on whether to retain the existing organizational functions and decisions made or change the method of operating in the new building. It would be rare for no change to occur and for the existing method of operation to be replicated. Even the act of moving from one building to another will alter, and improve, the way the organization has been operating.

To produce a balanced brief conflicts of requirements will have to be resolved while excessively expansionist views of particular individuals and departments will require curtailment. Close response will also need to be paid to the requirements of specific users unsympathetic to the layout.

The users need to define their function, the space they need to carry out their activities, the equipment they require and how they relate to other functions. Such information can be extracted by:

- direct involvement of all users in the briefing process through discussion;
- questionnaire survey of the users;
- observation by the brief-writer of activities and operations.

Experience elsewhere from similar building types can provide additional information, act as a check on the internal study of user requirements and may be a source of alternative ways in which certain functions can operate.

For buildings which exclusively or occasionally host touring companies, such companies need to be identified at this stage and their requirements for the delivery of scenery and costumes, performance (stage size, equipment, lighting and sound) performers (number and type of dressing rooms, rehearsal requirements), management and storage can be ascertained. Such studies should be carried out systematically, including the context of the experience of touring companies approached, by direct involvement by the companies, questionnaire survey and observations of their operations elsewhere.

When the proposal is for an unknown organization then the particular users cannot be identified until completion. In this situation it is necessary to rely on studies of comparable built examples elsewhere and the experience of others in the design and management of such buildings. Studies of comparable buildings should be carried out in a systematic manner and include a description of the context, expressed deficiencies and the advantages. Where a client is developing a building to be used by an organization other than themselves, at least the artistic director and/ or executive director should be appointed early within the design process so that the objectives can be determined against their artistic/financial policy. Specific user requirements can be then identified against a known set of objectives.

The client should consider the organization of the brief and the identification of the user requirements. The briefing process can be carried out by the client, with a member of the client organization given the responsibility of gathering together the information. If a client does not have experience in briefing and the practice of running a building for the performing arts then they should consider the employment of a brief writer, who can be:

- an architect, appointed to provide a briefing service either separately or as part of the full design service;
- a professional brief writer, who has specialized in the type of client organization;
- a theatre consultant, as specialist in the category of building being proposed.

The professional brief writer specializes in assisting a client to determine and describe their requirements, and can carry out objective studies of the user requirements and design implications.

The construction of a building for the performing arts has its own peculiar problems. Unless the client is familiar with all aspects of the practice they should employ a theatre consultant.

The brief writer will need to carry out the following processes:

- consultation with individuals and groups as eventual users of the building, if known, or in comparable facilities, if not.
- collection of information in a systematic manner.
- establishment of priorities and resolution of conflict.
- clear presentation of requirements and relationships.
- identification and classification of management structure.
- an indication of the overall image of the proposed building.

Information gathered as user requirements needs to be formally recorded and the content needs to be carefully examined so that duplication can be avoided and certain areas reduced or reconsidered.

Design process

The design of a building is, at its simplest, the creative development of an idea, in three-dimensional form, to solve problems. Design includes comprehending a multiplicity of information, the resolution of apparently conflicting issues and the application of appropriate technologies to satisfy particular social aims. Most situations are complex and the design of a building for a performing art is no exception. Indeed the geometry of the auditorium and platform/stage, the extent of servicing and technical necessities, and the public expectations makes such a building type even more complex than the majority of buildings.

The *design process* refers to those activities necessary to solve the problems from the understanding of the client's brief to the finalized design. The methods adopted can range from those based on intuition and experience on the one hand, to formal approaches on the other. Each method has to deal with measurable items – structure, ventilation, acoustics, audience sightlines and so on – and those essential qualitative aspects of design such as the external image, conducive atmosphere in the auditorium, welcoming public entrance and so on.

The process is not a linear sequence of logical steps leading from one stage to another by finding the correct answers at each stage before progressing to the next, but rather a series of actions comprising decisions grouped for convenience into stages, some or all of which may occur at the same time. The design of the auditorium and platform/stage may precede, say, the acquisition of the site and funds, while detailed studies of the public facilities may not emerge until a later stage within the design process, although initial assumptions will have to be made. Ultimately the design of a building needs to satisfy all the

requirements simultaneously. There may be a conflict of requirements requiring an acceptable level of compromise which will necessitate bargaining between the various interests. This process of bargaining is an inevitable aspect within the activity of designing a building: no systematic design process eases the bargaining. Also as new information becomes available, so ideas that seemed correct at an earlier stage may have to be changed. Indeed, the complete cycle of actions may have to be reconsidered on various occasions. Broadly the stages in the design process are:

- The process commences with a full appraisal of the detailed brief and the client's intentions by the appointed architect and other members of the design team.
- The development by the design team of a *scheme design* showing the layout of the building, relationship of the layout of the site, architectural character and cost estimate, responding to the stated standards of finishes, equipment, services and so on.
- The adjustment of the scheme design in the light of the client's comments and the development of the spatial arrangements including structure and services, construction method and appearance in sufficient detail to submit the scheme for detailed planning permission and for the client to approve the design.
- The detailed design of all aspects of the scheme including coordination and integration by the architect of work produced by the other consultants in the design team and specialists and an application for approval under the building regulations or codes. Application under building regulations or codes covers structure, ventilation, construction, energy, fire and provision for disabled people. Detailed drawings, specifications and energy and structural calculations need to be submitted and approval given before construction begins.
- A detailed estimate of costs can also be determined.

Once the design is finalized and approved by the client information requires to be produced by the design team so that building contractors may tender for the building works and for those works to be carried out in accordance with the design intentions in all aspects of detail. There are two further stages therefore within the design process before the building work can commence on site:

- *Production information*: the documentation in the form of specification, bills of quantities and working drawings produced by the members of the design team, as an accurate and explicit description of the building works in order to construct the design.
- *Invitation of tenders*: possibly 4–6 contractors (the number depends of the scale of the project) are asked to price for the carrying out of the building works, from which usually the lowest is selected.

This description of the design process outlines the common, or traditional, method for the design and construction of new building work i.e. design by consultants followed by the client employing a contractor to build the project as a result of a formal tendering process. An alternative is to consider the telescoping in time of the design and construction periods by negotiating with a contractor early within the design process. This allows work on site to commence before the design by the consultants is complete.

The traditional method has several advantages: it allows freedom to obtain competitive tenders for the construction based on the same production information. The alternative method has the benefit of involving the contractor in the design process to advise on buildability and sequence of operations implied in the design. This is particularly applicable when the proposed timetable is short or limited by circumstances, and where the project is a conversion of an existing building putting on performances, to reduce the time period for construction and limit closure.

The fitting out of the building, which may include fittings, fixtures, equipment and decoration, may be carried out by a separate and subsequent contractor following the same tendering process.

Specialist firms, such as suppliers and installers of auditorium seating and stage machinery, can be brought into the early stages of the design process to provide specific information and design input. Such firms can become nominated sub-contractors within the main contract.

Building process

The initial stage is the need for the client and the selected contractor to exchange signed contracts, of which standard formats are available for this purpose.

The actual execution of the construction works is the responsibility of the contractor, within a time period laid down in the contract, including the building sequence, coordination of the specialist sub-contractors and ensuring the full implementation of the production information.

During the construction period, inspection of the works is carried out by the architect and other members of the design team, as appropriate. For large projects, a clerk of works, appointed by the client, can also inspect the works as they progress to ensure proper execution: the scale of the project may suggest a resident architect and engineer on site for full or partial duration of the construction.

Commissioning is the testing of certain aspects of a building before completion. For a building for the performing arts there are four main areas where tests can establish if the building is achieving the design criteria:

- acoustic performance of the auditorium and other acoustically sensitive spaces;
- sound insulation between spaces;

- use and balancing of ventilation and heating systems;
- platform/stage sound, lighting and machinery and communication systems.

Hand over and opening night

On completion of the construction works, the finished building is handed over to the client with an explanation of the workings of the spaces, equipment and services.

Prior to the hand-over the client may need to *employ staff* for a new venture or an expanded existing organization sufficiently early for them, and existing staff, to become conversant with the workings of the building. As well as rehearsal for the first performance, the technical aspects also need to be rehearsed.

The opening of a building for a performing art differs from other building types as the opening can coincide with the first performance of the new season. The season will have to be planned well in advance with the appointment of performers, directors and other staff. If the building is for a resident company then there needs to be a period of time for rehearsal and preparation of scenery, properties and costumes (if opera, dance, musicals or drama) between hand over and opening. If the building is for touring companies then a shorter period of time will be necessary. There is also the need for the building to obtain a licence as a place of assembly before the public is allowed into the auditorium, and approval from the Environmental Health department for the areas for eating and drinking. The working areas of the building also require approval by the Health and Safety Inspector.

The implication is that the construction work requires to be complete in time for the preparations for the opening night as postponement of opening night arrangements is not good publicity and is also likely to incur cancellation costs.

Building in use

The maintenance of a building over its lifetime in use requires regular and systematic planning and expenditure. Neglecting a building will ultimately be more expensive to rectify with the possibility of a re-furbishment programme. Such a situation would probably mean closure during the construction period with the loss of income as a consequence. A set amount, increasing in line with inflation, requires to be set aside annually as part of the revenue cost.

Maintenance covers cleaning, checking equipment, servicing equipment and replacement of worn, broken or out-of-date items. It is desirable to keep a stock of items which are likely to be replaced, such as auditorium seats. Stage machinery should be inspected on a regular basis as should bleacher seating.

A member of staff should be given responsibility as a shared function of a small facility or a sole function of a large facility. Particularly large facilities with complex stage machinery and multi-purpose auditoria may require more than one person.

Part Three
Specific Studies

10

10 Audiences, companies and staff

Audiences: assessment of demand

The essential component of the feasibility study is the assessment of the demand for the performing arts within the community the proposed facility is to serve. The aim is to establish if there are *audiences* for the proposed programme of use as well as defining the catchment area from which the audiences are drawn. A market survey can identify such a potential audience, including how the numbers may be expanded and stimulated to attend a new or changed facility. Relocating existing facilities and even expansion of the public facilities will necessitate identifying future audience numbers.

Assessment requires the following studies of the area under consideration:

- population characteristics;
- transportation networks;
- potential audiences;
- local cultural traditions;
- existing provision;
- actual audiences;
- pilot scheme.

A similar set of studies can be undertaken to assess demand for non-performance activities, such as conferences, lectures, social events, meetings, eating and drinking, and so on.

Population characteristics

The present and projected size of the population and, where applicable, the tourist and other short-stay visitors in the area under consideration should be studied. Information gathered should include age, sex, marital status, parent responsibilities, car ownership, educational attainment and socio-economic structure. Census statistics and the local planning department can be sources of population figures and details, both present and projected. Tourist and conference information may be also available.

For 'captive audiences' in institutions such as universities, present and future numbers must be determined.

Transport networks

Present and future public and private transport patterns including car parking provision, road layouts and pedestrian routes for the area under consideration must be taken into account. Local planning and highway departments can be sources of information.

Potential audiences: Fig. 10.1

Audience surveys of comparable facilities elsewhere can be studied to establish the characteristics of

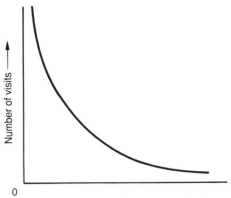

(a) Distance/ travel time from proposed site →

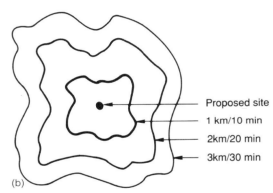

Proposed site
1 km/10 min
2km/20 min
3km/30 min

(b)

Fig. 10.1 *Demand studies. (a) The percentage of people visiting a proposed building for the performing arts diminishes as the distance/ travel time from the building increases. The attraction will vary according to type of production, reputation of touring company, and so on, at the same building. This demonstrates a typical urban 'gravity model' travel function. (b) The actual distance/travel time to a proposed site, as opposed to concentric circles, will be dependent on the specific road layouts and public transport routes. The distance/travel time pattern will resemble more the bands in this diagram. The percentage of population from each band who will visit a building will diminish as distance increases, as shown in (a).*

potential audiences. Audience surveys should cover the personal characteristics of those who attend comparable provision (age, gender, occupation and social grade), the frequency of their attendance, their reasons for attending particular performance, and including travel method, distance and – most important – time. The numbers with comparable characteristics within the area under consideration can be calculated and the maximum travel distance/ time can be established. Local surveys of the population can supplement this information to confirm potential audience numbers and also to establish those reasons for non-attendance at performances, especially among the non-traditional audience types. Non-attendance may be due to location, costs,

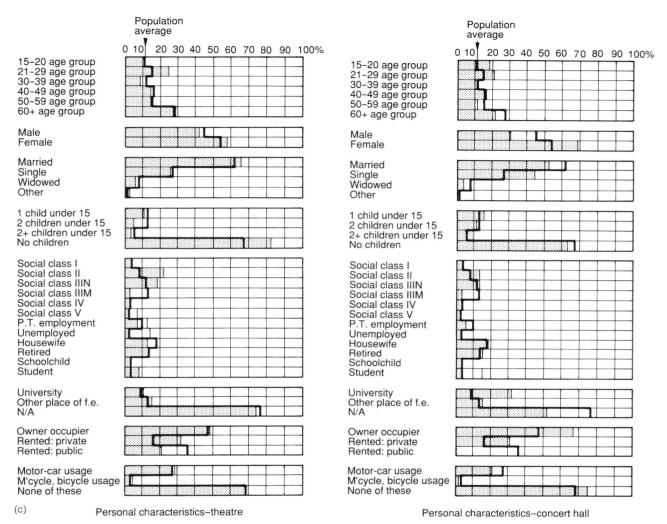

(c)   Personal characteristics–theatre   Personal characteristics–concert hall

Fig. 10.1 continued *Demand studies. (c) The actual number of people from each band shown in (b) will depend also on the percentage of the population with the characteristics of those who would be attracted to the proposed building. The figures show some examples of the characteristics of theatre – and concert – goers, against the overall characteristics of the population*

attraction, staff, lack of car parking, and timing of performances, as well as personal constraints such as young children.

The Arts Councils are sources of information on audience characteristics as they hold data from market research commissions.

Local cultural traditions

Demand is affected by a relevant, but difficult to quantify, understanding of a local tradition of involvement in, and support for, particular types of production: choral music tradition in a region is an example. This may be measured by investigating the local cultural history and traditions and frequency of attending, or participating in, performances.

Existing provision

An audit of existing and proposed facilities, promoting organizations and companies in the area, which may complement, or compete with, the client's proposal. The aim is to establish if there is a gap in the market. A client may wish to compete directly with an existing facility, which they consider inadequate. Existing organizations may be approached to consider combining in the new venture: for example, amateur companies hiring church halls may combine as users of a purpose-built facility. There may be under-used provision which, through physical and/or management change, may increase use and maybe satisfy the identified increase in demand.

Existing and proposed facilities of compatible functions (conference, lectures) and supplementary functions (restaurants, art gallery) should be also identified.

Actual audiences

While studies will indicate the potential demand in a population within a catchment area defined by the maximum travel distance from a building, the success of a building in terms of the *actual audience* numbers will depend on the attractiveness of the supply and the physical constraints on the auditorium size.

Attractiveness of the supply refers, among other factors, to:

- cost of a visit including travel costs, local taxation, price of admission and other attendant costs;
- quality of the competing attraction for the use of free time from other leisure activities;
- level to which the existing supply satisfies demand;
- quality of the performances, reputation of the performers and distinct appeal of the facilities;
- effectiveness of the publicity and marketing policy.

The physical constraint on the auditorium size refers to the visual and aural limitations which condition the maximum size of the auditorium. The audience will be limited by the size of auditorium. If demand exceeds this size then this will encourage longer runs of the same production or the construction of more than one auditorium.

Pilot scheme

Demand, and marketing effectiveness, may be tested by a *pilot scheme* whereby a suitable building is converted for performances demonstrating the artistic policy within the client's proposal. Such a programme would last for a sufficient period of time to establish response. A temporary building, the initial phase of the large proposal or a one-off event such as a festival may also be considered. This approach provides evidence of demand to assist funding applications, avoids the larger financial commitment if demand is not shown and is particularly useful in areas without a local tradition of interest in the proposed performing art.

Companies and staff

For buildings hosting touring companies, the type, availability and cost of such companies to satisfy the proposed programme and pattern of use needs to be established. For a programme which will rely on pop/ rock groups for a minimum of 200 performances a sufficient number of touring companies prepared to travel and perform must be identified. Similarly for a one-off event, as at an international festival, an orchestra, for example, may have to be booked years in advance. Promoters will have to be approached, and preferably contracts established before commencement of the construction of the building: financial arrangements may insist on a programme guarantee and formal agreements may be necessary.

For buildings to house a resident company, yet to be established, the client needs to identify the availability of appropriate performers, artistic directors and other staff to satisfy their objectives. Of these, the artistic director may be critical to the success of the proposal, and if so needs to be identified early on in the process.

11

11 Site considerations

This section identifies information relating to the characteristics of the site, as a checklist for the finding, evaluation and eventual acquisition. The topics covered are:

- *Location*: the position within the urban or rural area of the proposed building, its linkage to other activities within the catchment area, and possible wider development policy.
- *Parking*: the need for public car parking and also for coaches, off-site parking and TV and radio vans.
- *Site survey*: size and shape, access and entrance, outdoor areas, acoustics, conditions, constraints, characteristics and costs.
- *Building survey*: evaluation of an existing building if to be re-used and converted.

Location

The location of the site is a critical issue and requires to be:

- In an appropriate position to attract the anticipated visitors (audiences and others) within the metropolitan/regional/town/district/neighbourhood centre, rural/resort location or parent organization.
- Safely and easily accessible – by foot, bicycle, car, taxi coach and public transport – from all parts of the catchment area it is to serve. Public transport needs to be available after evening performances. As buildings for the performing arts are open late in the evening then the location should be safe.

For a new major building in a *metropolitan or regional centre*, there will be competition with commercial activity and associated high land values. While such a building for the performing arts requires to be easily accessible, it is doubtful if a prime core site would be economical. Studio and experimental theatres, which benefit from the large catchment area that a metropolitan centre can offer, can be located in secondary or transitional areas of lower land values but near to the core of the centre.

Awareness of a facility is an element of the marketing of performances. The visual impact of a building by its location should be considered including opportunities for external signs and posters, and other visual displays.

Existing buildings for the performing arts may find themselves located on expensive land when a city centre expands. Commercial pressures may suggest relocation, with the sale of the land and building for retail or office development.

The demolition of old buildings for the performing arts without replacement, especially in Britain, has been halted mainly by conservation policy.

The location should be considered in terms of its *functional linkages* with other activities within the catchment area (Fig. 11.1). These include:

- Linkages associated with a visit to a performance:
  - restaurants;
  - car parking;
  - coach parking;
  - public transport.
- Facilities which generate potential audiences:
  - conference facilities;
  - tourist attractions;
  - places of higher education;
  - hotels;
  - halls of residence;
  - residential areas.
- Production and administration services:
  - specialist shops;
  - rehearsal spaces;
  - printing and publicity facilities;
  - materials for scenery and costumes.
- Performers' linkages:
  - accommodation for visiting performers;
  - film, television, radio and recording studios.
- Associated facilities:
  - other buildings for the performing arts;
  - arts buildings: art gallery, arts centre, arts workshop;
  - cultural buildings: museum, library;
  - cinemas;
  - information centre;
  - ticket purchase outlets;
  - drama and music colleges (dual use).

If a building is open during the day for the public to benefit from restaurants, bars and other provision such as art galleries then proximity in a city and town centre to *shops* and *offices* encourages use.

Where the programme of use includes a *drama and/or music festival* then overnight accommodation – hotels, vacation use of halls of residence, hostels and so on – is an essential component. A visit to a primary function – tourist attraction, conference facility – also requiring overnight accommodation can include a visit to a building for the performing arts as a complementary activity and attraction.

There is an economic and functional convenience in the linkage with film, television, radio and recording studios for performers who can combine these other activities with evening performances.

At the scale of *town, district and neighbourhood centre* the functional linkages with other activities include:

- Linkages associated with a visit to a performance:
  - restaurant;
  - car-parking;
  - coach parking;
  - public transport.
- Production and administrative services:
  - rehearsal spaces;
  - printing and publicity facilities;
  - materials for scenery and costumes;
  - hiring costumes and scenery.
- Performers' linkages:
  - accommodation for visiting performers.
- Associated facilities:
  - other buildings for the performing arts;

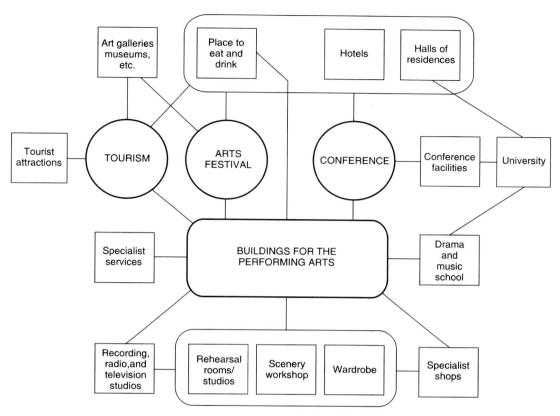

Fig. 11.1 *Functional linkages: buildings for the performing arts, especially at the city scale, are part of large functional groupings of conference, tourism and education as well as linkages associated with a visit to a performance and local services*

– arts buildings: art gallery, arts centre, arts workshop;
– cultural buildings: museum, library;
– other leisure facilities: sports hall, ice rink, swimming pool;
– schools and colleges (dual use).

Concentration of buildings for the performing arts such as the Lincoln Centre in New York and the South Bank Centre in London, where the major national facilities are located within a single site, have advantages and disadvantages. These issues are applicable also to regional centres. Advantages include management convenience if in single ownership, operational advantages by sharing resources (such as rehearsal rooms and workshops), proximity of artistic community can encourage creative links, and an area of city or town becomes associated with performing areas. Disadvantages include congestion before and after performances, dead areas through the day, ghetto association, loss of opportunity to use individual facilities to regenerate various parts of a city or town, and less scope for specialist shops and complementary activities to develop.

A building for the performing arts may be subject to a *development policy* where they effectively form a basis for a larger comprehensive programme of urban

revitalization, as a catalyst for further adjacent commercial growth and/or residential developments. A developer may be granted planning permission for a larger commercial development in return for constructing, or at least providing a site for, a building for the performing arts, or a lump sum contribution. A building for the performing arts may be part of a *larger complex* such as an institutional complex (university campus), other functions (offices, retails, residential) or an arts complex (facilities for painting, sculpture and crafts). If so, ensure that access for public and staff during performance times is retained if remaining parts of the complex are closed, that there is no conflict with the other uses, and that the facility for the performing arts is clearly and easily identifiable by the public. Investigate the potential of combining functions (parking, servicing, entrances, heating) to make savings to the capital and running costs.

Parking

Parking provision is essential and covers the following:

● *Public car parking* close to the public entrance, with the number of car park spaces as 25 per cent of the seating capacity in the auditorium: buildings in city centres, which are served by good adjacent public transport, can have less provision, while in rural areas the number of spaces should be increased to 40 per cent minimum. It is normally uneconomic to provide public car parking in urban areas for the exclusive use of those attending performances, especially if predominantly an evening activity. Car parking can be combined with complementary day-time activities, such as retail and offices.

- Designated areas for *coaches* for disembarking near the public entrance and their parking, which should be conveniently located rather than immediately adjacent to the building.
- Convenient *on-site parking* for staff cars and company vehicles. Also, when applicable, vans, containers and lorries of touring companies.
- Parking for *TV and radio vans* for occasional live broadcasts adjacent to the building with convenient cable access into the auditorium from an external parking position.

Site

Various factors condition selection and suitability of a site in terms of:

- *Size and shape*: Clearly a small studio theatre will require less land than an opera house. The estimated accommodation, expansion proposals, outdoor activities, parking and landscaping will indicate size and preferred shape. The position and orientation of the site needs to be easily identifiable by the public and easily serviced.
- *Access and entrances*: There are four broad categories of access to, and egress from, a building:
  - Public pedestrian and vehicular entrance and exit. The main public entrance should be readily accessible to all public coming to the building including disabled and infirm persons, and those alighting in inclement weather who wish to be dropped off close to the public entrance. Local planning requirements may require disabled parking immediately adjacent to the entrance.
  - Emergency exits in case of fire from all parts of the building. Legislation requires separate egress from all parts and levels of the auditorium for the public, with the disabled in wheelchairs able to egress on the same level from the auditorium to a safe external area.
  - Access for service vehicles for the delivery of goods: food and drink to the public area; materials, scenery and costumes to the stage areas and workshops.
  - Rear of stage pedestrian and vehicular entrance and exit for performers and back-stage staff (traditionally the stage door). Depending on the scale and style of the organization, the management may also have a separate entrance.

This extent of access/egress, plus the requirements of daylighting, suggests an island site or at least clear access all round a facility at ground level.

- *Outdoor areas*: gathering area in front of public entrance;
  - external performance area;
  - landscaping: where appropriate the building can be set within landscaping (an aim could be to retain such valuable features as trees, shrubs, and natural ground conditions wherever suitable);
  - future development and phasing as additional accommodation.

- *Acoustics*: Auditoria for the performing arts must be isolated from external noise sources. Sites with adjacent noise sources such as motorways and railways, or under a flight path, should be avoided to minimize the level of sound insulation. Otherwise the solution to the problem of sound penetration can be expensive. A site noise level survey must be carried out to determine the design of the enclosing elements and location of the acoustically sensitive areas.

  Facilities for the performing arts are also a source of noise: the arrival and departure of an audience, the loading of scenery and costumes from the stage areas.
- *Site conditions*: Site conditions for buildings for the performing arts vary greatly. For every building, large or small, a full site survey is necessary and includes:
  - levels and configuration;
  - trial bores to establish geology;
  - existing services: gas, electricity, water, drainage, telephone, refuse collection.
- *Constraints on development*:
  - availability of the site and time-scale to acquire land for development;
  - ownership of the site: leasehold or freehold (leasehold may include constraints on the development);
  - planning policy covering density, height, materials, functions, parking and transport proposals. The local plan should be checked to establish land use and if the proposal will be in accordance with the design policy of the planning authority. Outline planning permission should be obtained before progressing onto scheme design.
- *Site characteristics*:
  - pedestrian and vehicular approaches including possible approaches for service vehicles: density of movement;
  - frontage: convenient frontage onto recognized route;
  - climate: direction of prevailing winds and sun; intensity of winds, snow and rain;
  - prospect: views to, and from, the site; evaluation of the quality of the views;
  - character of features within the site;

- character of buildings and/or landscape surrounding the site.
- *Costs*: When considering the cost of the site, consider the following:
  - initial outlay;
  - rates and taxes;
  - effect of topography, soil conditions, etc. on building and landscape costs;
  - possible cost of providing certain services such as sewers and roads within the site;
  - possible demolition and excavation costs.

Sources of information on sites, availability and characteristics include local planning department, transport department and estates department; local estate agents and solicitors; local environmental and amenity groups; statutory undertakers, cleansing departments, and public utilities.

Building survey

If the proposed project is the re-use or adaptation of an existing building then consider the following:

- investigation of the fabric to establish age, condition and defects, including dimensional survey drawings;

- evaluation of the existing building in terms of image;
- the fit between the proposed accommodation and the existing building to evaluate suitability (particular reference is made to the large volume of the auditorium and stage/platform);
- the ability of the existing structure to take an increase in loading, and ease of incorporating additional services especially the ventilation ducting and plant;
- cost of changes against re-building;
- location characteristics suitable for building category, with appropriate access, frontage and acoustic conditions;
- conservation policy governing external fabric, interiors and any proposed extension;
- consent from local planning authority for change of use and proposed alterations.

Specialist assistance may be required to carry out the survey of an existing building in order to open up and examine foundations and structure, to identify services and to investigate any timber rot and woodworm. Consultants therefore may include a building surveyor, structural engineer and conservationist.

12

12 Initial brief: auditorium and platform/stage

The *auditorium* is the container for the audience, focused on the *platform/stage* upon which the performance occurs. The *platform* is usually found in the concert hall and recital room associated with classical and choral music, while the *stage* is associated with the other performing arts. The aim within the feasibility stage is to establish the overall volume and requirements of the auditorium and platform/stage, and the *actual* seating capacity. Below are listed the main factors to be considered in the design of the auditorium and platform/stage.

- Type(s) and scale of production;
- Auditorium and platform/stage formats:
  - predominant type of production;
  - multi-purpose formats:
      multi-form: single production type,
      single-form with flexibility,
      multi-form: various production types,
      multi-use,
      un-committed space;
- Auditorium design:
  - aural and visual limitations;
  - levels in the auditorium;
  - auditorium acoustics;
  - sound insulation and noise control;
  - seating layout;
  - means of escape;
  - circulation within auditorium;
  - wheelchair location within the seating;
  - broadcasting requirements;
  - latecomers;
  - attendants;
  - adaptation;
  - sightlines;
  - standing: pop/rock concerts;
  - standing room;
  - promenade performance;
  - cabaret layout;
  - air-conditioning, heating and ventilation;
  - lighting;
  - sound equipment;
  - fire protection;
  - structure;
  - ceiling zone;
  - seating capacity;
  - auditorium character.
- Platform/stage design:
  - platform: orchestral and choral music;
  - proscenium format: stage with or without flytower;
  - open stage formats;
  - stage: pop/rock music;
  - stage: jazz music;
  - multi-use stage;
  - combination with flat floor.

Type(s) and scale of production

The first decision is the selection, or confirmation, of the type(s) of production as each has its specific characteristics – classical music, pop/rock, jazz, opera, dance, musicals, drama – and the scale of the production – large, medium, small. All decisions over the requirements of the auditorium and platform/stage follow from these, as do the requirements for the public, performers, technical and management staff, and production. The decision may refer to more than one type of production thereby requiring a level of physical adaptation: however there are limitations to the level of adaptation without compromising the requirements and/or encouraging high capital and running costs.

Auditorium and platform/stage formats

The relationship between the auditorium – the audience – and the platform/stage – the performance – is a fundamental requirement. The selected format affects the experience for both audience and performers, seating capacity and auditorium size and shape, from which follows the general arrangement of the building. The relationship may be summarized as either the *proscenium format* or *open stage format*: the proscenium format is as if the performance is seen through a 'window' or hole in the wall and there is a clear division between audience and performers; the open stage formats follow the concept of the auditorium and platform/stage being within a single volume with the seating confronting, partially surrounding or wholly surrounding the platform/stage.

Predominant types of production

The following relationships accommodate a predominant type of production in purpose-built facilities. Compatible secondary uses may be included in the brief but they do not require any physical adaptation of the auditorium and platform/stage, or only require a modest level of flexibility.

For *orchestral and choral classical music* in a concert hall or recital room, there are three broad categories: the audience focused towards the orchestra and choir on the platform, with or without choir stalls, in a single direction; the audience on three sides, semi-surrounding the platform; the audience surrounding the platform (Fig. 12.1).

Types of single direction relationship include the:

- rectangular box;
- variations on the rectangular box;
- fan-shaped auditorium.

The rectangular box is a simple well-established form, rectangular in plan and section. This form allows full

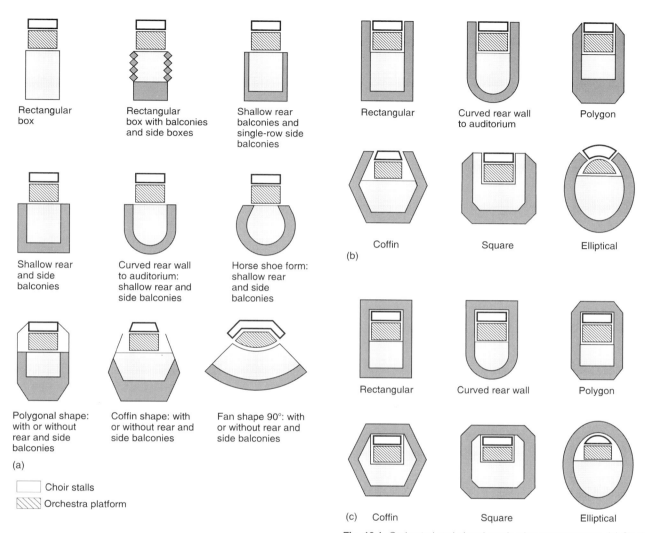

Choir stalls
Orchestra platform

(a)

(b)

(c)

Fig. 12.1 *Orchestral and choral music plan arrangements. (a) Single direction relationship. (b) Audience partially surrounding platform. With or without rear and side balconies. (c) Audience surrounding platform. With or without rear and side balconies*

cross-reflection of sound from the orchestra and choir between the side walls: the audience is central to the platform and achieves a good sound balance: the orchestra and choir are set within an architectural background.

The variations on the rectangular box are attempts to increase audience capacity, reduce the apparent blandness of the side walls by adding seating, and decrease the scale of the larger auditorium. Variations include side and rear galleries, geometric shapes on plan and sub-divisions within the seating areas. The fan-shaped auditorium is a particular variation on the rectangular box which increases the seating capacity by widening the side walls away from the stage. This shape, apparently reflecting the horn of a trumpet, does not necessarily produce an even sound across the audience and suffers from lack of side- and cross-reflection, as the acoustically useful side walls are pushed apart.

Extensions of these variations place sections of the audience along the sides of the stage thereby partially surrounding the platform by audience.

The platform may be surrounded by the audience, with the platform placed either in the centre or eccentrically along the long axis. The benefits include an increased proximity of the audience to the performance, reduction of the perceived division between audience and orchestra and conscious production of a unity within the interior of the auditorium. The audience can surround the platform by the use of galleries or by sub-division into terraces: each offers balcony fronts and walls for sound reflection. The setting for the orchestra is the audience.

Auditorium shape and size for classical music is acoustically sensitive and the selection of type of auditorium/platform relationship is conditioned by aural limitations, the quality of sound required and seating capacity. Concert halls may incorporate the ability to change the acoustic character of the space according to the music performed. Compositions were written within an acoustic at the time and can have a range in reverberation time of 1.5 to 2.2 seconds. Variability may be *either* mechanical, using retractable or movable elements, *or* electronic assisted resonance.

For *opera, dance and musicals* the formats are restricted to the proscenium and end stage. The *proscenium form* is defined as the audience facing the stage on one side only viewing the performing area through an architectural opening, which may have an elaborate architectural frame. This is a conventional arrangement and offers the maximum confrontation of performers and audience. It creates a limited, unified fixed frame for the pictorial composition of the performance. Scenery can be developed as a major design element. The traditional position for opera, dance and musicals is for the orchestra pit to be positioned between audience and stage with the conductor in the pivotable location of controlling orchestra and singers. The proscenium form has been sustained, in part, from the need to make rapid changes of scenery, which require side and rear stages, and a flytower over the performance stage. The auditorium forms include the *horse-shoe, courtyard* and *fan* with or without balconies. The *end stage* is similar to the proscenium form but without the architectural opening, placing both the performance and audience in the same rectangular box, suitable for small-scale productions (Fig. 12.2).

For jazz/pop/rock (formal setting) the audience/performance formats include (Fig 12.3):

- single direction: rectangular box;
- partial-surround, including amphitheatre form with a thrust stage;
- 90° encirclement.

The performance may be seen against a formal architectural background so that the description of the concert hall would apply. However there is an increasing theatrical nature in the presentation of pop and rock concerts, and also scale of production has grown. The staging has developed with adoption of lighting and sound effects as well as scenic devices which require side and/or rear stages for setting up and scenery changes.

These suggest, as described under opera, dance and musicals, the proscenium format, with or without flytower, and the end stage.

The formal setting for jazz suggests the format associated with the concert hall and, more likely, the recital room.

Amplification requires loudspeaker locations on the stage.

For *drama* there is a wide variation, and therefore choice, of relationship between auditorium and stage. The initial distinction lies between the proscenium format and open stage format, with a revival of historic forms as an additional category (Fig. 12.4).

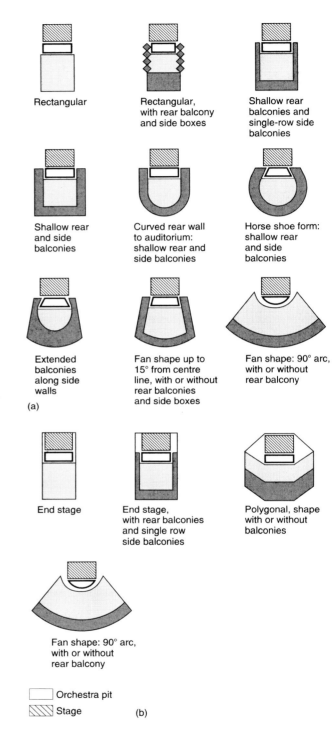

Fig. 12.2 *Opera, dance and musicals. (a) Proscenium formats. (b) Open stage formats*

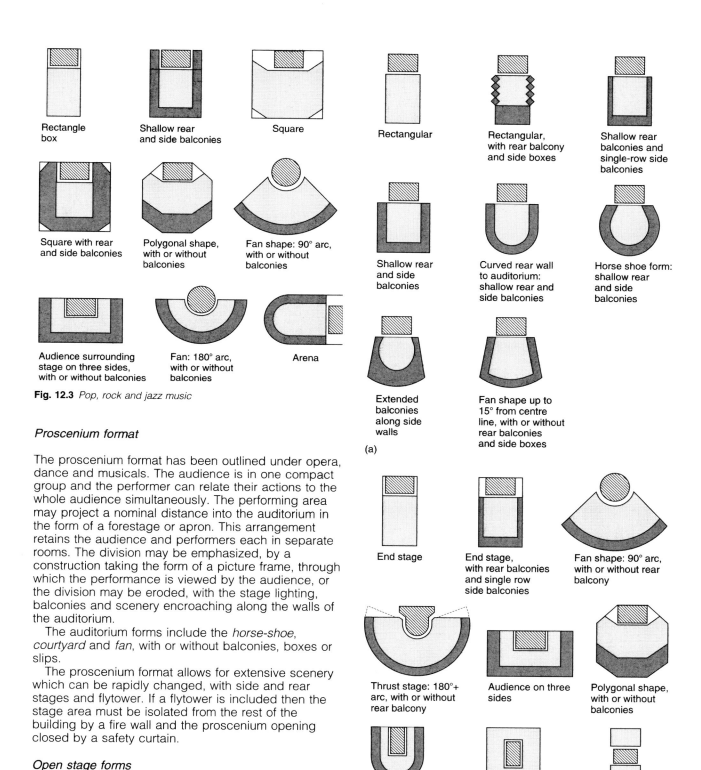

Fig. 12.3 *Pop, rock and jazz music*

Proscenium format

The proscenium format has been outlined under opera, dance and musicals. The audience is in one compact group and the performer can relate their actions to the whole audience simultaneously. The performing area may project a nominal distance into the auditorium in the form of a forestage or apron. This arrangement retains the audience and performers each in separate rooms. The division may be emphasized, by a construction taking the form of a picture frame, through which the performance is viewed by the audience, or the division may be eroded, with the stage lighting, balconies and scenery encroaching along the walls of the auditorium.

The auditorium forms include the *horse-shoe*, *courtyard* and *fan*, with or without balconies, boxes or slips.

The proscenium format allows for extensive scenery which can be rapidly changed, with side and rear stages and flytower. If a flytower is included then the stage area must be isolated from the rest of the building by a fire wall and the proscenium opening closed by a safety curtain.

Open stage forms

The open stage forms may be classified into five broad categories:

● *End stage*: the audience focused towards the stage within a rectangular box: the stage at the narrow end, with stage and audience in the same space.

Fig. 12.4 *Drama. (a) Proscenium formats. (b) Open stage formats*

- *Fan-shaped*: the stage is encircled by the audience by 90°. This level of encirclement allows the performer to command the audience and for the performer to be seen against a scenic background by the audience.
- *Thrust stage*: with the audience on three sides, semi-surrounding the stage.
- *Theatre-in-the-round*: the audience surrounds the performance. Entrances by the performers are through the audience. Acoustically the performer needs to project to the whole audience in every direction, which implies a limit to the maximum distance from stage to rear row.
- *Traverse stage*: the audience either side of the stage.

Historical forms

In addition, there is the re-establishment of historical forms, either as an archaeological reproduction, or interpretation, alluding to previous periods in the development of drama presentation.

Multi-purpose formats

As opposed to an auditorium and platform/stage for a predominant type of production in a purpose-built facility, the brief may refer to more than one type of production to be accommodated within a single format. Also productions may require combination with non-performing arts activities. Each of the alternative uses will require specific provisions to be made in its design and equipment; in platform/stage space; in orchestra space and modification of acoustics; in scenery storage and workshops; in stage lighting and sound. While some degree of flexibility can be accommodated at reasonable cost and with success, there is a limit to the multiplicity of use. Apart from design difficulties, the cost of providing for the different requirements and of operating a multi-purpose form may become disproportionately high. The success of a multi-purpose format depends upon the compatibility of the various activities and the designer must be rigorous in the assessment of the activities.

Multi-purpose use is usually considered for economic reasons where demand does not justify separate facilities. To ensure that auditoria are adequately used and to minimize capital expenditure it may be useful to combine *users* as well as *uses*. An example is the combination of local government, local education authority and a local amateur company to provide a single facility with a predominant type of production.

There are various categories of multi-purpose layouts which are outlined below:

- *Multi-format: single production type* (Fig. 12.5): The same type of production with more than one arrangement for the relationship between audience and performance.
- *Single format with flexibility* (Fig. 12.6): Reference to a relationship between audience and performers

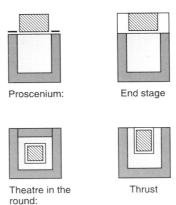

Proscenium: End stage

Theatre in the   Thrust
round:

Fig. 12.5 *Multi-form with single type of production: e.g. drama with more than one type of format within the same enclosure*

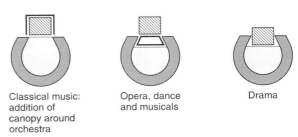

Classical music: Opera, dance   Drama
addition of   and musicals
canopy around
orchestra

Fig. 12.6 *Single form with flexibility: combination of opera, dance, musicals and drama and also classical and other music*

which accommodates more than one type of production and requires some physical adaptation.
- *Multi-format* (Fig. 12.7): More than one type of production and format, such as both opera and drama combined in a single auditorium and stage arrangement.

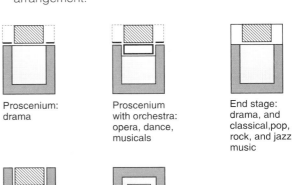

Proscenium: Proscenium   End stage:
drama   with orchestra: drama, and
                     opera, dance,   classical,pop,
                     musicals   rock, and jazz
                                         music

Audience semi   Theatre in the
surrounding the   round: drama
platform/stage:
classical, pop,
rock, and jazz
music

Fig. 12.7 *Multi-form: various productions within the same enclosure*

- *Multi-use* (Fig. 12.8): Combination of one or more type of production with activities which are not performing arts such as indoor sports. These include:
  - activities with compatible requirements requiring a modest level of physical change of the auditorium and stage (this relates to those

activities which benefit from a raked floor such as conference, lectures, films and slide shows);
  - activities which require adaptation of the auditorium and stage to satisfy their requirements (adaptation tends to relate to the accommodation of those activities requiring a flat floor, where the raked seating needs to be removed: such activities include dancing, banquets, exhibitions, indoor sports and keep fit classes).

- *Un-committed space or found space* (Fig. 12.9): An approach whereby there is no specific or predominant form of audience/stage relationship but which provides an enclosure into which seating and staging can be constructed according to the proposed production. This implies a simple square or rectangular enclosure with a flat floor, upon which the raked seating for the audience can be built by rostra or framing, but with a comprehensive ventilation system and heating provision. This format allows the whole setting – staging and audience – to be designed as a unique experience for each production.

  This category includes the re-use of an existing building: creating a stage and auditorium in a space offering a basic enclosure, with the designer of the space for theatrical purposes responding to the specific characteristics of the space, with possibly some adaptation, using inherited features of the interior as part of the setting of both performance and audience.

Rectangle box, with removable raked seating on flat floor

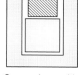

Square box, with fixed perimeter seating and removable central seating on flat floor

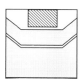

Square box, with rear seating and removable front seating on flat floor

Square box, with removable seating on flat floor

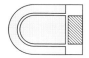

Arena format, with fixed perimeter seating and removable central seating on flat floor

Fig. 12.8 *Multi-use: e.g. combination of provision for performing arts with indoor sports facilities*

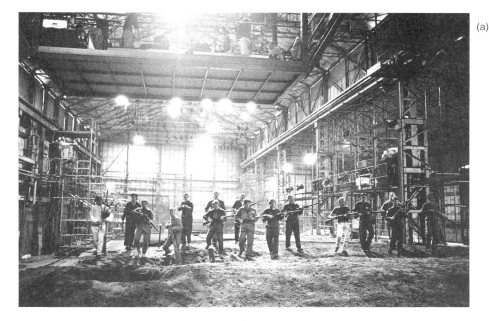

(a)

Fig. 12.9 *Harland and Wolff Shipyard, Glasgow. Adaptation of the disused Harland and Wolff ship maintenance shed in Glasgow for a performance space. The auditorium and stage followed the line of the main work area with fixed galleries on one long side for standing audience and raked seating on the other, on a tracked unit which could follow the action on the long central stage (for the production of The Big Picnic, a play about the First World War). The gantry over the stage followed the movement of the performance accommodating musicians, singers and stage lighting. (a) View of stage, with gantry over and audience structures, either side.*

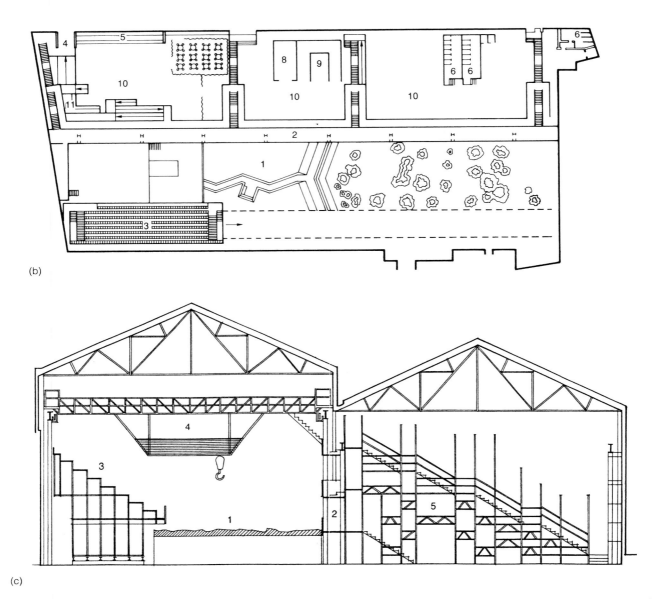

(b)

(c)

Fig. 12.9 continued *Harland and Wolff Shipyard, Glasgow. (b) General plan showing: 1 stage constructed for the particular production, 2 fixed galleries for standing audience, 3 mobile raked seating, 4 entrance, 5 bar, 6 toilets, 7 dining, 8 VIP room, 9 exhibition areas, 10 circulation, 11 box office. (c) Traverse section through, 1 stage, 2 audience structures, 3 mobile raked seating, 4 mobile crane, 5 public spaces*

Adaptability from one format to another is often a necessary study within the initial brief. If the level of adaptation is relatively minor such as the formation of a forestage for drama productions over an orchestra pit for opera, then it does not set insuperable problems of sightlines. Greater degrees of adaptability means alterations of seating and staging. On a small scale such changes can be achieved manually or mechanically with little consequence: on a large scale the problems become more challenging, both economically and technically if all formats are to perform satisfactorily. If there are problems of compatibility, economy and/or technical performance, then more than one auditorium should be considered.

Auditorium design

The three-dimensional volume of an auditorium is conditioned by the limitations set by all members of the audience able to hear and see a performance, and for the performers to be able to command the audience. Seating density, floor rake and seating layout are covered by legislation to ensure a satisfactory means of escape in case of fire, and by an appropriate level of comfort for the audience. Performance organization requires lighting, sound and broadcasting positions within the auditorium and a view of the whole performance area from control rooms.

Aural and visual limitations (Fig. 12.10)

Aural limitations

There are limits to the distance across which speech, singing and music can be clearly heard in an auditorium, without the assistance of amplification, and this has a bearing on the maximum distance from performance to the rear row of seats. Beyond these limits the lack of audibility gives the audience less than the basic requirement to clearly hear a performance. The distance varies according to type of production.

Other factors include the articulation of the spoken work by an actor or the sound quality, including loudness, from a musical instrument. An aspect of intimate drama is for the actors not necessarily to speak loudly and project some distance, while certain

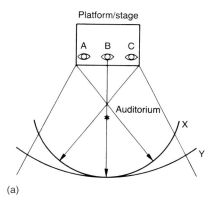

(a)

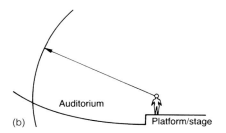

(b)

Fig. 12.10 *Aural and visual limitations. (a) Plan. A performer at position (B) creates a simple curve (Y) with a single arc to determine the maximum visual or aural distance from the performance. However the calculation from the performers at the side of the platform/stage (positions (A) and (C)) produces a more restrictive curve. (b) Section. Strict adherence of the visual or aural limitations on section follows a curve centred on the performer on the platform/ stage*

musical instruments such as an acoustic guitar may not be sufficiently loud to transfer long distances. These limit the maximum distance from performance to audience.

Acoustic limitations refer only to those performing arts which do not rely on amplification. Jazz/rock/pop music and musicals tend to use amplification as an integral part of the performance.

Visual limitations

There are visual limitations that determine the maximum distance from the performance area beyond which the audience is unable to appreciate the performance adequately and for the performers to command an audience. The distance to the furthest seat varies according to the type and scale of production:

- In order to discern facial expression – essential with drama – the maximum distance from the point of command on the stage should not exceed 20 m. The point of command is the geometric centre of an open stage or the setting line of a proscenium stage.
- For opera and musicals discerning facial expressions is less critical and the distance to the rear row can be 30 m.
- For dance, the audience needs to appreciate the body and feet of the dancers, *and* also to discern facial expressions: the maximum distance from the point of command on the stage should not exceed 20 m.
- For full symphonic concerts the visual definition may not be a critical factor with the rear row being more a function of acoustic limitation rather than visual. For chamber concerts the acoustic limitations predominate but it may be considered that the visual definition is a factor as part of the aim to provide an intimate setting.
- For jazz/pop/rock concerts the visual limitations seem not at all critical particularly with the addition of video screens to aid vision especially from the rear sections of the auditorium. However the aim for jazz may be to produce an intimate setting where discerning facial expressions may be a factor: if so, then the limit of 20 m applies.
- If an auditorium is to accommodate more than one type of production then the most onerous condition applies.

The greater the encirclement of the audience of the platform/stage, then the greater the number of people who can be accommodated within the aural and visual limitations, up to an encirclement which places the audience on three sides of the platform/stage. With theatre-in-the-round the aural and visual limitations restrict the distance from the stage, with drama, to not more than six rows.

Levels in the auditorium

With a single level only, the pitch of the rake requires particular attention to achieve a sense of enclosure. The Greek amphitheatre is the exemplar of the single tier auditorium, with its seating built onto the side of the hill. An example is the amphitheatre at Epidaurus, Greece, with a pitch of 26°. The Olivier Theatre at the Royal National Theatre, London, is an interpretation of this form, with a single tier where the central section is dropped: the upper level drops down either side of the central section (Fig. 12.11). The benefits of the single tier include: the improved sightlines (an introduction of one or more balconies will reduce the pitch of the lower level (the stalls) to the minimum sightline calculation, if not below; the 'wholeness' of the audience within one bowl, with every member of the audience seeing all others; the performers able to look only at the audience, except for gangways, without interruption of rear walls and balcony fronts.

Seating capacity can be increased by the addition of one or more balconies within the aural and visual limitations which determine the overall permissable volume of the auditorium. Similarly boxes, side galleries, and loges can be added to the side walls, especially in the case of the proscenium format. If the maximum number of seats within the permissible volume is to be achieved then the inclusion of at least one balcony will be necessary. Balconies may be considered for other reasons: to increase, for example, the intimacy of the auditorium by bringing a given seating capacity closer to the performance area. Balconies had become associated with social distinctions within an auditorium; such distinctions are no longer valid but balconies can concentrate seating within the vertical plane thereby increasing numbers close to the performance.

Deep balconies require compromise of the sightlines at the lowest level of seating with the rake reduced to restrict the height of the auditorium, while acoustic requirements may limit the depth of a balcony. Disadvantages may also lie with the vertical division of the audience (especially as seen by the performer), the increased number in the audience above the horizontal eye line of the performer and the cost of the balconies and associated public circulation areas.

The shallow balcony (one, two, or three rows of seats), as distinct from the deep balcony, allows more levels and provides the opportunity to 'paper the auditorium walls with people'. The courtyard theatre – e.g. the Georgian Theatre in Richmond, Yorkshire – is an example of the shallow balcony on the three sides of a rectangular auditorium: the Barbican Theatre, London, is a further example where the rear wall of the auditorium is covered in shallow balconies, each cantilevered over the one below (Fig. 12.11).

Sightlines from boxes along side walls to the auditorium may not be satisfactory but lack of perfect viewing positions could be justified by the character of the enclosing side walls and seating embracing the stage. Unpopulated blank side walls, especially with proscenium and end stage formats, distract from the

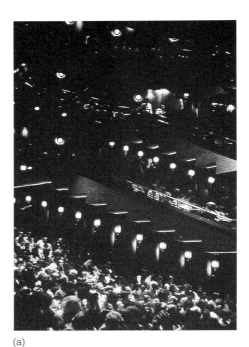

(a)

(b)

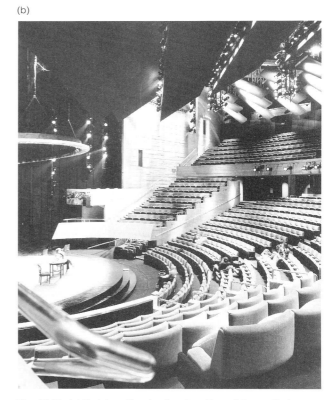

Fig. 12.11 *(a) Barbican Theatre, London. View of the auditorium showing shallow balconies, and also side slips. (b) Olivier Theatre, Royal National Theatre, London*

auditorium character. In the case of the concert hall, boxes, such as those in the Royal Festival Hall, London, fulfil an acoustic function, as well as visual and social, as they assist in breaking up the wall surfaces. Examples are shown in Fig. 12.12.

Balcony handrails are specified by legislation covering their height, width and structure. They must be located in such a way so as not to interfere adversely with sightlines (Fig. 12.13).

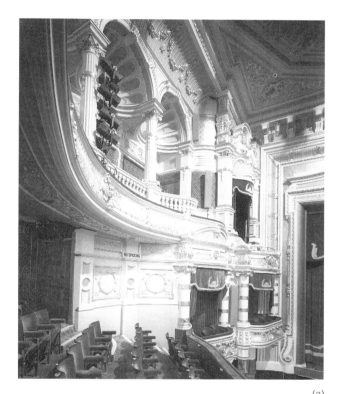

(a)

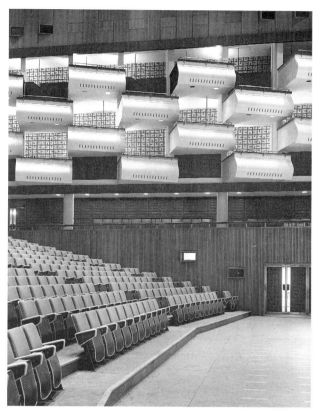

(b)

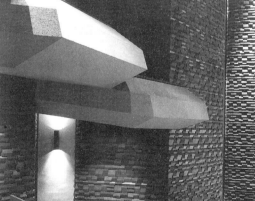

(c)

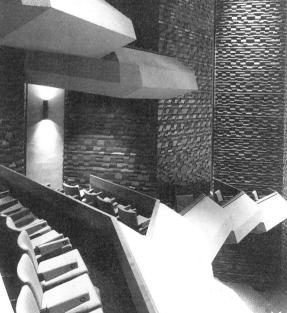

Auditorium acoustics

The acoustic performance of the auditorium is a critical design requirement and needs to be considered as part of the initial brief. Acoustic performance refers to the quality of the sound – music or speech – heard by each member of the audience, and also the performers on the platform/stage. Design considerations for the acoustics of an auditorium, when the sound is *not amplified*, include:

- Type of production: each type has its own requirements with different characteristics for music and speech.

Fig. 12.12 *Examples of the side boxes in an auditorium. (a) Traditional boxes to the auditorium side walls, with ornate framed enclosure and loose seats (King's Theatre, Glasgow). (b) Individual cantilevered boxes. The curved fronts and configuration of the boxes are part of the acoustic requirements (Royal Festival Hall, London). (c) Stepped and raked boxes extending the balconies along the side walls of the auditorium (Festival Theatre, Adelaide)*

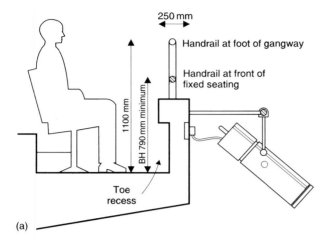

(a)

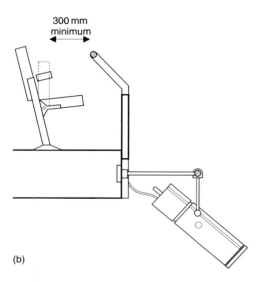

(b)

Fig. 12.13 *Balcony handrail height (BH) is determined, as a minimum height, by legislation, and can be as low as 790 mm in front of fixed seating, rising at the end of gangways to 1100 mm. (a) Traditional balcony front with shelf of 250 mm minimum width below handrail and allowance for feet positions when seated. (b) Simple balcony front for side galleries with the audience able to lean on the handrail, with minimum clearway. The whole front can be removed if it is part of a flexible auditorium. Balcony fronts are convenient and useful locations for performance lighting and lighting bars, and socket outlets may need to be incorporated into the design*

- Shape and size of the auditorium: the extent to which the audience surrounds the platform/stage; seating capacity; number and depth of balconies; rake of the seating; for concerts, the proportion of length to width and height to width; for opera, dance and musicals, the location of the orchestra pit; location of performance lighting and sound equipment and lighting bridges.
- Setting for the performance; such as permanent architectural setting, within audience, proscenium stage and so on.

- Volume of the auditorium; calculated as the number in the audience multiplied by a ratio of volume to person, according to the type of production: 3.4 m^3 per person for music and 9 m^3 per person for speech within the auditorium enclosure: for opera the ratio is between 7 m^3 and 8 m^3 per person.
- Reverberation time: the difference in time between direct sound to each member of an audience and the reflected sound from all surfaces of the auditorium, which requires to be short for speech and long for music. The aim is to balance these two sound sources by eliminating distortion and distributing sound evenly across the audience.
- Finishes: extent, size, shape and location of surfaces required for reflection, absorption and diffusion of sound to the walls, ceiling and floor, including the seat design, which can all affect the reverberation time.
- Quality of the sound: expectations vary according to speech and different types of music, and relate to such factors as the extent to which each member of the audience may feel surrounded by sound, respond in an intimate or detached manner, and experience a balance between sounds from different performers.

Model or computer simulation may be necessary to test the auditorium form against the design considerations: the more sensitive the acoustic performance such as opera and classical music, the greater the need for simulation as part of the design process (Fig. 12.14).

Auditoria for classical music may incorporate the ability to change the acoustic character of the space according to the music performed. Compositions were written within an acoustic at the time and can have a range of reverberation time of 1.5 to 2.2 seconds. Variability may be either mechanical, using retractable elements to change volume and formation of finishes, or electronic 'assisted resonance'.

Physical adjustment of the auditorium (Fig. 12.15) includes:

- increase of the volume by use of chambers in the walls and ceiling, with the opening of panels or doors;

(a)

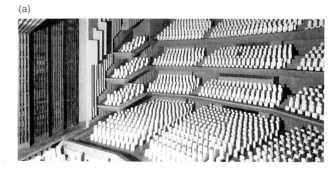

Fig. 12.14 *(a) Model simulation. Example of a physical model of an auditorium simulating the acoustic characteristics, by Sandy Brown and Associates.*

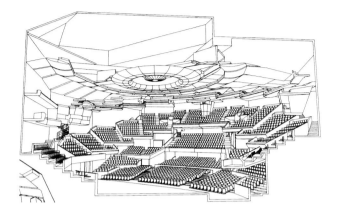

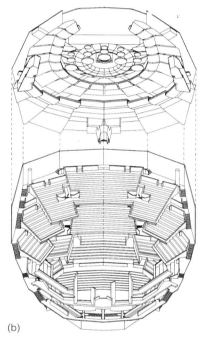

(b)

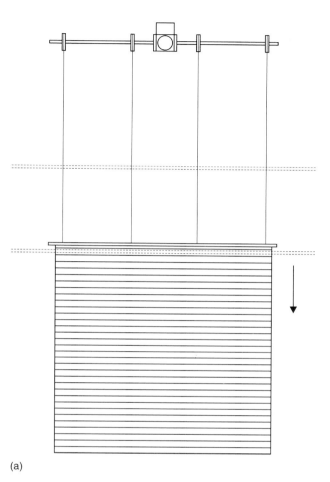

(a)

Fig. 12.14 continued *(b) Use of computer-aided design to simulate interior of Belfast's new concert hall to test acoustic performance as well as sightlines*

- adjustment of the ceiling and wall characteristics by hinged panels, dropped sound-absorbent banners or changed ceiling panels;
- change of volume and seating capacity by physical adaptation by lowering ceiling or a section of the seating curtained off.

Physical problems arise with the combination of different types of production in a single multi-purpose auditorium. Variation in volumes and reverberation times for speech and music implies difficulties when combined in a single auditorium. Volume can be adjusted physically by, for example, the lowering of the auditorium ceiling while changing the surface treatment to walls and ceiling and incorporating the

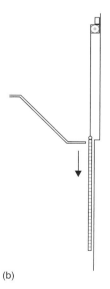

(b)

Fig. 12.15 *Physical adjustment. The acoustic characteristics of an auditorium can be adjusted by alterations to the volume and surface treatment. The illustrations show an example of insulated banners which have been dropped across the wall surface to provide an absorbent, rather than reflective surface. (a) Elevation; (b) Section*

electronic 'assisted resonance' can alter the reverberation times.

For performances which are non-amplified then the form of the auditorium on plan and section and its volume is considerably influenced by the acoustic requirements. For *amplified* performances these requirements are less significant. A potential problem lies with the possible dual system of direct sound and amplified sound, where for jazz concerts, for example, the auditorium may be required to have a dead acoustic, i.e. no reflected sound from the stage, relying exclusively on amplification, or a low reverberation time, and the need for the loudspeakers positioned to provide full and even coverage of the audience. Similarly for an auditorium for electronic music the condition of the dead acoustic will be a probable requirement.

Sound insulation and noise control

The auditorium needs to be insulated from sources of noise beyond its enclosure such as external traffic noises and from adjacent functions. An acceptable background noise level within the auditorium as heard by members of the audience needs to be identified: standards are expressed as Noise Rating (NR) and recommended levels vary according to the type of production. These include NR 20 for classical music, opera and dance and NR 25 for drama and musicals. If recording of live performances is part of the brief then the recommended level may be as low as NR 15. The lower the NR then the more difficult it is to achieve. With each rating there is an effect on the design of the enclosure, openings within the enclosure and the air-conditioning/heating/ventilation systems, which may suggest the following:

- isolation of the auditorium structurally from the adjacent spaces and/or a double wall, especially if external: double skin roof construction, especially if subject to aircraft noise; foundation of the structure on anti-vibration mounts to avoid ground-borne noise.
- sound locks to all doors at point of entry into the auditorium.
- services acoustically sealed when they penetrate the walls and floor of the auditorium.

Seating layout

The seating layout in an auditorium depends mainly on the selection of format – the relationship between audience and performance – and the visual and aural limitations associated with a particular type of production as well as the number of levels and sightlines. Other aspects which influence the layout, and thereby condition seating capacity, include factors in the following sections.

Design of the individual auditorium seat

The design aim is to provide an appropriate standard of comfort during a performance. The range of human body dimensions is wide, while a single, or restricted, size of seat is normally provided. Also tolerance levels vary between generations and indeed between different performing arts: the young can tolerate simple seating found less comfortable by older age groups, whereas those attending concerts of classical music appear to expect a level of comfort higher than those at a drama performance. The dimensions of a seat are generally based on a median characteristic of the anticipated users, which varies by age and also by nationality. Minor variation is achieved by the upholstery and adjustment of the back and seat pan material when the seat is occupied: otherwise the seat selection is a common size within the whole, or part of, the auditorium layout. Probably the best that can be achieved is in the order of 90 per cent of the audience within an acceptable range of comfort.

The working dimensions (Fig. 12.16) of an auditorium seat are:

- Seat width, with or without arms: the minimum dimension with arms is 500 mm and without arms, 450 mm, as stipulated by legislation. For seats with arms a width of 525 mm may be regarded as a minimum to offer reasonable comfort.
- Seat height and inclination: height of 430–450 mm and angle to the horizontal of 7–9°.
- Back height and inclination: height 800–850 mm above floor level (the height may be increased for acoustic reasons), with a back angle of 15–20° to the vertical.
- Seat depth: 600–720 mm for seat and back depth, reduced to 425–500 mm when the seat is tipped. The seat depth varies and depends on the thickness of upholstery and backing and whether the rear of the seat contains the air-conditioning. For a modest seat, with arms, the dimensions can be as low as 520 mm deep and 340 mm when the seat is tipped. The seat is able to tip, activated silently by weights when not occupied, and thus allows a clearway (which is a critical dimension) to pass along a row while limiting distance between rows. Conversely a static seat means an increased row to row distance.
- Arm rests: 50 mm minimum width, with the length coinciding with the seat in a tipped position to avoid obstruction to those passing along a row of seats; the height tends to be 600 mm above floor level, with the upper surface either sloping or flat.

Fixed seats can have side supports (legs shared by adjacent seats), pedestal (single vertical support to each seat), cantilevered (brackets shared by adjacent seats fixed to riser if they offer sufficient height) or a bar supporting a group of seats with leg or bracket support.

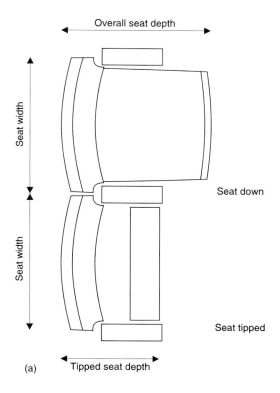

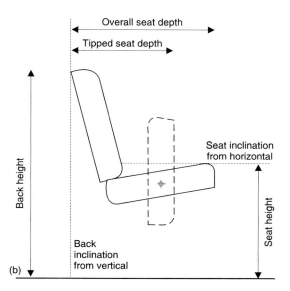

(a)

(b)

Fig. 12.16 *Seat variables. (a) Plan; (b) side elevation*

Other factors include:

- Acoustics: upholstery must satisfy the acoustic requirements, usually the level of absorbency when unoccupied; this is especially the case with music.
- Ventilation/heating: for air supply or extract under a seat, space should be allowed in the floor or riser to receive a grille.

- Upholstery: thickness of padding should provide comfort and avoid fatigue, but should not encourage excessive relaxation; the material of the padding and finish must satisfy fire regulations.

For choice of type of seat see Fig. 12.17.

Number of seats in a row

With *traditional seating* the maximum number in a row is limited to 22 if there are gangways at both ends of the row, and 11 if a gangway is on one side only. In following these guidelines, the seating, other than in the smallest rectangular auditoria, is divided into blocks by the gangways. Rows with more than 22 seats can be allowed if the audience is not imperilled. *Continental seating* refers to rows of seats with more than 22 seats extending to side gateways and more exits than with traditional seating. Continental seating is more appropriate with the proscenium format to achieve side wall to side wall rows of seats. With formats where the audience surrounds the platform/ stage it is less applicable and gangways within the seating become inevitable.

Row to row spacing

Spacing is conditioned by the distance between the leading edge of the seat (in an upright position, if tippable) and the rear of the back of the seat in front (Fig. 12.18). The critical dimension is the vertical clearway which enables people to pass along the row. For traditional seating the minimum is 300 mm and this dimension increases with the number of seats in a row. For continental seating the clearway is to be not less than 400 mm and not more than 500 mm. Legislation also dictates the minimum row to row dimension at 760 mm: this is usually not adequate and the minimum should be 850 mm for traditional seating.

Gangways

The widths of gangways within seating layouts at each level within an auditorium are determined by their role as escape routes and the number of seats served. The minimum width is 1100 mm. Gangways can be ramped up to a ratio of 1.10 and 1.12 if used by persons in wheelchairs. Steeper slopes must have regular steps extending the full gangway width. Steps should have a consistent tread and riser in each section of the gangway: the row to row spacing and row rise should be compatible with a convenient ratio of tread to riser. A uniform pattern of steps and row risers means that the shallow curve formed by the sightline calculation should be aggregated into a regular profile.

Seating geometry

Seating is usually laid out in straight or curved rows focused towards the performance. Further forms are the angled row, the straight row with curved change of

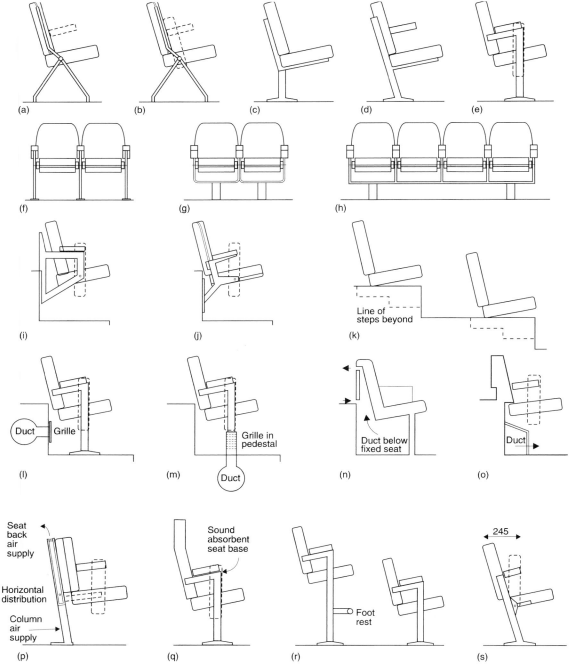

Fig. 12.17 *Seat: choice of type. (a) Loose seating: upholstered individual seats or short sections of seating, capable of being removed (to clear floor or rostra for other purposes, to allow use of seats elsewhere, for flexible seating arrangements); loose seating needs to be fixed firmly to the floor or riser when in public use; seats may be with or without arms, and stackable. Storage space is required for seats when not in use: various trolley systems are available for moving large numbers of seats. (b) Loose seating as (a), with tip-up seat. (c) Fixed upholstered continuous bench seating. (d) Fixed upholstered individual seating, with or without arms. (e) Fixed upholstered individual seating, with tip-up seat, with or without arms. (f) Fixed seating with side support, off floor or tread. (g) Fixed seating with pedestal support, off floor or tread. (h) Fixed seating with bar support, off floor or tread. (i) Fixed seating with cantilevered support, off high riser, without overlap of riser. (j) Fixed seating with cantilevered support, off high riser, with overlap of riser. (k) Seat fixed directly to tread, with a stepped tier; fixed seats, either continuous or individual. Note that the gangway steps have to be inset into the profile of the stepped tier to achieve ease of access into each row from the gangway. (l) Ventilation grille below seats, in riser (or in floor). (m) Ventilation grille below seats incorporated into pedestal. (n) Riser and ventilation integrated into seat design: fixed seating. This arrangement allows continuous seating per row, with or without arms, and ease of cleaning floor. (o) Riser and ventilation integrated into seat design: tip-up seat. (p) Air-conditioned seat: with seat-back air-supply providing low pressure, low volume air. Preferred method of locating outlet for air-conditioning. Note though the possible increased depth of seat back which may affect row to row spacing. (q) Acoustic seat, incorporating high seat back and perforated base to seat to absorb sound when not occupied: applicable mainly in concert halls. (r) Elevated seat raising occupant to allow view over row in front while retaining a flat floor, suitable for shallow balconies. (s) Slim 'studio' seat with arms and tippable seat, suitable where space and comfort requirements are limited.*

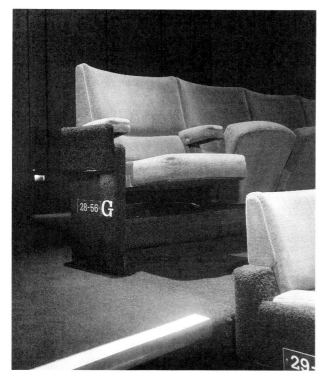

Fig. 12.17 continued *Seat: choice of type.(t) Example of auditorium seat (Royal National Theatre, London)*

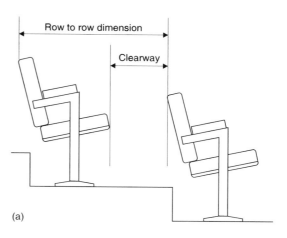

(a)

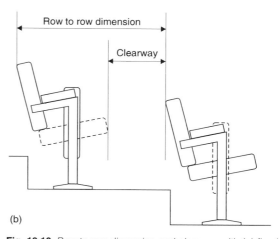

(b)

Fig. 12.18 *Row to row dimension and clearway with (a) fixed seating and (b) tipped seating*

direction (Fig. 12.19). Curved rows are slightly more efficient in terms of numbers within a given area but may increase construction costs. An example of the curved row is the Olivier Theatre at the Royal National Theatre in London, which evokes the predominant Greco-Roman outdoor auditorium. The Berlin Philharmonic is an example of straight rows where blocks of seats are also emphasized to reduce the scale of a large auditorium (see page 134). The angular nature of the straight rows is seen in the Tyrone Guthrie Theatre in Minneapolis, USA.

Seating density

Density of seating can vary (Fig. 12.20): seats with arms and a tippable seat can occupy an area as small as 500 mm wide, and less with seats without arms, with a row to row dimension of 760 mm, but can be as large as 750 mm wide by 1400 mm. This is a variation from 0.38 m^2 to 1.05 m^2, with these examples, and the increased dimensions means fewer seats within a given area and reduces the seating capacity. The minimum dimensions laid down by legislation offer a low standard of comfort for the audience. Comfort needs to be considered, especially knee room, and these dimensions should not be taken as the norm. Social cohesion of the audience may be lost if the space standards are too high, with the performer

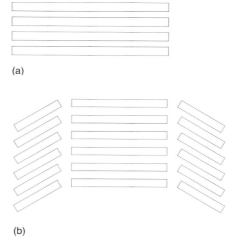

(a)

(b)

Fig. 12.19 *Seating geometry. (a) Straight rows. (b) Straight rows, with side blocks of seats angled and focused towards the platform/ stage: blocks of seating defined by gangways.*

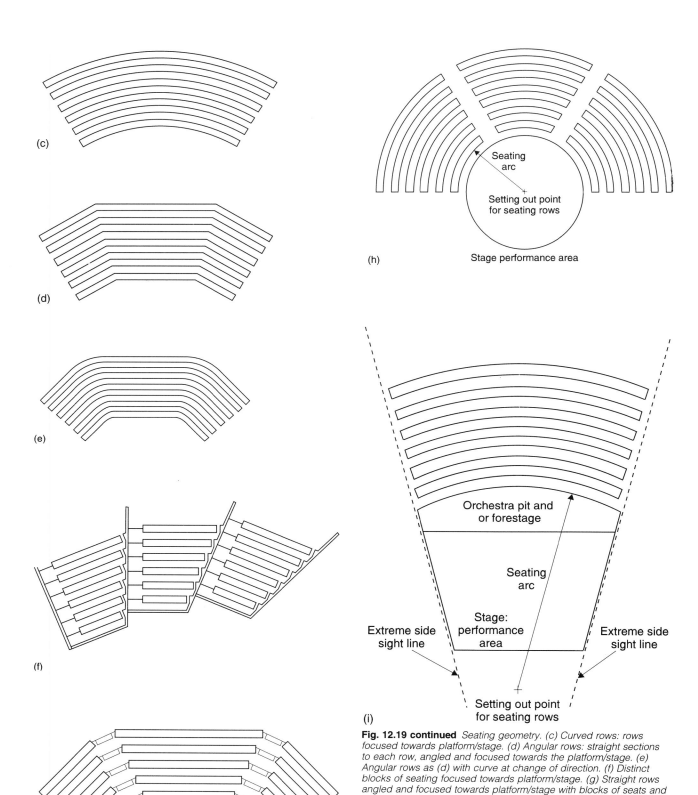

(c)

(d)

(e)

(f)

(g)

(h)

Seating
arc

Setting out point
for seating rows

Stage performance area

(i)

Orchestra pit and
or forestage

Seating
arc

Stage:
performance
area

Extreme side
sight line

Extreme side
sight line

Setting out point
for seating rows

Fig. 12.19 continued *Seating geometry. (c) Curved rows: rows
focused towards platform/stage. (d) Angular rows: straight sections
to each row, angled and focused towards the platform/stage. (e)
Angular rows as (d) with curve at change of direction. (f) Distinct
blocks of seating focused towards platform/stage. (g) Straight rows
angled and focused towards platform/stage with blocks of seats and
gangways located at change of direction. (h) Setting out point for
seating rows same as centre of performance area: this coincidence
of seating out points tends to be a characteristic of open stage
layouts. (i) Setting out point for seating rows distinct from geometry
of performance area and extreme side sightlines: this arrangement
tends to be a characteristic of proscenium formats.*

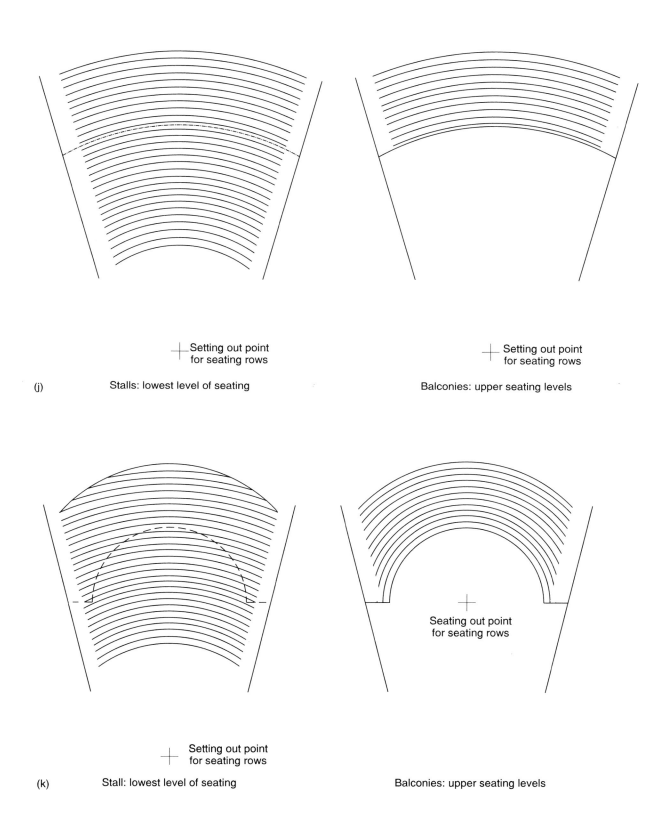

—┼— Setting out point
for seating rows

(j)   Stalls: lowest level of seating

—┼— Setting out point
for seating rows

Balconies: upper seating levels

—┼— Setting out point
for seating rows

(k)   Stall: lowest level of seating

—┼—
Seating out point
for seating rows

Balconies: upper seating levels

Fig. 12.19 continued *Seating geometry. (j) Proscenium/end stage formats: geometry of the various levels in an auditorium to have the same setting out point for the seating rows. (k) Proscenium/end stage formats: distinct setting out points for seating rows according to level within auditorium*

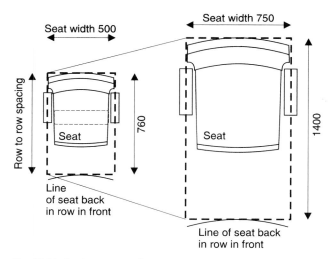

Fig. 12.20 *Seating density. Sizes of seats and area allocated to each seat can vary. The plans show the range from 0.38m² (and less) to 1.05 m² (and more)*

being less aware of the grouping and more the individuals.

Standards may vary in different sections of the seating layout reflecting pricing variation, distance from the performing area and status distinctions.

Means of escape

The aim is for everyone in the auditorium to be able to egress to a place of safety within a set period of time. The escape route is from the seat, along the clearway and gangway and through exit doors immediately, or through an enclosed corridor, to a place of safety. The time restriction provides the maximum travel distance from seat to exit within the auditorium, and the number of seats provides the width and number of exit routes.

Travel distance

The evacuation from each level of the auditorium within a limited period of time is required in case of a fire. For traditional seating the travel distance is 18 m measured from the gangway: for continental seating, 15 m from any seat. The aim is to evacuate the audience of each level within 2.5 minutes.

Exit numbers

At least two separate independent exits must be provided from each level within the auditorium. The exits should be located with sufficient remoteness from each other to allow alternative directions of escape. The number of exits per level are two for each level within an auditorium with the seating capacity up to 500: an additional exit is required for every further 250 seats as defined by legislation. Egress in case of emergencies should follow the natural flow of movement from the seats away from the platform/stage.

Exit widths

The exit widths are laid down by regulations. The base calculation is 45 persons per minute per unit width of 520–530 mm. The minimum total exit widths required are outlined in Table 12.1.

Table 12.1 Minimum total exit widths

Number of persons	Metres
up to 200	2.2
201–300	2.4
301–400	2.8
401–500	3.2
501–999	4.8
1000–1999	6.4
2000–2999	14.4
3000	20.8

Exit route

The exits from the auditorium must lead directly to a place of safety. The exit route must be the same width as the exit and be a consistent width avoiding bottlenecks. The exit doors from the auditorium, any doors within the route and the final exit doors must open in the direction of egress. Staircases within the route are subject to the following conditions: the maximum number of steps, 16: the minimum number, 2; tread/riser to be 275 × 180 and consistent.

Ramps are to be a maximum pitch of 1.12, in lengths of 4.5 m. Exit routes for wheelchair users are required to be on the flat or ramped if there is a change of level, and may be required to be separate from the other routes. Routes are to be enclosed by fire-resistant material within the building.

Circulation within auditorium

Audience entry points into the auditorium from the foyer can be at the rear or sides of the seating, or within the banks of seating, and should be related to the gangway positions (Fig. 12.21). While gangways are primarily calculated as part of the escape route in case of fire, they also act as circulation routes through the auditorium, with possible additional gangways, from the audience entry points to the particular row and seat. Access through banks of raked seating – vomitories – remove seats, and thereby reduce the potential seating capacity (Fig. 12.22). A threshold space at the entry points for ticket checks, programme sales and for members of the audience to orientate themselves should be considered.

Handrails will be required to a stepped gangway adjacent to an enclosing wall; to a stepped gangway if a drop at the side; at landings, rear of rostra and where there is a drop of more than 600 mm; where the rake is above 25° to a gangway the ends of the rows

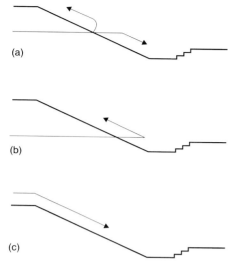

Fig. 12.21 *Points of entry into auditorium. (a) Entry to block of raked seating at an intermediate level, either at the sides of or within (vomitory entry), the seating. Vomitory entry displaces centrally located seats. (b) Entry to block of raked seating at the bottom level, either at the sides of, or within (vomitory entry), the seating. Vomitory entry at this level erodes particularly valuable seating. (c) Entry at the top level, or rear of blocks of raked seating. This allows easy access at various points of entry into blocks of seating*

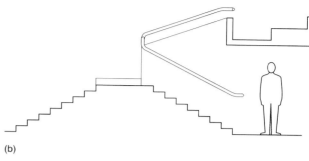

Fig. 12.22 *Audience vomitory. A public entrance into the auditorium through a block of seating as distinct from through the side enclosing walls to the auditorium. (a) Diagrammatic projection showing a simple form of vomitory within a seating area: the gangway is to one side serving rows above the vomitory and central to the vomitory below; the example shown displaces some 20 seats. The actual number of seats displaced and the complexity of vomitory design will depend on size and spacing of the seats, the general layout and the pitch of the raked floor. (b) Section through the vomitory, with staircase access: a sound lobby is necessary between public spaces and auditorium. The access from the public spaces can be on the flat or ramped: the effect is an increase in lost seats*

served by the gangway *may* require a loop rail (Fig. 12.23).

Rails are usually 900 mm above the pitch line and 1200 mm above landings, with panels either solid or sub-divisions which may require a 100 mm maximum gap.

Performers' access through the auditorium

Performers may have access to the stage through the auditorium during a performance by way of:

- access along the gangways, with step access onto the stage if raised;

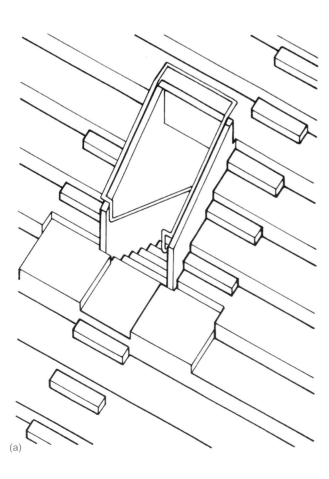

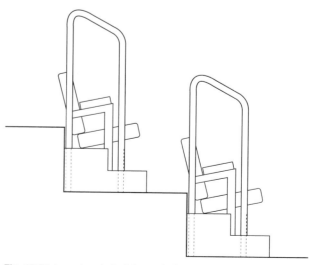

Fig. 12.23 *Loop handrail at the end of each row where the rake is steep, either of gangways within seating areas*

● access through vomitories exclusively for performers. Details of a performers' vomitory are shown in Fig. 12.24. The performers' vomitory can be filled to accommodate auditorium seating if not in use.

Wheelchair location within the seating

Regulations require a minimum of six places for wheelchairs or 1/100th of the audience capacity whichever is the greater. Wheelchair locations, as discrete areas, can occur at the rear, front, side or within the seating. Wheelchairs can be centrally positioned by forming a bay off a cross gangway. The actual location will be conditioned by the particular seating layout, the convenient points of entry from the public areas and the escape arrangements in the case of fire. Separate entrances into the auditorium as well as escape routes should be considered.

The dimensions for wheelchairs are shown in Fig. 12.25. A wheelchair user should be able to sit with a party of friends who may not be in wheelchairs. Sightlines for the wheelchair should be checked, as should the sightlines of those audience members behind.

Some wheelchair users can transfer into auditorium seats: the following should be noted:

● the wheelchair should be able to be located adjacent to the auditorium seat for ease of sideways movement from the wheelchair;

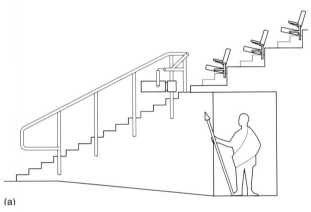

(a)

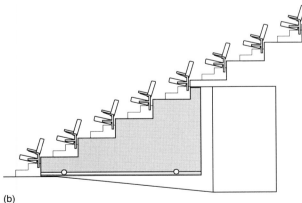

(b)

Fig. 12.24 *Performers' vomitory. A performer's entry onto the stage through a block of seating. Access through the audience may supplement other access points onto the stage for the performers. Such vomitories are used in open stage formats rather than with a proscenium stage. (a) Section through vomitory. The head room must allow performers in costume ease of access from a corridor below the auditorium seating to the stage. The floor, if ramped, requires to be no steeper than 1:12. A stage lighting position is shown allowing low level illumination of the stage. (b) Section through vomitory showing removable seating unit in position if vomitory not in use for a production. The example shown is fixed seating on a mobile unit, with channels on side walls along which the unit can be wheeled. The handrails and stage lighting positions are removed, possibly stored in the seating unit*

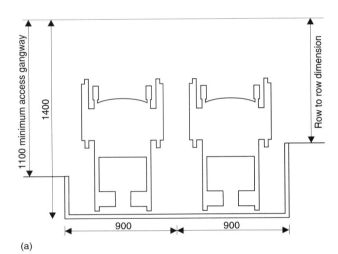

(a)

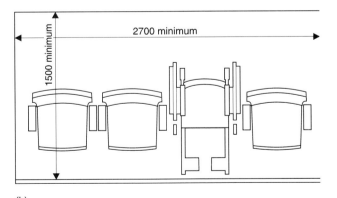

(b)

Fig. 12.25 *Wheelchair positions. Designated areas within the seating blocks in an auditorium providing a space for persons to sit in wheelchairs to see and hear performances. Such areas may be permanent, occupied only by wheelchair users, or able to take loose seats or fixed seats. (a) Plan of an area within a seating block showing minimum dimensions for a wheelchair and access. (b) Plan of a box at the rear of the auditorium for wheelchair users, accompanied by friends who can use the loose chairs. The box can be used by non-disabled persons only if necessary. The dimensions show the minimum requirements for a box*

- the seat should not be tippable and should be strong enough, especially the arms, to receive the weight of the user when transferring;
- a position for the folded wheelchair when not in use during the performance should be provided.

The management has a role during emergencies to assist egress.

Broadcasting requirements

Television cameras

External broadcasting – television and radio – and recording in auditoria my be a requirement especially in those buildings for the performing arts housing or hosting national and regional professional companies. Television cameras (Fig. 12.26) require to be located in the seating areas either in specific locations, on platforms, or by displacing seats.

Sound control room

In large auditoria with amplified sound and/or sound effects the sound control room may be located within the seating area to benefit from being in the acoustic volume of the auditorium (see page 183 for the discussion of sound control location).

Latecomers

Latecomers may be obliged to wait at the entrance points into the auditorium until a convenient time in the performance when they can be ushered to their seats: waiting can be in an area within the auditorium out of sight of the seated audience or a separate enclosed space at the rear of the auditorium with a viewing panel and tannoyed sound of the performance.

Attendants

Legislation dictates the minimum number of attendants to be present during a performance; each attendant requires a seat in the auditorium.

Adaptation

In multi-purpose auditoria where different formats or uses are combined then all or part of the raked seating will require to be movable. This can be achieved by forming a structure off a flat floor, and include (Fig. 12.27):

- *Bleacher seating*: Telescopic structure with tippable upholstered seating with backs, able to be retracted into the depth of a single and highest row. The rows are straight and the extended structure is a simple rectangular block, which places a discipline on the seating layout.

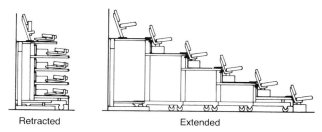

Retracted   Extended

(a)

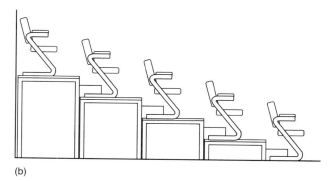

(b)

Fig. 12.27 *Temporary seating with raked floor. (a) Retractable, or telescopic, seating (bleachers) as proprietary systems: each row retracts into row behind until the stored unit is one rear row deep. The seating – continuous bench, fixed individual seats with tip-up seats (with or without arms) – is hinged to lie flat in a stored position. Unit widths are restricted to 6 m and the number of rows up to 30 m. The stepped floor and seating can be pulled out and retracted electrically, by towing bracket or manually according to size. For seating with arms and tip-up seats, the minimum riser height is 250 mm. The seats can be loose, with a secure fixing to the riser when in use, on the stepped floor which can be retracted only: the addition of loose seats will take time to set up, but the seats can be used in other situations when the bleachers are retracted. (b) Rostra: a set of metal/timber units able to be built up to form a stepped floor on a flat floor, with loose seating secured onto floor or riser, or fixed seating on upper units. Each rostra unit can be collapsed by hinged legs or sides to reduce storage requirements.*

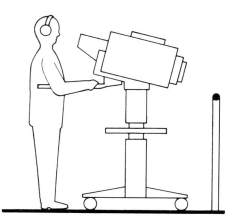

Fig. 12.26 *Television camera position, with operative. The area required for each position is 1.5 m × 1 m minimum*

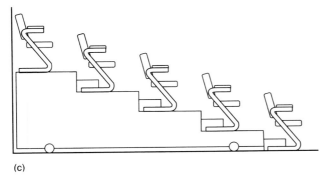

(c)

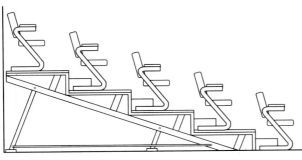

(d)

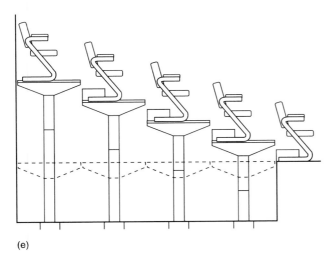

(e)

Fig. 12.27 continued *Temporary seating with raked floor. (c) Seating units: large units on braked casters or air cushion with either loose seating secured onto floor or riser, or fixed seating. Large storage area required to accommodate the units when not in use. (d) Demountable kit of parts: proprietary system to form stepped floor or scaffolding built up to form stepped floor. Trolleys are available to move kit of parts to and from storage areas. (e) Hydraulic method: sections of a flat floor capable of being raised to varying heights to form a stepped floor; loose seating can then be secured onto the risers*

- *Rostra*: Complete raked units with either permanent or removable seats, on wheels or air pallettes for ease of movement into storage areas when not in use.

- *Sectional rostra*: A set of boxes able to be built up to form raked units with removable seats. The storage requirements are less than complete rostra.
- *Kit of parts*: Scaffolding or equivalent set of components able to form raked levels to receive seating. This is the most flexible system, it has efficient storage requirements, but is labour intensive.
- *Hydraulic lifts*: Mechanical method of raising sections of the flat floor to form a rake floor to receive seating.

Loose seats, secured in position when required for performances, can be used with functions requiring a flat floor.

Sightlines: seated audience

For the whole of the audience to have an uninterrupted view of the performance and its setting over the heads in front and clear of overhangs, the section and plan of the auditorium needs to conform to certain limitations set by vertical and horizontal sightlines.

Vertical sightlines

Vertical sightlines may be calculated by establishing:

P   Lowest and nearest point of sight on the platform/ stage for the audience to see clearly. The platform/stage height, when raised, can range from 600 to 1100 mm above the lowest level of the auditorium and point P can be the leading edge, or setting line for the performance, at or above the platform/stage level. If a forestage is part of the proscenium or end stage formats then point P needs to relate to the forestage. If an orchestra pit is included between stage and seating then point P may be regarded as the conductor's head.

  With a symphony orchestra in a concert hall, the ability to see each musician at the front of the stage (who partially masks the other musicians) may not be critical and point P may be taken as over 600 mm above the platform level at the front edge. For dance the audience requires to see the feet of the dancers so the point P needs to be taken from at least the setting line at stage level. For opera, musicals, and drama, point P should be not more than 600 mm above stage level.

HD   Horizontal distance between the eyes of the seated members of the audience, which relates to the row spacing and can vary from 760 to 1150 mm and more.

EH   Average eye height at 1120 mm above the theoretical floor level: the actual eye point will depend on seat dimensions.

E   Distance from the centre of the eye to the top of the head, taken as 100 mm as a minimum dimension for the calculations of sightlines. For assurance that there is a clear view over the heads of those in the row in front, this dimension should be at least 125 mm.

D   Front row of seats: the distance from point P to the edge of the average member of the audience in the front row. The closer the first row to the platform/stage, the steeper will be the rake. For orchestral and choral music, the area immediately in front of the platform may be required to be clear for acoustic reasons. For

rock concerts a rail and space may be required for security reasons between audience and stage.

The relationship is shown in Fig. 12.28. The position of the eye of seated user to seat and stepped floor is shown in Fig. 12.29.

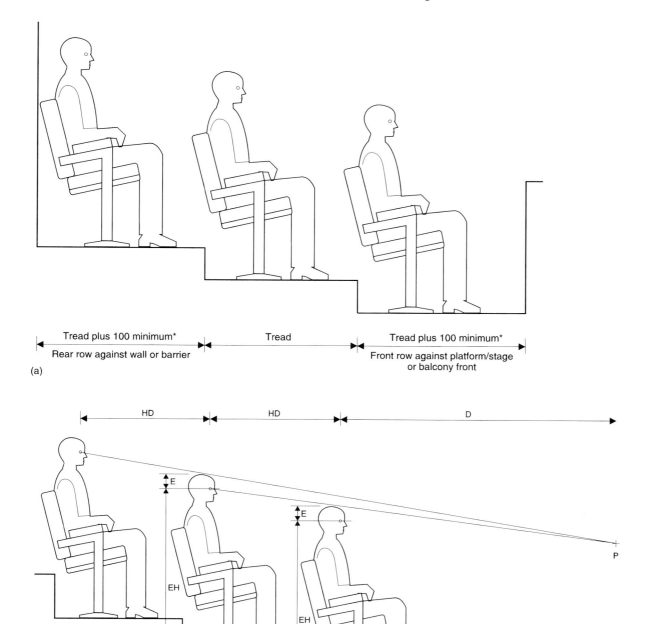

(a)

Tread plus 100 minimum*

Rear row against wall or barrier

Tread

Tread plus 100 minimum*

Front row against platform/stage or balcony front

(b)

Fig. 12.28 *(a) Rear and front rows. (*indicates working dimensions. The actual dimensions will depend on the design of the individual seat and will vary according to the thickness of the upholstery to seat back and inclination of the seat back.) (b) Graphic representation of vertical sightlines*

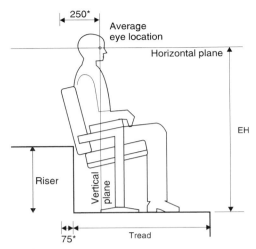

Fig. 12.29 *Position of eye in relation to seat and stepped floor (*indicates working dimensions. The actual dimensions will depend on the design of the individual seat and will vary according to thickness of upholstery to seat back and inclination of seat back)*

The longitudinal section is a parabolic stepped floor as the theoretical rake produced by the sightline calculation. This gives every member of the audience similar viewing conditions. This may be reduced to a single angle or series of angles.

When applied as described the rake will also be steep. This is satisfactory for a single tier of seating with no balconies and is especially appropriate for open stage formats. If a balcony or balconies are introduced, as with proscenium formats, the rake of the lower bank of seats can be reduced, assuming vision to be every other row allowing for point P being seen between heads in the row in front. The vertical distance between a point from the eye to the top of the head for calculation purposes can be reduced to 65 mm. If the seats are staggered then the situation can be marginally improved. This is particularly applicable with the design of a large auditorium where, within the visual and aural limitations, the aim is to maximize the seating capacity. This implies a balance between sightlines, height of the auditorium and seating capacity: a reduction in the accumulative height of the lower level of seating allows more height for balconies.

With the smaller auditorium, especially with the audience partially or wholly surrounding the stage and a limited number of rows of seats, an increased height of the rake to the seating encourages a sense of enclosure of the stage, while providing good sightlines.

Where balconies are included, seated members of the audience need to see the full volume of the performance from the rear row of the highest balcony and from the rear row under the balcony. These extreme sightlines depend on the following limitations (see Fig. 12.30):

P   Nearest and lowest part of the stage which must be within the unrestricted view of all members of

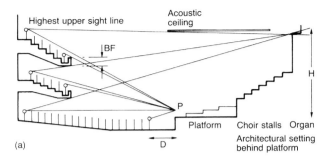

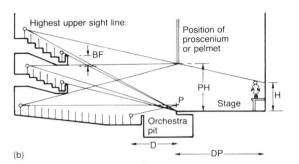

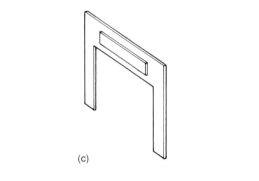

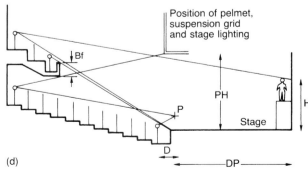

Fig. 12.30 *(a) Vertical sightlines through auditorium with concert platform: sightlines require to include choir stalls and any architectural setting behind the platform as well as the conductor, soloists and orchestra on the platform. Note, however, that acoustic requirements of direct and reflected sound may override sightline calculations. (b) Vertical sightlines through the auditorium with proscenium stage. (c) Subtitle panel over proscenium opening. If incorporated then the vertical sightlines require the panel to be seen by all members of the audience. (d) Vertical sightlines through auditorium with an open stage*

the seated audience as previously described. Point P may be located within the lower level of seating so that those seated in the balconies can be aware of the audience at this level: this is easier to achieve with shallow balconies.

DP Depth of the performance area.

HP Height of the performance area at the rear. For opera, musicals, dance and drama, this may mean the ability to see a performer, at least, standing on a balcony or second floor within the stage set, or, in the case of orchestral and choral music, the height of the setting which may include the choir stalls and organ.

HO Height of the proscenium opening, if applicable, for opera, musicals, dance and drama. The panel over the proscenium opening may require a sub-title panel: this raises the extreme upper sightline from the rear eyelines under balconies.

BF Height of balcony front. The placement of the balcony railings should not interfere with a clear view of the platform/stage.

D Distance to front row, as previously described.

Also the maximum rake is 35° and the highest seat in the auditorium should be on a sightline which is not more than 30° to the horizontal from point P.

Vertical sightlines require to be checked on several sections through the auditorium in addition to through the central line. The wrapping round of a balcony towards the platform/stage will change the sightline conditions to the extreme corner seats.

With cross gangways the line of the auditorium rake must continue so that the audience can see the performance area above the gangway as below. With stepped rows there will need to be a handrail to the

upper side of the gangway and, if a steep rake, a handrail to the lower side (Fig. 12.31).

The design of the auditorium on section is required further to accommodate the sightlines from the lighting and sound control rooms (Fig. 12.32), including projection, and stage management room (if at the rear of the auditorium) and the lighting angles from the lighting bridges and follow spot positions.

Sightlines should be considered also from the performance area of the auditorium by the performer. This is particularly critical for drama and the need for the actor to command the audience: less critical but remaining important is the condition for opera, musicals and dance as well as rock/pop and jazz. The orchestra and choir need to communicate but eye contact with the audience is not seen as critical, although soloists, as singers and instrumentalists may disagree. The zone of vision from the performer and effect of layouts in terms of extent to which audience faces are seen and 'gaps' are minimized: 'gaps'

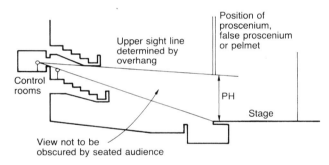

Fig. 12.32 *Vertical sightlines from control rooms at rear of auditorium*

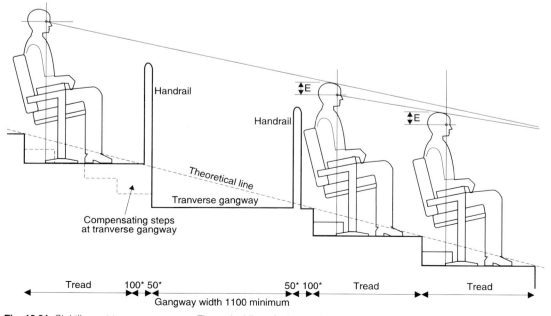

Fig. 12.31 *Sightlines at traverse gangway. Theoretical line of rake requires to continue across the gangway (*indicate mimimum dimensions. Actual dimensions will depend on seat and handrail design)*

include gangways, rear, and side walls and other forms of division within the auditorium such as balconies.

There is a distinction between the performer speaking or singing *at* an audience as opposed to *over* an audience in a dominant position, so dropping the lower level of seating to accommodate balconies with the audience below the eye level of the performer has this consequence.

Horizontal sightlines

Horizontal sightlines are to be considered only with a proscenium stage and possibly end stage and platforms for classical and choral music. Given a particular performance area, sightlines will limit the width of seating that can be provided in the auditorium. Conversely the sightlines from the side seats restrict the amount of the performance area that can be used. The narrowest dimension of the proscenium opening, if adjustable, should be taken as the basis of the calculations.

Each member of the audience should have a direct view of the performance focused towards the centre of the performance area. Curved or angled rows direct the focus of the audience towards the centre. The curved rows radiating from the circular stage of a Greco-Roman theatre is a clear and simple example of this form with the geometry emanating from a single point. With a proscenium stage the geometry of the performance area varies from the setting out point of the seating; the audience should be contained within a 130° angle peripheral spread of vision from the performer at the point of command on the performance area for opera, dance, musicals and drama (Fig. 12.33).

Without head movement the arc to view the whole of the performance area on plan is 40° from the eye. An acceptable degree of head movement is debatable, where the seat is focused away from the stage, as with side galleries, requiring the head to be turned by the member of the audience (Fig. 12.34).

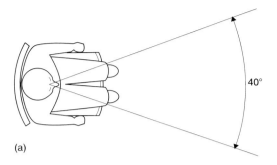

(a)

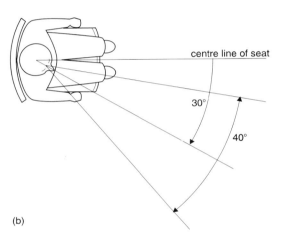

centre line of seat

(b)

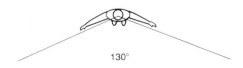

130°

Fig. 12.33 *Horizontal sightlines: performer*

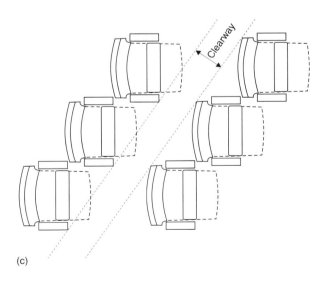

(c)

Fig. 12.34 *Horizontal sightlines: audience. (a) The angle of horizontal vision can be taken as a 40° arc. (b) The turn of the head to be directed towards the platform/stage may not exceed 30° from the centre line of the seat: beyond which angle the member of the audience can experience discomfort. (c) If beyond 30° from the centre line of the seat at right angles to the row then the seats can be set at an angle along each row, directed towards the platform/stage*

Standing: pop/rock concerts

There is a tradition at pop/rock concerts of standing on a flat floor or modest slope at the lower level, immediately in front of the stage. The standards are covered by legislation. Reference is made to:

- density: minimum 0.3 m^2;
- crush barriers at the front and pit in front (minimum width of 3 m, with non-slip finish) for stewards and television coverage. Crush barrier 'A' frame, with panels and tread plate; each section able to receive a force of 3 KN at a height of 1.2 m.
- crush barriers within audience to divide audience into separate areas;
- protection of ground within standing area, if open air;
- means of escape.

The scale may be well beyond the audience capacities found with a traditional concert hall, for example. A pop/rock concert can fill a football stadium and larger. The numbers involved require crowd control and the layout must be designed to avoid congestion, allow ease of movement and have clear signs, entry and exit points, and be well-defined. Stewards, emergency services, local licensing authority and management should develop such a facility jointly and agree such layouts as well as egress procedure in emergencies. A major influence is the type of performer and the level of excitement generated at a concert.

The aims should be: an individual must be able to move without hindrance on personal initiative from an occupied position to exits and other services; crowd management and medical personnel should be able to move without undue hindrance at any time to any individual.

Standing room

Standing room is not usually incorporated into the modern auditorium especially if a formal layout. Cabaret and less formal venues may include standing areas around the perimeter of the main body of seating. The standing areas need to be defined. The sightlines still apply, with the eye level though at 1500 mm.

Promenade performance

This requires no seats at all; the audience stands and moves within an area which also includes performance areas which are not in fixed positions. The local regulations may not permit a mixture of standing and seating at the same level. The standard calculation of space required is one standing person for every 1m^2 of space excluding the stage area. Requirements for gangways and exits will follow from this calculation.

Cabaret layout

Cabaret layout may consist of loose tables and chairs: there must be a provision for clear gangways through the area covered by this layout. Allow a minimum of 1.1 m^2 per person of a seated audience, excluding general circulation.

Air-conditioning, heating and ventilation

The design of the air-conditioning, heating and ventilation depend on the internal standards to be achieved within the auditorium, the thermal insulation levels to the walls, roof and floor, and the external climatic conditions during the times the auditorium is in use. Ventilation supply rates of air relate to the need to provide fresh air at a rate of change to achieve suitable comfort conditions: rates are subject to legislation expressed as a minimum fresh air supply per person, including a proportion of recycled conditioned air.

The design criteria of an auditorium ventilation system include ensuring that there is appropriate air movement which does not produce draughts and is distributed evenly to avoid stagnant pockets. The audience needs to experience a consistent temperature level. The visible components such as the supply and extract grilles should be considered in relation to the interior design. Similarly the external supply and extract grilles need to be integrated into the external fabric.

Full air-conditioning refers to a ventilation system with humidity control and filtration, heating and cooling of the air. Heat in an auditorium is generated from performance lighting at high level and, to a lesser extent, from the audience itself, which suggests cooling of the supply air, especially when in use at times when the external temperature is high. Fresh air mechanical ventilation, without cooling, may be considered when funds are limited, climatic conditions are favourable and standards are reduced.

The design of heating and ventilation must satisfy the performers' requirements during rehearsal on the stage when the director and others are in the auditorium.

Extract ductwork is usually at ceiling level and under balconies, with supply below the seating with grilles in the floor. In multi-purpose auditoria with movable seating units where air supply is not possible, it must occur in the enclosing walls or from above. Supply ductwork may serve a plenum (a large void) with a large number of outlets under the seats which assists in reducing noise levels. Similarly a plenum may be formed as a collector of extracted air through a large number of grilles.

An alternative method is to incorporate an outlet in the rear of each seat providing low volume and low pressure air directed towards the person sitting behind.

Ducts must be odourless and fire, rot and vermin proof. Fire protection will require shutters to be incorporated as ducts pass through the compartment walls: access to the shutters for maintenance is necessary. Ductwork for both supply and return of air is large and needs to be integrated into the auditorium design. Realistic sizes should be considered for vertical and horizontal ducts for the plant room(s) including external supply and extract grilles and access requirements at an early stage in the design process.

The plant should be remote from the auditorium to avoid noise transmission into the auditorium through the ductwork, and equipment vibration transmitted through the structure to the auditorium and other sensitive areas. Access is required to the plant for maintenance and eventual replacement of equipment: this suggests location of the plant room(s) at roof level or ground level. Access to the plant room(s) is necessary internally preferably without passing through public areas. Space may be required for more than one air-conditioning unit and silencers according to the size of the auditorium.

Lighting

Lighting within the auditorium covers the following:

- *Performance lighting* (Fig. 12.35): Lighting positions within the auditorium at ceiling level, on side and rear walls, balcony fronts and at low level within the seating; the lighting direction is towards the platform/stage with clear projection; each position requires ease of access for technicians to change and adjust, with lighting bridges at ceiling level and ladder access to wall locations; follow spotlights require a location at the rear of the auditorium or from a lighting bridge at ceiling level with space for an operator. Performance lighting is an integral part of the staging of all types of production, except classical and choral music, and is subject to changes within a performance controlled by operatives at the rear of the auditorium (see Control Rooms, under Performance Organisation page x). The tradition for classical and choral music is for the platform to be illuminated during the performance with a general and fixed level of lighting: however this may be changing with, say, follow spotlights as an increasingly common feature.
- *Auditorium lighting*: For illumination of circulation routes and seating areas for the audience to move

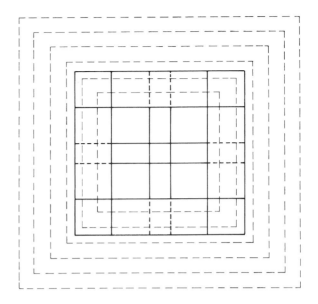

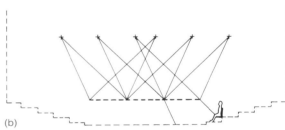

(b)

Fig. 12.35 *Performance lighting. The illumination of performers and their setting during a performance. (a) Theoretical position of fixed performance spot lights: method of locating theoretical positions of spotlights. Spotlights at A will light an actor at the edge of the stage at 55° in section, about 45° to 50° after crossing, but as the actor moves in from the edge the angle will decrease. At Q it is only 40° in section, about 35° after crossing and this is the minimum. It is therefore necessary to provide another lighting position B, which will cover the area Q to R within the same range of angles; and then positions C and D, lighting areas R to S and S to T. For proscenium and end stage formats, additional lighting positions may be required on the auditorium side walls and behind the proscenium opening. With extensive scenery on a stage then more positions than those shown in the diagram will be necessary. (b) On thrust and theatre-in-the-round stages, virtually all the performance lighting must come from overhead locations to avoid glare in the eyes of the audience. Other lighting positions are therefore limited, in particular flat angles. With a thrust stage, the use of performers' vomitories can be locations for low level lighting positions (see Fig. 12.24a). The plan and section show mounting positions for lighting equipment over a theatre-in-the-round stage: the approach is also applicable to thrust stages.*

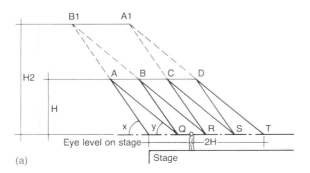

(a)

around the auditorium, read programmes, and so on; decorative lighting emphasizing architectural features within the auditorium. Auditorium lighting is usually dimmed and out during the actual performance for all types of production except for classical and choral music, where the tradition is to dim the lights only.

- *Emergency lighting*: An illumination of the circulation routes within the auditorium during a performance, with the luminaires located at ceiling level or/and at a low level incorporated into the design of the gangways; exit signs and emergency directions at points of egress in the auditorium; lighting of the auditorium at times of emergency.
- *Working lights*: general illumination of the auditorium for cleaning and maintenance as a separate system during times when the auditorium is not used for performance and rehearsals.
- *Director's desk lighting*: supply of power within the auditorium to serve temporary location of director's desk during rehearsals. This is not usually applicable for classical music.
- *Cue lights*: at entry points into the auditorium.
- *Blue lights*: areas within the auditorium which will be accessed during the performance by technicians and performers require lighting but at a low level with a blue light to avoid distraction to the audience. This covers lighting bridges and entry points into the auditorium.

Ease of access is required to service all luminaires.

Sound equipment

The sound equipment described in the following sections may be required to be incorporated into the auditorium design. Control rooms for performance sound, broadcasting and recording are discussed under Performance Organization, pp. 183–84.

Sound reinforcement

Location of loudspeakers for the amplification of music, voices or special effects, especially for those performances relying on amplification such as musicals and pop/rock concerts. The aim is to locate the main loudspeaker to distribute sound across the whole of the audience and can be:

- over the platform/stage along the setting line or above the proscenium opening;
- at the sides of the platform/stage as the traditional position for pop/rock/jazz concerts (often touring groups providing their own equipment);
- various positions within the auditorium to supplement main loudspeakers and for sound effects on side and rear walls, ceiling to auditorium and balconies and, possibly, under the floor. Location requires an uninterrupted line from speakers to members of the audience.

Public address

Loudspeakers may be required within the auditorium for announcements to the audience as a separate system.

Rehearsals

Loudspeakers may be required, usually located at the rear of the auditorium, for use during rehearsals on the stage, so that the director located in the auditorium can communicate with the performers on the stage. This requirement tends not to be applicable for classical and choral music rehearsals, or for small auditoria.

Broadcasting and recording

Consideration should be made of provision within the auditorium for television and radio transmission and for video, film and tape recording of a performance. Spatial requirements, beyond camera and operator locations, are nominal and mainly include access for cables and equipment.

Deaf aid

To assist the hard of hearing, consider the applications of one of the following:

- *induction loop:* magnetic field transmission looped around auditorium;
- *infra-red system:* modulated light signals, radiated from a number of sources;
- *hard-wired:* cable within floor trunking connected to panel in seat.

Fire protection

The enclosing walls and floors of the auditorium should be fire-resistant as should the doors and other openings in the walls. Other aspects to be considered, include:

- non-combustibility of materials including finishes and seating;
- *detector system:* smoke detectors in auditorium and associated voids;
- *extinguishers:* hose-reels, portable extinguishers; automatic sprinkler systems will not be allowed over seating areas;
- *alarms:* connected to automatic detector system and central indicator panel, and possibly, direct link to local fire station; alarms should be visual (flashing light) in auditorium and not audible.

Fire precautions should be discussed with the local fire authority and fire insurers.

Structure

A large span structure will be required, capable of carrying shaped ceiling, lighting bridges and ventilation ducts. Floors will be sloped, raked, dished or, if a multi-purpose auditorium, flat. Balconies introduce additional long spans able to carry heavy loads. For sound insulation purposes the auditorium walls will have to be substantial, which suggests load-bearing construction.

Ceiling zone

The ceiling and ceiling zone are mainly determined by functional needs and include the following requirements:

- *Acoustic requirements*: Profiled reflector panels and possible adjustable diffusers to ensure distribution of sound over the whole seating area. For non-amplified music the reflectors will need to be suspended over the platform as well.
- *Lighting requirements*: Lighting bridges for access and supporting framework for performance lighting, 'house' lighting and also working lights and emergency lights.
- *Ventilation requirements*: Air ducts and plenums, diffusers, noise attenuation and monitoring equipment, supporting hangers and means of access for servicing.
- *Production requirements*: If for opera, dance, musicals and drama, a grid and pulley suspension system for flying or suspending scenery over fore-stage, including access by technicians.
- *Fire control requirements*: Alarm system in voids; fire dampers in ducts.

Seating capacity

The *maximum* capacity within an auditorium depends on the selection of format and the aural and visual limitations set by the type of production. Other influences on the calculation include, as described, levels, sightlines, acoustics, circulation and seating density, as well as the size and shape of the platform/stage (to be described in the following section). To maximize the seating capacity within these limitations, sightlines may be compromised so that, say, 10 per cent of the audience experiences 90 per cent of the performance area. This is a debatable issue mainly associated with the proscenium format, where, to achieve an intimate character in the auditorium, a desire to provide perfect sightlines for everyone may have to be overridden.

The *actual* seating capacity depends on the ability to attract audiences which may be less than the possible maximum. Also the potential peak demand could exceed the selected capacity on a particular evening: the aim though should be to spread attendance across less popular days, or extend performances over a longer period of time rather than increase the capacity over a short duration.

Seating capacity is an important aspect of the financial appraisal, with income derived from ticket sales based on the anticipated attendance numbers. Level of attendance will not match the seating capacity for every performance and an average across a year, within a season or at an event will need to be taken. Financing suggests that the seating capacity should be as large as possible, consistent with the size of the

potential audience: however artistic policy may try to set the seating capacity as low as possible to avoid diminishing the experience of a performance with high numbers.

Broadly the range of seating capacities for different categories of building for the performing arts are as indicated in Table 12.2.

Table 12.2 Seating capacities by category of building

Metropolitan centre

Opera house	1600–2000
Dance theatre	1200–1500
Concert hall	1500–2000
Recital room	600–800
Experimental music workshop	varies
Commercial theatre	
Drama	750–900, with proscenium format
	500–1200 open stage formats
Musicals	1500–3000
Arena	2000 +
Drama theatre	750–900, with prosccenium format
	500–1200, with open stage formats
Small- and medium-scale drama	150–350, 350–500
Educational institution	150–350

Regional centre	
Concert hall	1200–1700
Touring theatre	900–1400
Drama theatre	750–900, with proscenium format
	500–1200, with open stage formats
Arena	2000 +
Small- and medium-scale drama	150–350, 350–500
Educational institution	150–350

Town centre	
Community theatre	150–350
Arts workshop	150–350
Amateur theatre	150–350

District centre	
Community school	150–350

Neighbourhood centre	
Multi-purpose hall	150–350

Auditorium character

The quality of an individual's response to a live performance depends partly on the corporate experience, with a reciprocal response between audience and performers. From the performers' viewpoint the audience should not be split into sections, while the audience should sense an atmosphere of expectation and excitement before a performance begins with the character not obtruding after it commences. The auditorium sets the mood and tone for the performance and may be expansive or intimate, formal or informal, angular or curved, may emphasize the blocks of seats or the wholeness of the interior, may reduce or increase scale, a sense of permanence or spontaneity, and so on. Examples are shown in Fig. 12.36.

It may be an architectural set piece reflecting a wider approach to the building design, with a distinct physical character using balconies, galleries, seating, enclosing elements and house lighting and colours. The ornate Baroque auditorium with its domed ceiling developed the set piece in the most distinctive manner. This approach contrasts directly with the neutral space which can be designed for each production so that the setting for the performance can be extended into the auditorium. Other approaches include putting the emphasis on the audience and seating and the staging of the performance only where the physical elements (walls, ceiling, handrails, balconies and so on) are reduced visually. The 'black box' is the ultimate expression where the performance and audience only are illuminated. Lighting, materials and colour can offer either conspicuous glitter and a sense of affluence, or spartan, conspicuous thrift.

Much depends on the selection of format, traditions of the type of production and context: the proscenium format for opera is more sympathetic to the set piece, with a colourful and sparkling interior, while the open-

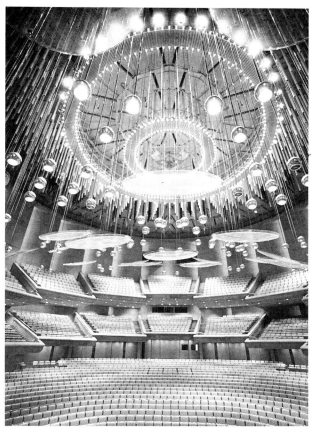

(b)

Fig. 12.36 *Interior views of auditoria showing examples of approaches to the design and character. (a) Birmingham Symphony Hall 1991 (Seating capacity: 2200) Rectangular box with shallow balconies on three sides, with curved rear wall (Architects: Percy Thomas Partnership). (b) Roy Thomson Hall, Toronto, 1982 (Seating capacity: 2812) Elliptical form, with two balconies. The central ceiling feature includes lighting, sound systems, ventilation and acoustic banners (Architects: Arthur Erickson/Mathers and Haldenby Associated Architects).*

(a)

stage formats for drama are more susceptible to the emphasis on the audience and performance.

For concerts and chamber music the interiors can take light colours. The lighting may have its intensity lowered during a performance but the auditorium as an overall setting retains its architectural character.

Platform/stage design

The size and shape of the platform or stage are determined by the type of production, the relationship between the audience and the performance and the scale of the selected production.

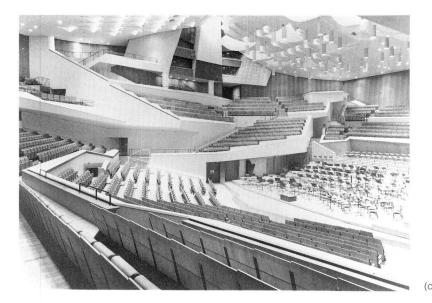

(c)

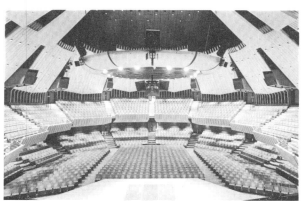

(d)

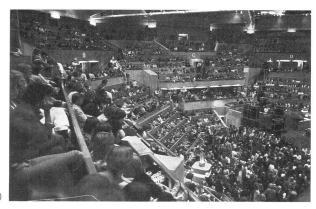

(e)

(f)

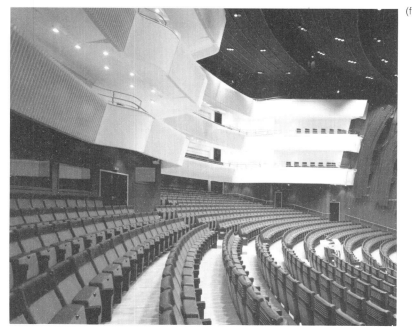

Fig. 12.36 continued *Interior views of auditoria showing examples of approaches to the design and character. (c) Berlin Philharmonic 1963 (Seating capacity: 2200) An auditorium with a small raked tier broken up into distinct blocks of seating – the vineyard approach – each offering a grouping of seats (about 300 in each section) at ever increasing pitches of rake as the distance from the platform increases (Architects: Hans Scharoun). (d) Christchurch Town Hall, 1972 (Seating capacity: 2338 plus 324 in choir stalls) Single balcony surrounding platform and lowest level, within an elliptical form: suspended acoustic reflectors form tent-like ceiling (Architects: Warren and Mahoney). (e) Music Centre, Vredenburg, Utrecht, 1979 (Seating capacity: 1700–1900) Square plan, for orchestral and choral concerts and other activities (Architects: Herman Hertzberger). (f) Opera House, Essen 1988 (Seating capacity: 1600) Eccentric fan proscenium format, with shallow rear balconies, each cantilevered over those below (Architects: Alvar Aalto).*

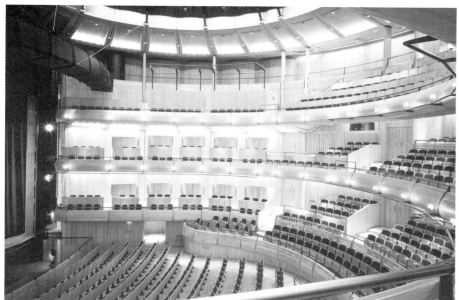

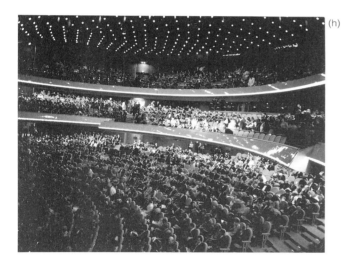

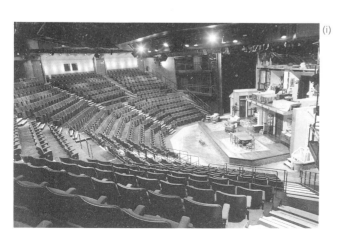

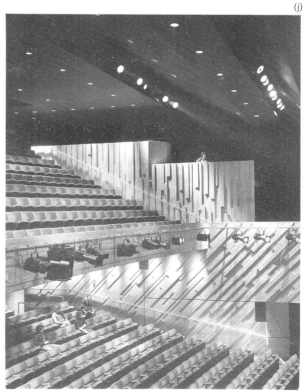

Fig. 12.36 continued *Interior views of auditoria showing examples of approaches to the design and character. (g) Glyndbourne Opera House 1994 (Seating capacity: 1200) Horse-shoe form, with side balconies extended to proscenium opening (Architects: Michael Hopkins and Partners). (h) Opera House, Amsterdam, 1986 (Seating capacity: 1614–1689) Wide fan, with 2 balconies. Architects: Wilhelm Holzbauer and Cees Dam (Courtesy of Kors van Bennekom). (i) Quarry Theatre, West Yorkshire Playhouse, Leeds, 1990 (Seating capacity: 750) Drama the predominant production type, with a 90° fan auditorium on a single raked level (Architects: The Appleton Partnership). (j) Lyttleton Theatre, Royal National Theatre, London, 1976 (Seating capacity: 895) Proscenium theatre, within a rectangular box with a single balcony. The division between the proscenium opening and auditorium is effectively eroded as is the line between the enclosing auditorium walls and ceiling (Architects: Denys Lasdun & Partners).*

(g)

(h)

(j)

(i)

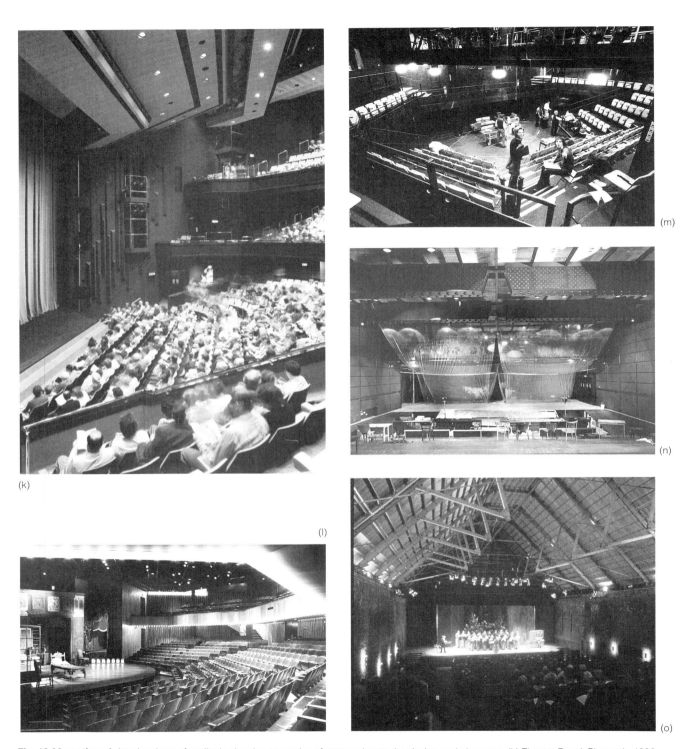

(k)

(l)

(m)

(n)

(o)

Fig. 12.36 continued *Interior views of auditoria showing examples of approaches to the design and character. (k) Theatre Royal, Plymouth, 1982 (Seating capacity: 1296, able to be reduced to 764) Combined music and drama proscenium theatre with two balconies, the lower balcony drops on one side. The division between the proscenium opening and auditorium eroded with an emphasis on long lines of seating rows, straight with a gentle curve at the change of direction, with their colour set within a black finish to walls (Architects: The Peter Moro Partnership). (l) Center Stage, Baltimore, 1978 (Seating capacity: 500) Medium-sized theatre with 90° fan and a shallow balcony (Architects: James R. Grieves Associates). (m) Studio Theatre, Theatre Royal, Bristol, 1973 (Seating capacity: 212) Small flexible theatre, as a black box, with removable rostra able to be laid out in different configurations and loose seating (Architects: The Peter Moro Partnership). (n) Theatre, Staatgallerie, Stuttgart, 1983 (Seating capacity: 350 maximum) Rectangular box with flat floor and flexible seating: gantry at ceiling level includes control rooms and performance lighting positions (Architects: James Stirling, Michael Wilford and Associates). (o) Maltings Concert Hall, Snape 1967 (Seating capacity: 824) Conversion of an existing building: narrow shape, large volume, admired acoustic, exposed roof trusses (Architects: Arup Associates).*

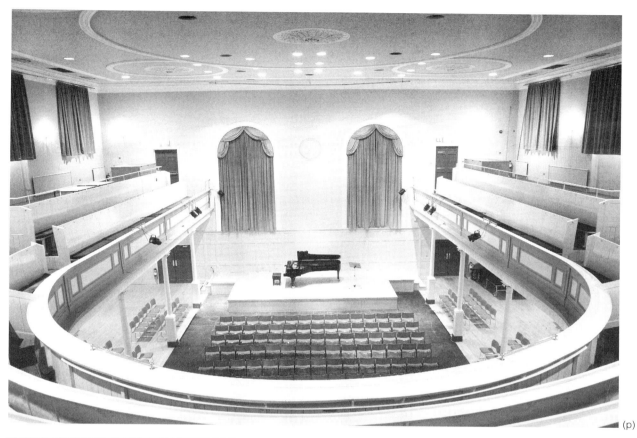

(p)

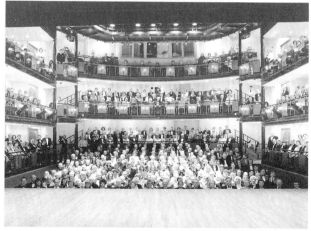

(q)

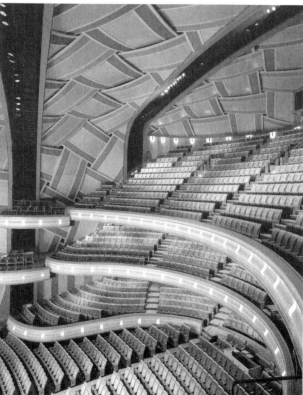

(r)

Fig. 12.36 continued *Interior views of auditoria showing examples of approaches to the design and character. (p) Queens Hall, Edinburgh 1980 (Seating capacity: 800) Conversion of an existing church building into a recital hall: relatively modest adaptation to create an auditorium for music (Architects: Hurd Rolland). (q) Lawrence Bately Theatre, Huddersfield, 1994 (Seating capacity: 450) Conversion of an existing chapel building into a flexible theatre: careful adaptation of chapel interior to theatre auditorium. The flat floor is on sectional lifts which can form a raked floor for seating (Architects: Kirklees Metropolitan Council: Design Practice). (r) Silva Hall, Hult Centre for the Performing Arts, Eugene, Oregon, 1982 (Seating capacity: 2537) Proscenium form with two balconies: the balcony geometry contrasts with the lower level seating. The sweeping lines of the balcony fronts and seating are the main visual characteristics of the interior (Architects: Hardy Holyman Pfeiffer Associates)*

Platform: orchestral and choral music

The music components include orchestra platform, choir stalls and organ (Fig. 12.37). The design of the platform relates to the size of the orchestra type: symphony orchestra and choir; symphony orchestra, 80–120 musicians; chamber orchestra, 40–50 musicians; small ensemble.

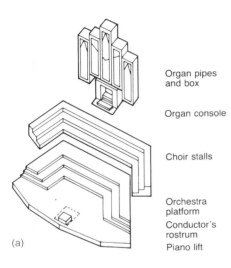

Organ pipes and box

Organ console

Choir stalls

Orchestra platform
Conductor's rostrum
Piano lift

(a)

(b)

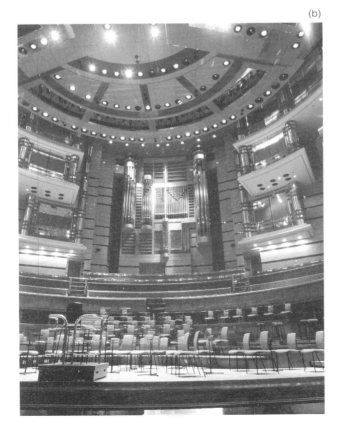

(c)

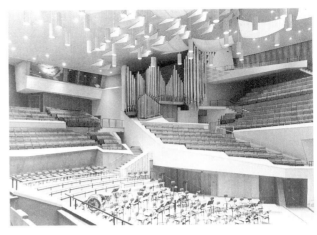

Fig. 12.37 (a) Platform design: music components. For classical orchestral and choral music, the platform components include the orchestra platform on various levels, the conductor's rostrum, the piano lift, the choir stalls, organ console and organ pipes and box. (b) Birmingham Symphony Hall. The formal setting in the Birmingham Symphony Hall shows the orchestra platform focused towards the conductor's rostrum, the choir stalls and organ. (c) Berlin Philharmonic. The orchestra platform is centrally located, focused towards the conductor's rostrum. The organ is to one side, which avoids underlining the formality of a concert hall and allows the audience to more easily encompass the platform

For chamber orchestras the platform can be 6 m deep, 9 m wide and 900 mm high. A full orchestra requires an area of 12 m × 12 m with a platform height of 1000 mm: such an area would also accommodate a choir of 220 with 60 players. Layouts vary and examples are shown in Fig. 12.38.

Areas for individual musicians are:

- violin players and small wind instruments 1000 mm × 600 mm: the horns and bassoons, larger areas at 1000 mm × 800 mm; 1200 mm tiers for string and wind players including cellos and double bases;
- tiers of up to 2 m for percussion;
- concert grand piano: 2750 mm × 1600 mm;
- choir: 0.38 m^2 minimum per singer in choir stalls with seats (as auditorium seating, if used by audience when choir is not present).

The longitudinal section can be flat and stepped traversely, rising from the conductor's rostrum. Risers should not exceed 450 mm because of the difficulty of carrying heavy instruments.

The platform should be kept as small as possible. Size and shape affect tone, balance and homogeneity due to the variation in the delay with the location of different musicians on the platform. The shape of the platform should not vary from the square, with the choir embracing the orchestra at the rear.

The height of the platform determines the focus for the sightlines. Recommended heights have been given. It should not, however, be less than 600, nor higher than 1.1 m to avoid a complete screening of the

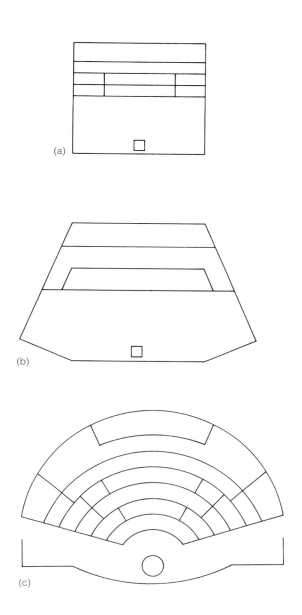

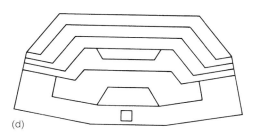

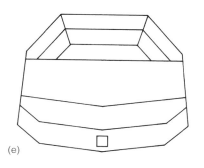

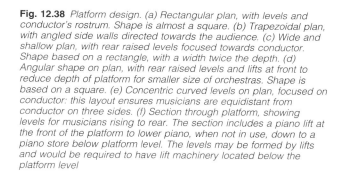

Fig. 12.38 *Platform design. (a) Rectangular plan, with levels and conductor's rostrum. Shape is almost a square. (b) Trapezoidal plan, with angled side walls directed towards the audience. (c) Wide and shallow plan, with rear raised levels focused towards conductor. Shape based on a rectangle, with a width twice the depth. (d) Angular shape on plan, with rear raised levels and lifts at front to reduce depth of platform for smaller size of orchestras. Shape is based on a square. (e) Concentric curved levels on plan, focused on conductor: this layout ensures musicians are equidistant from conductor on three sides. (f) Section through platform, showing levels for musicians rising to rear. The section includes a piano lift at the front of the platform to lower piano, when not in use, down to a piano store below platform level. The levels may be formed by lifts and would be required to have lift machinery located below the platform level*

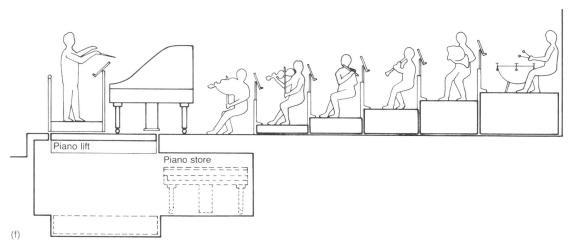

platform by those in the front rows of the audience. The tiers may be permanent, formed from rostra or formed by lifts: use of rostra and lifts allows a flexibility in the layout of the orchestra. Apron flexibility may necessitate exchanging the front platform area for seating if the size of the platform needs to reflect the size of the orchestra. A sub-platform store for seating units and platform rostra served by apron lifts has been incorporated into the Royal Glasgow Concert Hall.

Construction of the floor should be hardwood on timber joists which will respond to cellos and double bases: the floor structure has to support the point load to the piano legs, when static and when being moved. The platform must be fully serviced with floor sockets for electrical light and power, microphones and communications. Such outlets can be within the platform floor finish and/or grouped in panels in the adjacent platform walls.

Access to the platform from the assembly area is required for the musicians, soloists and conductor. Entry to the platform should be on the same level and any change of level from the assembly area to the front tier of the platform should be avoided. The choir can have a separate entrance into the choir stalls: the larger numbers imply more than one entrance. Access is also required for musical instruments not carried on by the musicians. This can be through the same entrance for the musicians from the assembly area. The piano can be rolled off to its off-platform store or dropped by lift at the front of the platform to a below platform store. Fire escapes from the platform will be required with entry points to the platform also being used for escape.

The placing of a pipe organ requires a large volume, either as part of the architectural setting behind the platform or to one side, especially if the audience surrounds the platform. A console may be detached from the pipe box.

The setting, walls and ceiling to the platform, is intimately connected with the acoustic design. The primary function is to reflect the sound of the orchestra to the audience and also to the orchestra and choir. The profile is to direct the sound to the whole of the audience in a diffused manner. This is easier to achieve with an end-on form: balcony fronts and immediate walls aid the reflection of the sound. These points are also applicable to both outdoor and indoor temporary facilities.

The ceiling over can be part of the main ceiling line or a suspended reflector: an advantage of a reflector includes the space over being part of the overall volume of the auditorium.

The platform for orchestral and choral music will be within the same volume as the auditorium and the conditions of structure, air conditioning, heating, ventilation, fire protection, acoustics and noise control remain as described under the section on the auditorium: attention though should be also given to heating during rehearsals, to provide comfortable conditions for the musicians, singers, soloists and conductor.

Proscenium format: stage with or without flytower

The term 'stage' refers to the main performance area and also its associated flytower and wing space, basement and orchestra pit. Examples are shown in Fig. 12.39.

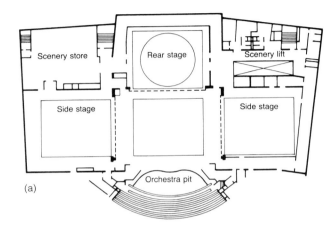

(a)

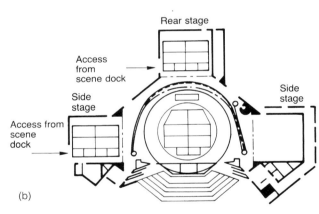

(b)

Fig. 12.39 *Stage layout: proscenium stage with flytower. (a) Stage layout for opera and dance, showing side stages and rear stage and double-purchase flying system over the performance area. The side and rear stages can be closed off, with vertically sliding shutters. Access for performers is at each corner of the performance area with a cross-over corridor behind the rear stage and corridor access to a down-stage position independent of a side stage. Example: Opera House, Essen. (b) Stage layout for drama and dance, with side stages and rear stage, and double-purchase flying system over the performance area. The layout offers a wide structural proscenium opening, able to be reduced in width, a revolve and cyclorama. Example: Civic Theatre, Helsinki.*

Performance area

The size and shape of the performance area – the section of the stage visible to the audience – is determined by the type of production, auditorium layout and sightlines. The dimensional decisions are focused on the proscenium width which are summarized as in Table 12.3.

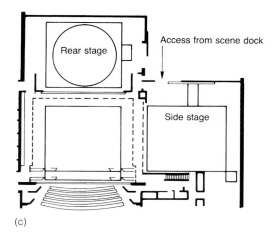

(c)

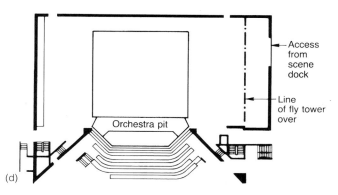

(d)

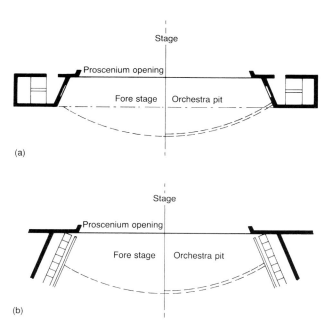

Fig. 12.39 continued *Stage layout: proscenium stage with flytower. (c) Stage layout for drama, with one side stage and rear stage and double-purchase flying system over the performance area. The side and rear stages are able to be closed off, with vertically sliding shutters. Example: Lyttleton Theatre, Royal National Theatre, London. (d) Stage for touring opera, dance, musicals and drama as well as concerts. Rectangular stage with single-purchase flying system and extended side stage on one side. Access for performers on the stage is at each corner with a cross-over corridor beyond the stage enclosure. Example: Theatre Royal, Plymouth*

Fig. 12.40 *Proscenium opening. With the proscenium format, an aspect of the design of the auditorium is the zone around the proscenium opening and the division between auditorium and stage. This division may be emphasized or eroded. The area immediately adjacent to the proscenium opening is claimed for a set of functions which may be in conflict: performance lighting, acoustics, scenery, performers' balconies, decorative features, loudspeakers, public boxes or balconies and structural edge to the proscenium opening as well as the fire separation requirements. The figures show some of the approaches. (a) The proscenium opening emphasized as a 'picture window' with decorative frame, through which the audience views the performance on the stage. The splayed opening emphasizes the perspective. Such a design is associated with the illusionary approach to presentation, traditionally associated with opera productions. When a fore-stage is in use it remains within the depth of the opening: the side walls to the opening can consist of architectural elements such as doors, balconies and windows which may incorporate discretely located lighting positions. (b) The immediate side walls populated with the audience in boxes, or balconies, extending balconies to the rear of the auditorium, thereby placing a social priority on the layout with the audience overlapping the orchestra pit/fore-stage.*

Table 12.3 Recommended dimensions for stage areas

Type of performance	Small scale m	Medium Scale m	Large Scale m
Opera	12	15	20
Musical	10	12	15
Dance	10	12	15
Drama	8	10	10

The depth of the performance area may be calculated as the same as the proscenium. opening.

The height of the stage can be between 600 mm and 1100 mm with a straight, angled or curved front edge. The proscenium opening itself can be emphasized as a picture frame or alternatively the division between stage and auditorium can be eroded visually (Fig. 12.40).

The floor to the performance area, in part or total, may be a series of traps: modular sections which can be removed selectively to provide entrances and exits to and from the stage basement. Each trap is usually 1200 × 1200 mm. The stage may consist of a series of lifts for raising and lowering sections of the stage to provide multi-levels traps and ramps. Lifts may be operated by ropes and winches, screw jacks or hydraulic rams.

The stage floor needs to be timber and to satisfy the local fire-resistant requirements: this may be achieved with hardboard on 25 mm plywood (the hardboard can be easily replaced over time). Dancers require softwood and a resilient floor: the floor finish can be linoleum sheet or foam-based rubber.

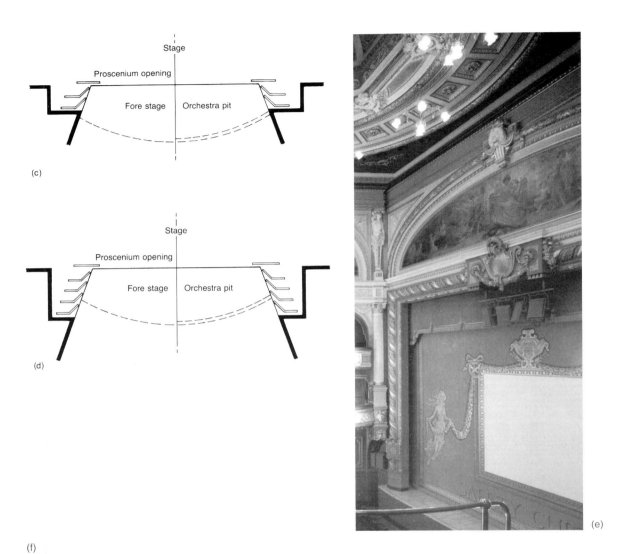

(c)

(d)

(e)

(f)

Fig. 12.40 continued *Proscenium opening. (c) The proscenium opening visually eroded, with stage lighting slots and allowance for performers access onto the fore-stage. (d) The division between auditorium and stage visually eroded further, bringing the staging requirements of lighting and performance further into the seating areas. (e) An example of an emphasized proscenium opening: Alhambra, Bradford. (f) An example of an eroded proscenium opening: Lyttleton Theatre, Royal National Theatre, London*

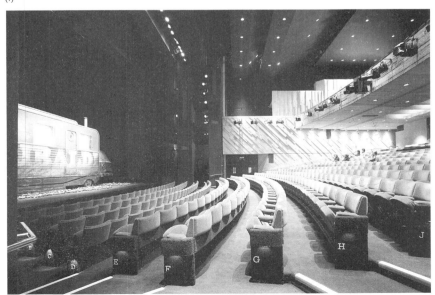

Stage basement

The basement requires a minimum headroom of 2500 mm: if used for the storage of sets on lifts, 7–10 m will be necessary. When the basement is used in connection with a performance it must be provided with a fire-escape independent of the stage.

Side and rear stages

The dimensions on plan relate to the size of the performance area: the side and rear stages need to accommodate a stage set as on the performance area, with circulation all round. The clear height should accommodate the highest scenery plus 1 m.

Walls should be clear to receive leaning scenery, etc. Services can be concentrated over the entrance and exit doors or under galleries, as necessary.

Scenery may be moved to the side or rear of the performance area, by: stacking, manually dismantling and stacking on the side or rear stages; through movable stage sections, large sections of the stage on trucks or wagons moving to either side or to the rear, on casters or air pallets; revolving stages, two or more revolves allows rapid changes of scenery.

Safety curtain

In case of fire on the stage it is necessary to separate the stage areas from the auditorium, with the proscenium opening being closed by a safety curtain. The normal form of safety curtain is a rigid type which is suspended immediately behind the proscenium opening, running between side tracks and dropping onto the stage front from the flytower (Fig. 12.41).

The safety curtain can be on the straight line of the stage separating the orchestra pit, as part of the auditorium from the stage, or on the line of the rail to the orchestra pit so that when the pit is exchanged for an apron stage it is accommodated within the stage area. If there is a curved or angled pit rail then the safety curtain should follow the same line.

Access to the stage: performers

The door leading from the dressing rooms for the performers should be located down stage of the prompt side (PS) as the primary point of entry to the stage, with a cross-over behind the stage, and at least a second point of entry on the non-PS side. All entrances to the stage require lobbies as sound and light locks. The entrances should be located so as to leave a maximum amount of clear wall space. Access is also required to the sub-stage by performers from both sides of the performance area and possibly also from the auditorium, which may require steps at the side of the front of the stage.

With opera, there are a large number of performers including principals, chorus and dancers: separate access points should be considered for each group.

At least one fire escape will be required from the stage areas directly to the outside.

Access to the stage: scenery

Access for the delivery of scenery through the scene dock onto the performance area is necessary.

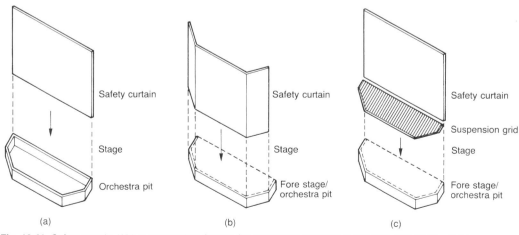

Fig. 12.41 *Safety curtain. With a proscenium format, fire separation between auditorium and stage will be necessary. There are three situations: (a) A simple flat safety curtain capable of being dropped to separate auditorium from stage in the case of an emergency. The orchestra pit remains on the auditorium side of the safety curtain. (b) An auditorium, with an orchestra pit for opera, dance and musicals, which can become a fore-stage for drama and its attendant scenery. The flytower needs to cover the fore-stage and the safety curtain needs to be located on the auditorium edge of the orchestra pit to descend onto the pit rail, or the fore-stage leading edge when in position. (c) The line of the safety curtain lies behind a fore-stage which has a grid over for the suspension of scenery and stage lighting. There would be a distinction between scenery used in front of the safety curtain, on and over the fore-stage, which would require to be fully incombustible*

Flytower

The flytower allows scenery, and also stage lighting and sound, to be suspended over the performance area, off bars capable of being raised so that they are out of sight of the audience. Scenery can be lowered into positions as part of the stage set. This system has the advantage that scenery can be moved quickly and does not take up floor space when stored in the flytower. In particular, it allows backcloths to be suspended and dropped into place during a performance. The flytower can also accommodate the false proscenium, which can be adjusted to change the height of the proscenium opening, curtain tracks, pelmets, marking and borders as well as lighting bars and projection screens.

Scenery is hung and balanced against a set of weights suspended on wire ropes which pass over pulley blocks above the grid at the head of the flytower and the side walls. Scenery is fixed to a suspension barrel which has to travel from the stage floor to the underside of the grid. There are two types of manual operation (Fig. 12.42):

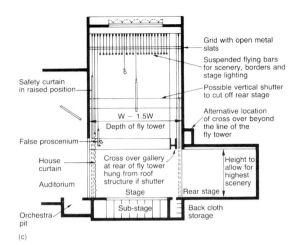

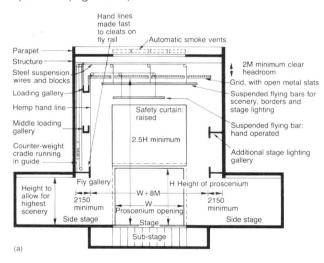

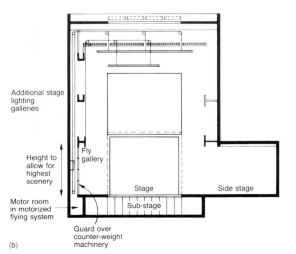

Fig. 12.42 *Flytower. The diagrams indicate the main dimensional requirements and components of a flytower to a proscenium stage. Access is required to the galleries and the grid, and to the roof, by catladder or staircase. A small lift from the stage to the various operational levels is desirable. An emergency exit must be provided from the grid and other levels by a protected staircase and there must be a means of escape to the outside of the building. (a) Section through flytower and stage, showing layout with a double-purchase flying system and side stages. (b) Section through flytower and stage, showing layout with a single-purchase flying system. Such a system restricts the size of the side stage on the operational side and allows operation only one full side stage. Single-purchase systems can be operated from the stage floor but this uses valuable space. The operator has a better view from the raised gallery. (c) Cross section through flytower and stage, including rear stage*

- *Single purchase counter weights*: The travel distance is equal to the height of the grid above the stage. A continuous vertical wall running higher than the grid is required for the guides. The operation can be from the stage level.
  Single purchase is a more accurate system as there is less friction to overcome. The operation at stage level benefits the operator, especially in small theatres, who may have other duties during a performance.
- *Double purchase counter weights*: The distance travelled by the counter weights is halved in relation to the distance of the suspension. This allows the operation to occur from a gallery above stage level: an extra loading gallery is necessary between the flying gallery and grid.
  Double purchase requires less width of flytower and releases the stage area.

Electric and hydraulic systems are available where the ropes are mechanically wound onto a drum.

The grid is a framework of steel fixed above the stage floor and used to support the sets of lines used in the flying of scenery. Blocks and tackle are suspended from the grid.

The minimum width of the grid should be the proscenium width plus an overlap on each side of 2 m, with a further 2 m beyond on each side for counter weights and fly gallery. This makes the width at least

W (proscenium width) + 8 m. However if the single purchase system is adopted then the width is determined by the requirements of a clear floor area to the stage plus 750 mm for counter weights and guard rail.

The depth requires to be as the performance area plus 3 m or $1\frac{1}{2}$ times the width of the proscenium opening as the internal dimension from front to back. The height of the grid, as a minimum, above the stage is $2\frac{1}{2}$ times the height of the structural proscenium opening: backcloths, curtains and safety curtain will be higher than the effective proscenium opening. A further 2.5 m above the grid, below the roof, will be required.

The lines, running parallel with the proscenium opening, require a minimum spacing of 150 mm and often 200 mm. The number of lines will depend on the size of the performance area to be covered.

An automatic smoke vent is required at the top of the flytower. If a fire occurs within the volume of the stage and flytower the smoke is drawn upwards through the flytower, which acts as a smoke stack. The vent opens automatically when activated by the increase in temperature, by the release of a fusible link or operated manually from the prompt corner (and possibly the firemen's entry to the building). Regulations require the cross-sectional area of the vent to be a particular proportion of the stage – usually 10 per cent. There are three categories of vent: sloping glazed panel, horizontal metal vents and powered exhaust system.

Access is required to all levels, on both sides of the flytower, by staircase and/or cat ladder. For the higher grids a small lift from stage level to grid is desirable. A cross gallery at the rear of the flytower, either within or beyond the flytower, is essential. Escape is required from each level of gallery and the grid. The escape route may be into adjacent accommodation or, especially from the grid, via an enclosed staircase, which may also be the main access staircase.

Frame construction is preferred for the flytower as load bearing masonry places a weight on the lower structure which may be too large. Infill panels need to take into consideration thermal and sound insulation. The proscenium opening involves a large spanbeam with heavy supports either side of the opening, as does the opening at the back of the flytower if a rear stage. The rear and side stages need to be enclosed with fire protected walls and ceiling when they are adjacent to other accommodation.

Suspension

In addition to the flytower, the forestage and rear stage, being beyond the area covered by the flytower, can receive a winching system to suspend scenery. Suspension is supported by a structural grid at ceiling level which extends over these areas.

Orchestra pit: opera, musicals, dance

The orchestra for opera, musicals and dance is in a pit between the stage and the audience. The limiting factor is for the conductor to be seen by both the singers and dancers on the stage and the musicians. The audience requires to hear a balance of singers and orchestra, especially for opera. Amplification in musicals makes this requirement less of a necessity.

Allow 1.3 m^2 average per player, 5 m^2 for the piano, 10 m^2 for tympani and percussion and 4 m^2 for the conductor. The actual production will have specific orchestral requirements with variation in the size and composition of the orchestra. The conductor's eye level must not be lower than stage level when seated on a high stool.

To minimize the gulf between stage and audience the pit can extend under the stage front for a distance no greater than 2 m. The soffit of the overhang should reflect the sound outward into the auditorium.

For opera, the pit should be designed for a maximum of 100 musicians: for musicals, 60; for dance, 60–90. The numbers could be less with touring companies. The floor level of the orchestra pit should be adjustable, between 2–3 m, below the stage level to suit the different requirements of the musicians and directors. See Fig. 12.43 for an example of a flexible orchestra pit.

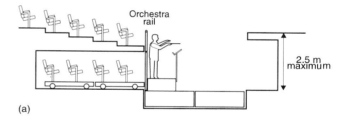

(a)

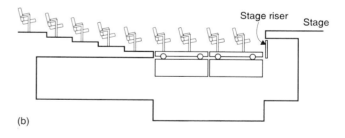

(b)

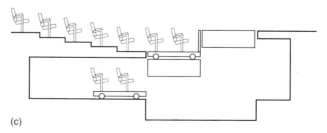

(c)

Fig. 12.43 *Orchestra pit lift detail. (a) Orchestra pit, with seat wagons in possible store under fixed seating and orchestra pit lifts in lowest position. (b) Rows of seating, with orchestra pit lifts partially raised and stage riser in position. (c) Half fore-stage, with one half of orchestra pit lifts raised.*

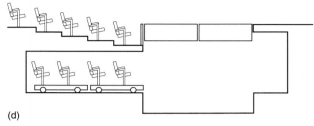

(d)

Fig. 12.43 continued *Orchestra pit lift detail. (d) Full fore-stage, with both sets of orchestra pit lifts raised*

The fire separation between auditorium and stage must be maintained including the entry point into the pit: access must be possible from both ends.

The *orchestra pit* requires its own independent ventilation system, locally controlled. Lifts may be required to reduce the size of the pit, and its acoustics. The orchestra pit requires acoustic treatment and working lights, as well as the socket outlets for lighting to music stands.

Orchestra: drama

Live musicians may be required in drama productions. The location can follow the orchestra pit as previously described above, or the musicians can be placed in alternative positions. As they are likely to be few in number, musicians can be located in a box or gallery at the side of the stage, or at the side or rear of the main stage level. A permanent structure may not be appropriate with the position created, as necessary, for a particular production.

Proscenium format without flytower

For the smaller auditorium (Fig. 12.44) where a rigid safety curtain is not an essential provision (as covered by legislation) due to the low seating capacity, and a flytower is not regarded as appropriate, it is still necessary to suspend scenery, curtains, pelmets,

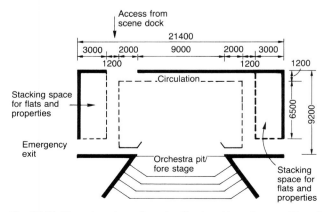

Fig. 12.44 *Stage layout: medium-size theatre without flytower. Plan of stage showing dimensional requirements and layout*

borders and lighting barrels above the stage. Lines can be fitted to pulleys hung on a grid with the flying from a side gallery above the stage or from the stage level.

Side stages are required for stacking spaces for flats, properties and rostra, and circulation routes within the stage area.

Open stage formats

Requirements as to the size and shape of the stage vary according to format. The four main formats are described in the following sections.

End stage

For dance, the minimum performance area is 10 m × 10 m, for drama 10 m × 8 m. Modest side stages, with masking, are necessary for dance and drama productions, for the storage of scenery, as well as performers' entrances. Entrance to the stage should be onto the side stages, with a crossover on stage behind backcloth, curtain or cyclorama, and/or behind the rear wall of the stage. Doors should be located in the corners of the stage. An orchestra pit can be formed between stage and audience, with access by the musicians from below stage level.

90° fan

The dimensions vary and are based on a circle or faceted circle, with diameters ranging from 8 m to 11 m. Modest side stages are a minimum requirement for the storage of scenery and performers' entrance, with a crossover on stage behind backcloth or curtain and/or behind rear wall to the stage. Entry can also be through the seating areas via the gangways and performers' vomitories: access would be necessary from the stage to the rear of the auditorium and vomitories (Fig. 12.45).

Thrust stage

The performance area is a peninsular projecting from a rear setting: an example, with dimensions, is shown in Fig. 12.46. The centre point is the centre of the seating geometry. The example shows a gangway between the performance area and the front row of seats, which may be regarded as part of the performance area. A raised stage is usually stepped along its leading edge to allow ease of movement through the audience onto the stage. The rear wall can be a permanent architectural setting or flexible structure, with access points at stage and upper levels for performers. A change of level will require at least one staircase within the rear wall. Access is necessary at stage level for the movement of scenery and props to and from the performance area, with a rear stage behind the rear wall for the storage of scenery for use during a performance and for performers to assemble (the rear stage should be at least the size of the performance area). Performers will need to enter through the rear

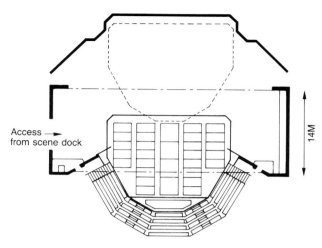

Fig. 12.45 *Stage layout: 90° fan. Plan of the stage at the West Yorkshire Playhouse in Leeds, where the auditorium encircles the stage by 90°. A wagon stage covering the performance area can be retracted to the rear stage: the wagon is at stage level, capable of being raised before being retracted with a compensating lift, which becomes a rear stage floor. Single-purchase flying system*

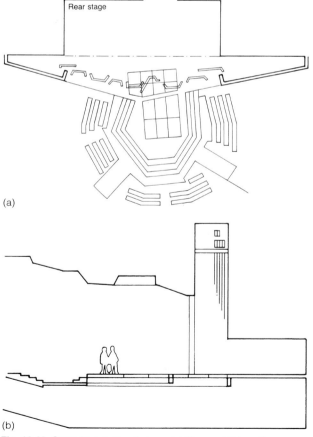

Fig. 12.46 *Stage layout: thrust stage. (a) Plan and (b) section through the thrust stage at Tyrone Guthrie Theatre, Minneapolis. The stage is raised with steps at the stage edge which allows performers access from various parts of the auditorium during a performance. The stage has traps, a rear stage and a flying system to allow backcloths behind the performance*

wall and also through the seating areas, via the gangways and performers' vomitories: access is required to the rear of the auditorium and vomitories from the rear stage.

Theatre-in-the round

Performance areas can be circular, square and polygonal: rectangular and eclipse, which provide a degree of direction to the staging (Fig. 12.47). Due to the movement of scenery and performers onto the stage during a performance, a raised stage tends to be inconvenient. An area behind the seating but out of view of the audience is required for the storage of scenery during a performance. Entry can be separate from the public entry points or combined: to minimize the intrusion into the seating areas surrounding the performance area, combined access is preferable. The entry points should not be directly opposite each other.

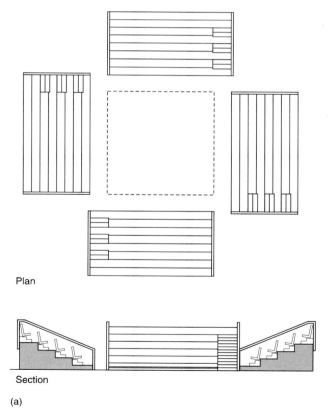

Fig. 12.47 *Theatre-in-the-round. The formats for theatre-in-the-round vary and depend on number of rows, size and shape of the stage, if the performers and audience can enter at the same or different points and if built off a flat floor or permanent structure. The diagrams illustrate different approaches. (a) Four simple units with single access to seating rows, built off a flat roof surrounding and defining performance area. Audience and performers can enter at the same points.*

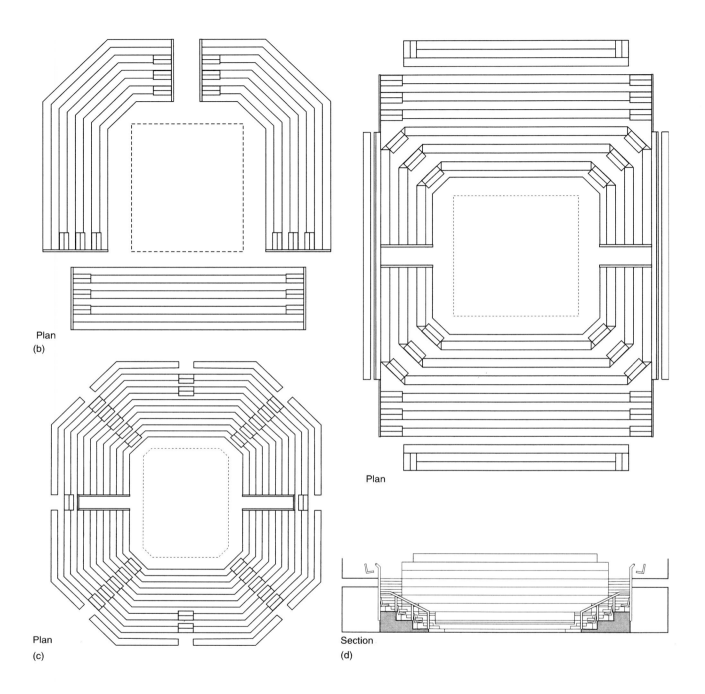

Plan
(b)

Plan
(c)

Plan

Section
(d)

Fig. 12.47 continued *Theatre-in-the-round. The formats for theatre-in-the-round vary and depend on number of rows, size and shape of the stage, if the performers and audience can enter at the same or different points and if built off a flat floor or permanent structure. The diagrams illustrate different approaches. (b) Three units defining a rectangular performance area, built off a flat floor, with access at each end of seating rows. Audience and performers can enter at the same points. (c) Rectangular performance area with separate entry point for performers – through vomitories at stage level – and audience – with gangway access from the rear of the seating. (d) Eccentric layout with a larger number of rows on two opposite sides, with balcony seating on the other two sides. Separate entry points for performers, at stage level, from audience.*

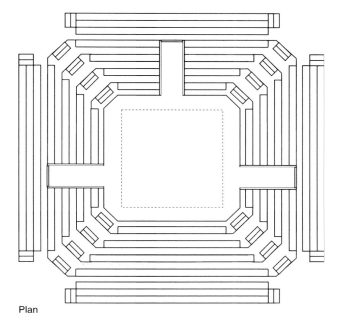

Plan

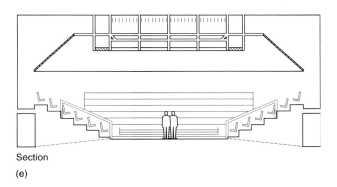

Section

(e)

Fig. 12.47 continued *Theatre-in-the-round. (e) Symmetrical layout with three performers' vomitories and audience entry from the upper level. The section shows performance lighting positions over the stage and a suspension grid which can be operated off a lighting bridge. Sound reflectors are also shown as a possible requirement to ensure all sections of the auditorium are able to hear the performers in the centre of the space, and achieve an appropriate volume*

The height of the performance area in open stage formats, if raised, tends to be low, ranging from 300 mm to 750 mm, with 600 mm an accepted dimension: the minimum clear height over the stage including suspension and stage lighting is 6.5 m. The whole or a part of the performance area can receive traps, as previously described, with a 'grave' trap (1200 × 2400 mm) as a minimum. The performance area will require a basement, if trapped, with access down for the performers and a minimum ceiling height of 2400 mm.

Scenery can be suspended from a grid over the stage as previously described, operated from a fly gallery at 6.5 m above the stage as a minimum height. The grid may be higher thereby increasing the height of scenery that can be suspended: this may be beneficial with the end stage and 90° fan formats. Also for these two formats, increased side stages and a rear stage may offer improved movement of scenery on and off the performance area, as shown under the proscenium format.

Stage: pop/rock music

There are four common situations for staging a pop/ rock concert:

- conditions comparable to the platform of the concert hall;
- the proscenium format, with a flytower but without orchestra pit;
- the arena format, with distinct conditions for pop/ rock concerts;
- the stadium concert: the temporary staging with distinct conditions for rock/pop concerts.

Distinct requirements include an average stage size of 12 m × 12 m, with a height of up to 2 m for reasons of security (to stop audience members climbing onto the stage) and visibility (when playing to mass audiences, mainly standing on a flat floor). In addition there are the following requirements:
- a metal structure along the line of the stage edge forming a 'proscenium' opening to receive stage lighting, framing the performance;
- a lighting grid over the stage to receive stage lighting;
- levels formed on stage, with rostra;
- a backcloth or curtain at the rear of the stage;
- masking at the side of the stage;
- side stages for musical instruments, and performers entry and assembly;
- sound relay positions at the side of the stage;
- video screen(s) (Fig. 12.48);
- performance sound, lighting and power outlets: temporary cable access with cable link to control rooms, relay towers, etc.

Access is required for performers, musical instruments and any staging: if a raised stage then staircase access is required on both sides. A revolve allows rapid changes of group or setting. If a temporary stage, then subject to legislation covering design and precautions, local fire officers and promoter should discuss and approve layout.

Stage: jazz music

The largest stage size for a jazz band, instrumentalists and singers is 6 m deep, 9 m wide and 900 mm high, with rostra built up according to the layout of the band. Smaller sizes are necessary for smaller groups and instrumentalists: the stage should always be kept as

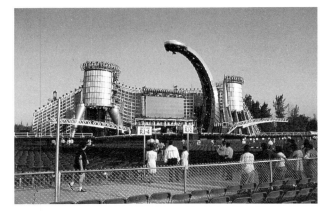

(a)

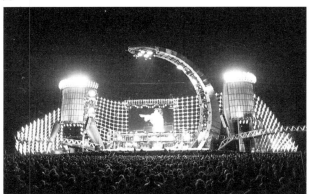

(b)

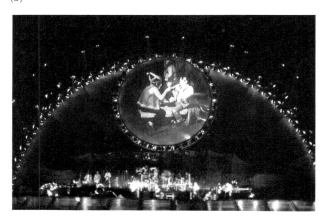

(c)

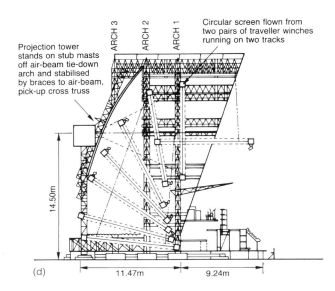

Projection tower
stands on stub masts
off air-beam tie-down
arch and stabilised
by braces to air-beam,
pick-up cross truss

ARCH 3 ARCH 2 ARCH 1

Circular screen flown from
two pairs of traveller winches
running on two tracks

14.50m

(d)   11.47m   9.24m

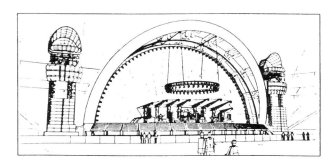

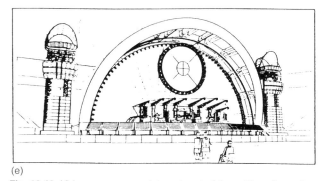

(e)

Fig. 12.48 *Video screen as an integral part of the setting of a rock concert; (a) and (b) the Rolling Stones tour 1994. (Architect: Mark Fisher)*
(c) Staging for the Pink Floyd concert tour (Architect: Mark Fisher)
(d) Cross sections through the stage showing the canopy and mobile screen. (e) Circular screen in horizontal and vertical position.

small as possible. Other conditions are described under Platform: orchestral and choral music (p.xx).

Multi-use stage

For those categories of building for the performing arts which combine uses, flexibility can be achieved by mechanical devices. In the case of combining opera, musicals and dance with drama within a proscenium

format, a fore-stage can be formed with a lift in place of the orchestra pit.

The fore-stage can be adjusted into three modes (Fig. 12.49):

● A fore-stage to the main stage created with the lift's highest position coinciding with the stage level.

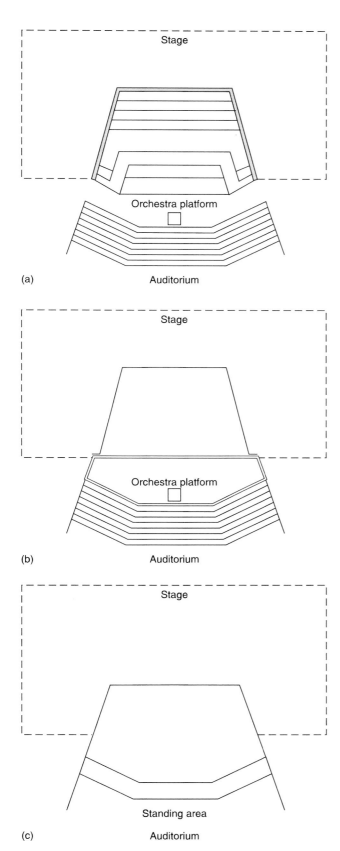

(a) Auditorium

(b) Auditorium

(c) Auditorium

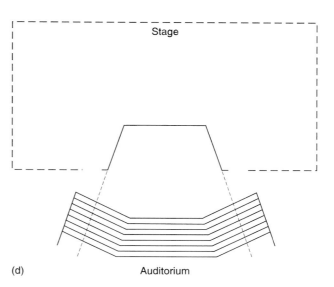

(d) Auditorium

Fig. 12.49 *A multi-use proscenium stage with flytower and a flexible proscenium zone in the tradition of lyric theatre which becomes concert hall, and can cover the following types of productions: (a) Orchestral and choral music. Acoustic shell around and over the platform and choir stalls, with fore-stage in position over orchestra pit. Side stages allow orchestra and choir assembly. The proscenium opening is at its widest. (b) Opera, dance and musical. Wide proscenium opening, with orchestra pit: side and rear stages serve the performance area. (c) Pop/rock and jazz music. Wide proscenium opening, with fore-stage in position, over orchestra pit. The seating to the lower level in the auditorium can be removed and a standing level formed with crush barrier in front of the stage. (d) Drama. Reduced width of proscenium opening, with fore-stage in position over the orchestra pit, bringing the performance area closer to the audience. Side and rear stages serve the performance area*

Banks of seats can be stored under the remaining front seats.
- Seating formed to continue auditorium level, with a stage riser added.
- Orchestra pit formed with lift at its lowest level. An orchestra rail needs to be added with the displaced auditorium seats stored under the remaining seating.

The fore-stage should include microphone points, electrical points and traps.

If a flytower is included then, as previously discussed (p. 144), the depth should cover the fore-stage/orchestra pit. Otherwise suspension over the performance area, including the fore-stage, for hanging scenery must be provided.

In the case of combining orchestral music with opera, musicals, dance and also drama, the comments outlined above on a flexible fore-stage will apply. In addition a ceiling to reflect sound requires to be flown over the stage, and possibly reflecting rear and side walls set up about the orchestra and choir.

Combination with flat floor

For those categories which combine performing arts with activities requiring a flat floor, a raised stage can be formed by (Fig. 12.50):

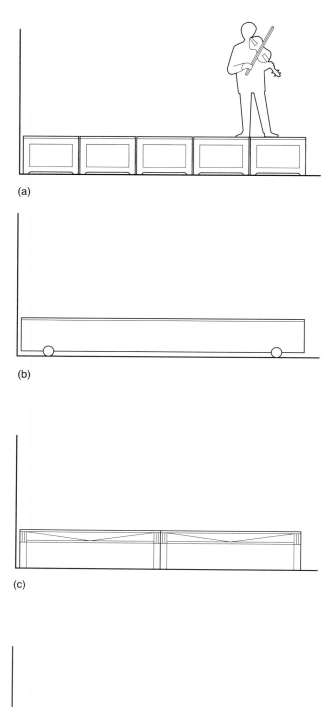

(a)

(b)

(c)

(d)

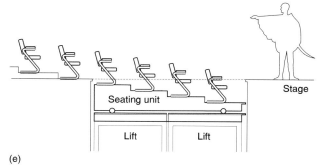

(e)

Fig. 12.50 *Temporary raised platform/stage. (a) Rostra: a set of metal/timber units capable of being built up to form a raised platform/stage: each rostra unit can be collapsed by hinged legs or sides to reduce storage requirements. Rostra require to be firmly clamped together to avoid movement and creaking in use. (b) Units: large units on braked castors or air cushion producing platform/stage. Large storage area required, immediately adjacent to auditorium. (c) Demountable kit of parts: proprietary system to form raised platform/stage, or scaffolding units built up to raised floor. Trolleys are available to move kit of parts to and from storage areas. (d) Hydraulic method: sections of a flat floor capable of being raised to form platform/stage. (e) Floor lift(s): section(s) of a flat floor able to drop to form a platform/stage front, with the addition of temporary raked seating or a raked floor formed by more than one hydraulic lift*

- the addition of rostra built up off the flat floor;
- sectional lifts which can be raised above the floor level;
- dropping the first few rows of the seating: a lift covering, say, the first few rows can be lowered and a section of raked seating added. The seating must be stored in the basement when not in use.

For sports, the flat floor must be absolutely flat without the possibility of the athletes tripping on the edges of lifts. In that circumstance building up a raised stage is preferable, unless accuracy of levels can be assured. A cloth can be laid across a playing area but will need to be stored and laid each time it is used for sports.

For opera, musicals and dance, an orchestra pit can be formed by a lift between stage and audience. The comments about the flat floor for sports remain.

For concerts, an acoustic reflecting ceiling and walls may need to be added to the stage. A flytower could be included, although structural problems may exclude this option. Suspension for hanging scenery for opera, musicals, dance and drama needs to be included.

Multi-purpose formats

Two examples illustrate flexible small-scale theatres offering different formats for the presentation of predominantly drama productions.

- Courtyard Theatre, West Yorkshire Playhouse, Leeds (Architects: The Appleton Partnership).
  This small theatre has a maximum capacity of 350

seats, with 2 shallow balconies and higher technical level: the raked seating at the lower level is formed by bleachers off a flat floor. The formats include theatre-in-the-round, end stage, proscenium stage and promenade productions as well as the use of workshops, cabaret and presentations (Fig. 12.51).

- Studio Theatre, Hong Kong Centre for the Performing Arts (Architects: The Peter Moro Partnership).

This is a small theatre with a maximum seating capacity of 240. The configurations include thrust stage, centre stage, end stage and promenade productions. The raked seating areas are made up of a series of rostra able to be located into the various layouts. There is a first floor which is either a balcony with a single row or links with the raked rostra built off the flat floor (Fig. 12.52).

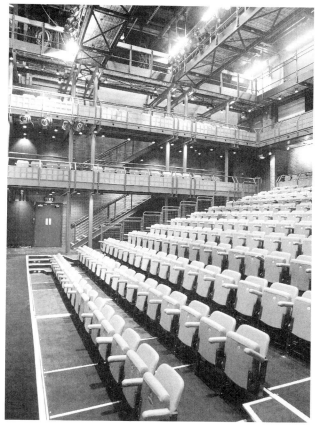

Fig. 12.51 *Courtyard Theatre, West Yorkshire Playhouse. (a) View of interior.*

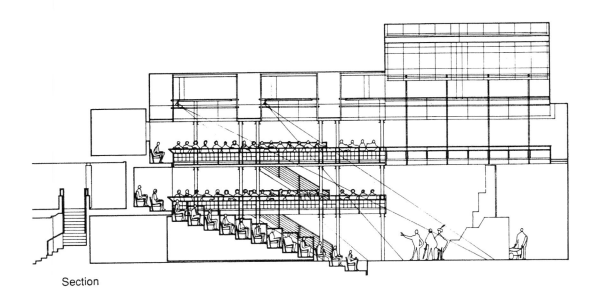

Section

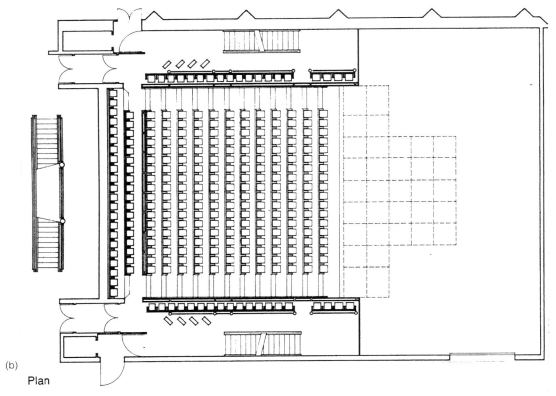

(b)

Plan

Fig. 12.51 continued *Courtyard Theatre, West Yorkshire Playhouse. (b) Plan and section of end stage layout.*

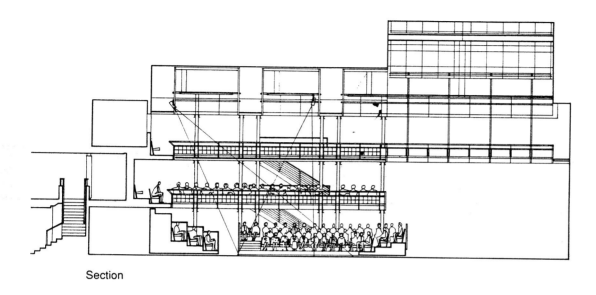

Section

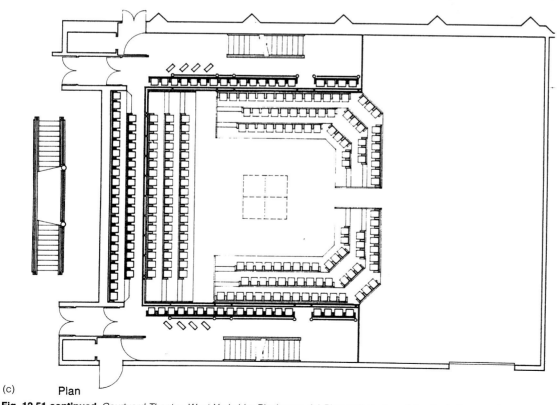

(c)   Plan

Fig. 12.51 continued *Courtyard Theatre, West Yorkshire Playhouse. (c) Plan and section of theatre-in-the-round.*

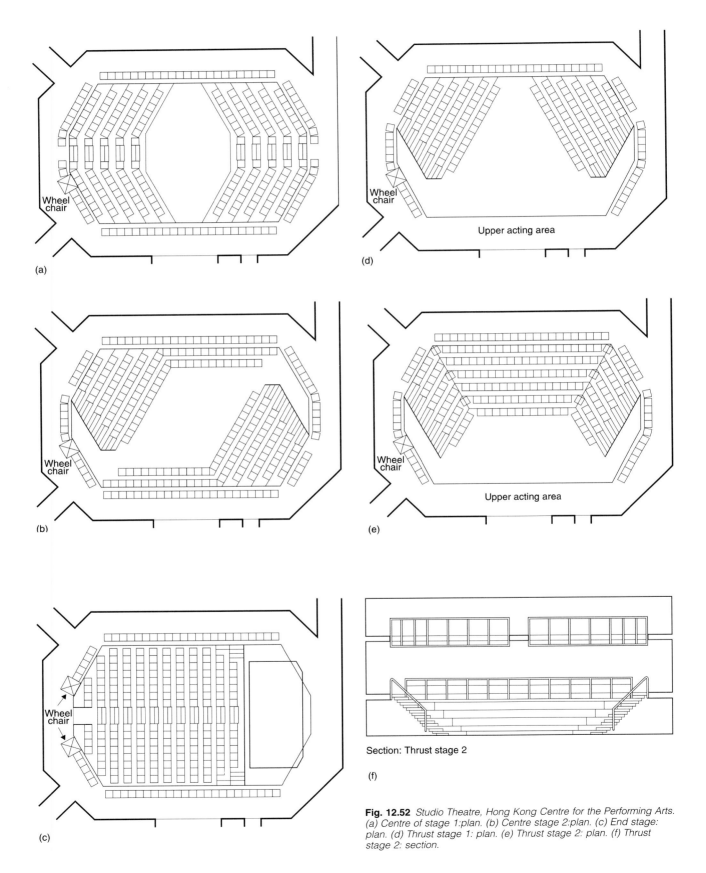

Fig. 12.52 *Studio Theatre, Hong Kong Centre for the Performing Arts. (a) Centre of stage 1:plan. (b) Centre stage 2:plan. (c) End stage: plan. (d) Thrust stage 1: plan. (e) Thrust stage 2: plan. (f) Thrust stage 2: section.*

(a)

(b)

(c)

(d)

Upper acting area

(e)

Upper acting area

(f)

Section: Thrust stage 2

Wheel chair

13

13 Initial brief: support facilities

A characteristic of a building for the performing arts is the distinct sequence of operations for each of the main functions. These essential patterns of operation, and also the relationship between functions, are common to the majority of buildings for the performing arts. Apart from the performance itself, the main functions are the:

- access and egress by the public and their welfare;
- organization of the stage/platform, and performance lighting and sound before and during a particular performance;
- preparation by performers for a performance;
- managerial functions of policy making and administration;
- delivery and removal of scenery, properties, costumes and/or musical instruments for buildings receiving touring companies;
- instigation and development of a production including company organization, rehearsal and, if applicable, the preparation of scenery, properties and costumes.

Each of the main functions may be regarded as distinct, linked by the ultimate focus of the performance on the platform/stage. The circulation within each should be for the particular users only, avoiding cross-circulation.

The emphasis will vary according to type and scale of production, the pattern of use, whether the company is professional or amateur and whether the building is for touring companies and/or a resident company.

Public spaces

Public spaces are those areas accessible by the public between the entrance and the auditorium. For those attending a performance, public spaces are part of the wider experience of a visit to a building for the performing arts. If the public spaces are attractive, and access to and through them are easy and pleasant, then this adds to the experience and encourages attendance. The public spaces may also be used by those not attending a performance, using facilities for eating, drinking, display, meetings and social activities. The public space could even serve as a performance space itself for, say, late night shows.

Public spaces may be subject to an open policy, with the public able to use the facilities without necessarily attending a performance, where control of entry into the auditorium is at the entry points. Or the policy may be to restrict the use of the public spaces to those attending a performance only with ticket checks at the entrance.

Increasingly, management policy encourages public spaces to be open during the day and evening for use by those not attending performances. Such use, especially of the refreshment areas, increases revenue and allows occupancy of spaces whose use is otherwise restricted to the short periods before a performance and during the intervals.

Management policy needs to consider:

- methods of controlling and directing the public from the entrance to the various levels in the auditorium, and to the other available facilities;
- whether the facilities are to be made available for those attending a performance only, or also for those not attending performances;
- the primary activities: ticket and programme purchase, circulation, toilets, cloakroom, and social and refreshment needs (before, during and after a performance);
- other amenities to be provided (such as places to eat and drink, display areas, meeting places and shop) and the extent to which these are income-generating (such as the meeting rooms for hire and the sales outlets);
- the pattern of use: opening hours (related to performance only or open during non-performance times), extent of multiple use of the foyer spaces (informal performance, displays, meetings, etc.).

The type and numbers of users of the public spaces need to be estimated:

- those attending performances in the auditorium;
- others visiting the building for non-performance activities which may include:
  - purchasing of tickets in advance,
  - having a drink or meal whether or not it is associated with a visit to the auditorium,
  - visiting other attractions: performances in the foyer, art gallery, exhibitions, talks,
  - attending meetings, receptions, etc. in meeting rooms,
  - depositing children in a crèche,
  - club members and sponsors accessing their separate facilities;
- members of the public visiting the management staff;
- access to the building by staff including management, performers, technicians, and production staff. Such staff may have a separate entrance – the traditional stage door – and not use the public entrance.

The public spaces may be open to all or selected groups. Each of the accessible spaces requires consideration of those with special needs such as:

- disabled persons in wheelchairs;
- ambulant disabled persons;
- visually impaired members of the public and those with hearing disabilities;
- the elderly and infirm;
- children;
- visiting dignitaries and royalty;
- the press;
- groups of visitors.

The numbers will be conditioned by the activities themselves: the maximum seating capacity in the auditorium, the number of seats in the restaurant and so on. Attention must be given to the access by the public arriving mainly through a period of time up to 30 minutes before the commencement of a performance, and leaving in a period which may be as short as 10 minutes. Cloakroom and toilets have to cope with such a concentrated demand. During the interval(s) there is a further concentration of use of the public spaces with a peak demand for bar and coffee services and toilets. Numbers are multiplied if there is more than one auditorium. Programming of performances can avoid simultaneous commencement, interval(s) and completion, so that the auditorium with the maximum capacity prevails. Restaurant provision, however, should relate to the seating capacity of all auditoria, while the foyer spaces and other public attractions, should acknowledge the larger numbers likely to be present than in facilities with only one auditorium.

The term 'public spaces' covers a range of facilities and areas, and these are discussed in the following sections.

Public entrance

The front entrance provides the main access into, and egress from, the building for the public. The entrance should be located along the main access route and be clearly visible: the public should be aware of the entrance by its location and signage. The entrance gives information about the attitude of the management towards the public and can be welcoming or intimidating, exclusive or embracing, clear or obscure. Examples of public forms of buildings for a performing art are shown in Fig. 13.1.

Requirements for public entrance areas include:

- *Access and parking*: Provision for passengers to alight at the main entrance by taxi, car or coach, with a discrete lay by or service road, especially if it is a large building complex, and close proximity to parking.
- *External display*: Name of the building and/or company as an illuminated external sign; posters and advertising material; current and future attractions on adjustable signs or electronic signs; banners and flags. The building itself, suitably artificially lit when dark, is also an external display.
- *Canopy*: Provision of shelter at the main entrance from inclement weather with a protective cover over, and across, the line of doors. A canopy is a useful device for gathering together pedestrian routes and dropping-off points if dispersed (Fig. 13.2).
- *Entrance doors and lobbies*: Two lines of doors reduce noise and draught penetration into the foyer; automatic doors are essential for wheelchair users. The distance between the lines of doors should be a minimum of 2 m: several pairs of doors with one or more lobbies will be necessary for the larger numbers arriving and departing, with the number of doors related to the estimated peak movement.

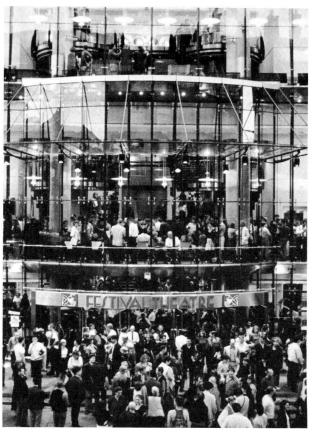

(a)

(b)

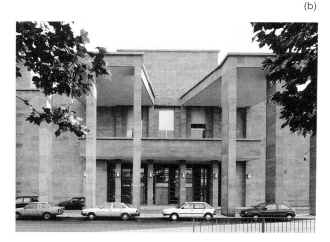

Fig. 13.1 *Public face. (a) Festival Theatre, Edinburgh. Fully glazed public face to the building in a predominantly commercial street. The entrance foyer and circulation are revealed through the transparent envelope. Modest threshold space between public entrance and general pedestrian route. (b) Royal Concert Hall, Glasgow. Emphasis on the canopy, or port cochere, raising the scale of the entrance, embracing the pedestrian route across the front of the building and providing a drop down area for vehicles. Formal entry into the building.*

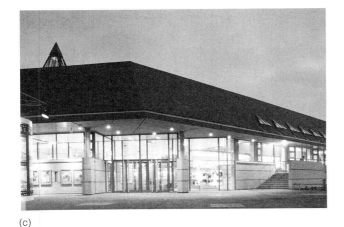

(c)

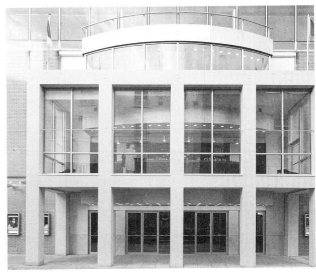

(f)

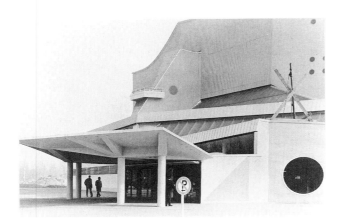

(d)

(g)

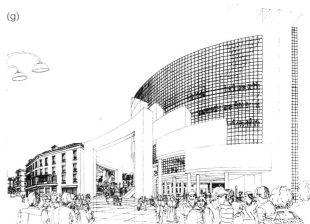

Fig. 13.1 continued *Public face. (c) West Yorkshire Playhouse, Leeds. Reduction in scale to virtually a single storey as the entrance into the public spaces. All the public amenities are visible from the entrances. (d) Berlin Philharmonic. The entrance is reduced in scale by a single storey canopy and box office. This addition to the back of the building beyond acts as a threshold or transitional space before entering the main public spaces. There is a predominant solid wall to the foyer and circulation providing a concealed public space. The emphasis is on the sculptural nature of the form. (e) Civic Theatre, Helsinki. The public entrance is a lengthy canopy, reducing the scale of the building, allowing for various vehicles to drop off their passengers at one time from a discrete road access, and a landscaped setting. The approach offers a threshold area as a transition from park to building. The entrance scale contrasts with the view of the main foyer spaces, on the axis of the principal auditorium and viewed across the park. (f) Abbey Theatre, Dublin. Simple street façade, offering canopy to public entrance and arcade to pavement and views into, and from, the first floor foyer. (g) Bastille Opera House, Paris. Original sketch of entrance of new Bastille Opera House in Paris. The ambulatory form of foyers are glazed, allowing views across the city. The actual entrance is increased in scale by an inclusion of an arch, which also adopts the height of the existing adjacent block*

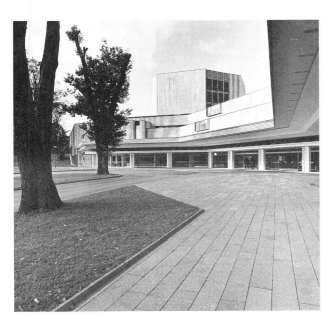

(e)

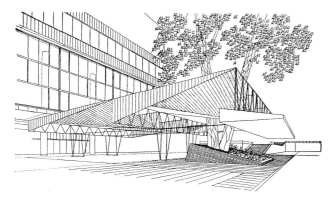

Fig. 13.2 *Canopy: Royal Festival Hall, London (original design)*

Egress at the end of a performance may be through doors distinct from, or in addition to, the main entrance doors.

Separate access for booking tickets or to the restaurant may be necessary for the public if the foyer spaces are only open during performance hours.

Entrance foyer

The entrance foyer may be required to accommodate the following:

- ticket check if at entrance, and not at points of entry into the auditorium;
- information in the form of leaflets and other hand-outs describing productions and events, notice boards providing information on events and, possibly, a reception/information desk;
- circulation and waiting area;
- seating (desirable for ambulent disabled);
- directional signage directing the public to the various facilities (consider carefully colour, size and type face for clarity and for the visually impaired/elderly, etc.);
- supervision: some consideration needs to be given to oversee the entrance area by the staff in order to offer assistance and exercise control;
- exhibition and display: space for temporary exhibitions or wall display; display cases for merchandise and crafts;
- access to box office, crèche, cloakrooms, toilets and sales, as well as meeting rooms and other public facilities.

The public needs to be able to easily identify visually the main circulation routes to the auditorium and other public facilities from the entrance foyer.

Box office

The box office refers to the point of contact between staff and public for the purchase, issue and picking up of tickets, and covers advanced booking for future performances and pre-performance booking of tickets.

Fuller details are given in the section entitled Managerial space.

Crèche

If facilities for child-minding are required, consider:

- the number of children to be provided for;
- special requirements: toilets and washing facilities, pram storage, storage for toys, etc.;
- shared use: with committee room or club room.

Such provision can be made to encourage use of the building by young parents especially if there is a day-time programme of events.
Standards include:

- at least 2.5 m^2 per child;
- separate toilets with one WC and wash basin per 12 children, with WCs and wash basins, and also coat hooks, at a low level;
- ceiling of sound absorbent material;
- adequate storage for tables, playmats and toys.

Shop

The area required for a shop will depend on the marketing policy, type and quantity of material to be displayed and its relation to the main circulation. The location should be adjacent to, and have access from, the entrance foyer, with a shop front or display to attract customers. Consider:

- *Method of display*: Display cases, shelves, free standing display; the lighting of items displayed.
- *Method of selling*: A cash point with a cash register at the entrance, and with a clear general view of the display units, assists control and supervision.
- *Security*: Display units capable of being closed off individually or an enclosed room with lockable doors, sliding doors or panel, or grille.
- *Circulation*: Allow sufficient space between shelving and display units for customers to browse.
- *Storage*: Lower section of the display units and/or separate store, with shelves.
- *Office*: The extent of sales may justify an office for administration; 10 m^2 minimum.

Cloakrooms

Cloakrooms are either attended or unattended. For attended cloakrooms provide a counter and hooks with a numbering system: hooks should be at 120 mm centres above open racks 500–600 mm deep, each in rows 3.6 m long: allow 0.09–0.1 m^2 per user including circulation.

For unattended cloakrooms consider the use of automatic locking systems, coin-operated storage boxes for valuables or lockers: locking hangers at 90 mm centres in rows 3.6 m long: allow 0.16–0.18 m^2 per user, including circulation. Locker floor area will depend on the type used – full height or half height:

locker size on plan ranges from 300 × 300 mm to 500 × 500 mm, with a height of 1.7 m.

Cloakrooms should be located directly off the main circulation route near the entrance. Allow space for queueing and for taking off and putting on coats. The location should allow, for open cloakrooms, a level of supervision from, say the box office or reception/information desk.

Toilets

Legislation provides a guide to the minimum provision: this is usually inadequate especially for women. A general guide to the minimum requirements is as follows:

Men WCs	minimum of 2 for up to 500 males, then one for each additional 500.
Urinals	minimum of 2 for up to 100 males, then one for each additional 100.
Wash basins	one for each WC plus one for each five urinals.
Women WCs	minimum of 2 for up to 75 females, then one for each additional 50.
Wash basin	one for each WC.

Also consider powder shelves, long mirrors and sanitary towel dispensers and disposal in women's toilets and provision for changing nappies. Allow for hand drying facilities: either electric warm air dryers, roller towels or paper towels with containers for disposal. Separate toilet or toilets for disabled persons, containing 1 WC and 1 wash basin in each toilet, are essential provision.

Toilets should be located off the main circulation near the entrance lobby and also at each level of the foyer in a multi-level auditorium.

First aid room

A separate room, with first aid equipment including a wash basin and bed, is required, preferably at street level near the public entrance. For a stadium concert the scale justifies the consideration of hospital conditions.

Foyer (Figs 13.3, 13.4)

The foyer provides the means of access to all parts of the auditorium and should have facilities for the public to sit, talk, walk about and meet friends. These social aims can include also a legitimate level of self-display from formal promenading to a general awareness of those attending a performance. The floor area is related to the capacity of the auditorium: allow a minimum of 0.6 m² per person for all the foyer areas, excluding toilets, cloakroom and vertical circulation. The form of the public spaces will be governed by the site, number of levels, and points of entry into the auditorium. The layout and atmosphere should perpetuate the sense of occasion according to the type of production, method of presentation and type of audience and other users: the foyer spaces can be formal or informal. If there is a pleasant external aspect or interesting view from the foyer, it can be incorporated into the design. Views also into the foyer spaces from outside should be considered. However

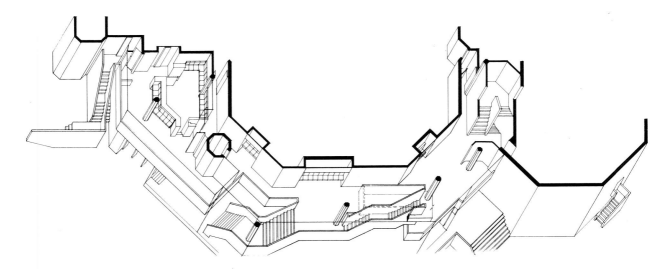

Fig. 13.3 *The organization of the public entrance and public spaces. The link is the circulation route from the entrance to the auditorium with the need to have control of the entry, contain entry requirements of the box office, cloakroom, toilets, shops and so on, and offer access to places to eat and drink while providing a clear route to the various levels of the auditorium. (a) Theatre Royal, Plymouth. The main public entrance and entrance foyer is to one side of the main axis of the building through the centre of the dominant auditorium, stage and flytower. The main staircase takes the public from the entrance foyer to the centre line from which point access is possible to the upper levels of the auditorium if necessary. (Architects: The Peter Moro Partnership)*

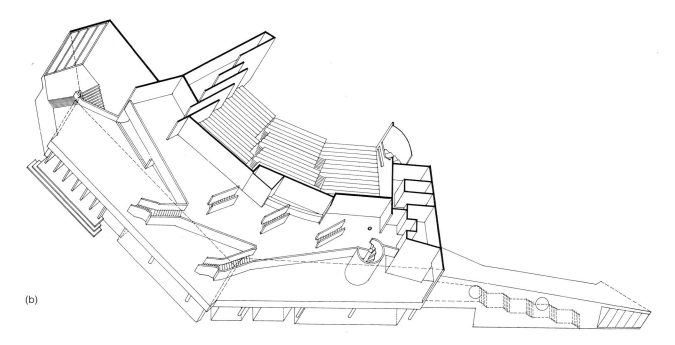

(b)

Fig. 13.3 continued *(b) Theatre, Mannheim. Eccentric location of the main public entrance with large 'bill-board' façade over. Access to the first floor is by a single wide dog-leg staircase, with a view of the city square from the intermediate platform. Access to the lower seating in the auditorium are from staircase vomitories serving particular blocks of seats from below: each block of seats and vomitory base have their own cloakroom below the auditorium. Staircases scoop up the public to the upper foyer levels. Restaurant and shops occur on the ground floor: a spiral staircase links the restaurant with the public foyer levels. The public spaces are pulled along the main elevation of the building to link the main entrances of the larger auditorium as illustrated and the adjacent smaller auditorium. Competition winning entry – not executed. (Architects: Hans Scharoun) (c) West Yorkshire Playhouse, Leeds. There are two public entrances (one for the pedestrians arriving from the city centre, the other for those arriving from the car park) with the intermediate external wall as a background for external performances in a civic square. The entrance foyer includes the box office and reception. (Architects: The Appleton Partnership)*

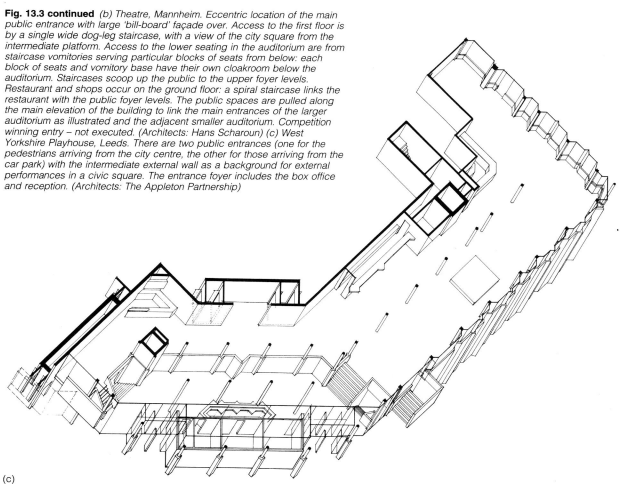

(c)

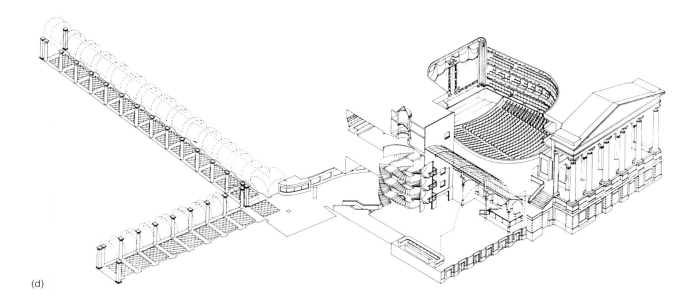

(d)

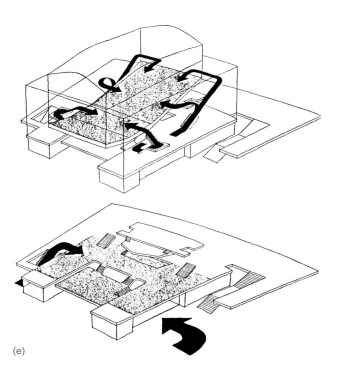

(e)

(a)

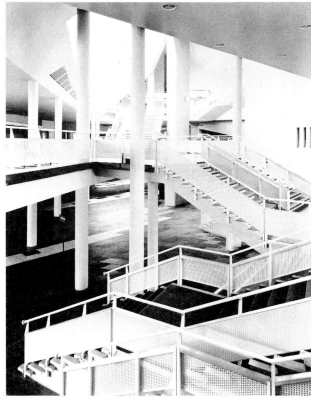

Fig. 13.3 continued *(d) Royal Opera House, London. Proposed main public circulation with two public entrances one from the principal street on axis with the auditorium and the other from the rear adjacent former market. A new double staircase links the various foyer levels. (Architects: Jeremy Dixon) (e) Royal Festival Hall, London. Staircase access from a common foyer below the auditorium to each part of the seating layout with a simple symmetrical distribution. (Architects: London County Council)*

Fig. 13.4 *Approaches to the foyer design and layout. (a) Berlin Philharmonic. Visually dramatic movement through a single volume using the angular nature of the staircases and direction of the platforms and stairs rising to the various levels of the auditorium.*

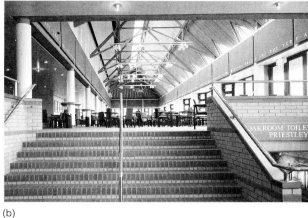

(b)

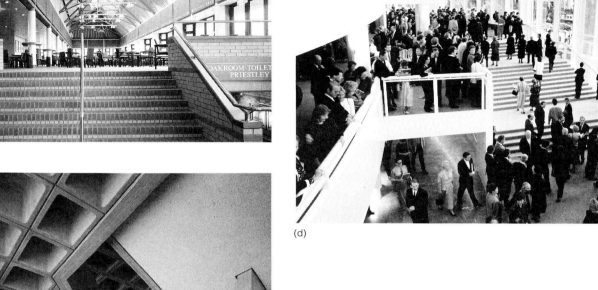

(d)

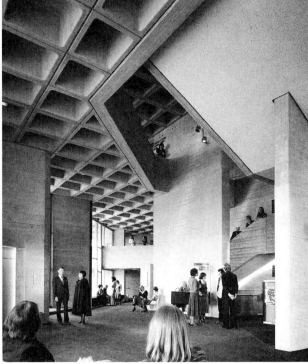

(c)

(e)

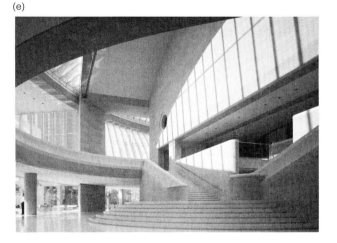

the outer walls may be considered suitable for display in the foyer, making glazed areas inappropriate.

Circulation

There are two main aspects of circulation to be considered.

Access to the auditorium

Main circulation routes are required for the public from the entrance to all levels and points of entry into the auditorium. These routes should be easily recognizable and free from cross-circulation: crowds gathered at

Fig. 13.4 continued *Approaches to the foyer design and layout. (b) West Yorkshire Playhouse, Leeds. Single room as a predominant space with refreshment and seating areas, seen as a further performance space and location for other social activities throughout the day and evening. (c) Royal National Theatre, London. Series of shelves and vertical planes providing spatial sequences, long vistas and voids with a unified foyer serving two auditoria and various levels. (d) Amsterdam Opera House. An ambulatory with a dominant level concentric to the form of the auditorium, with vertical access between auditorium and foyer. (Courtesy of Kors van Bennekom) (e) Morton H Meyerson Symphony Centre, Dallas. Interior in the Baroque tradition emphasizing the staircase and processional nature of the circulation route to the auditorium.*

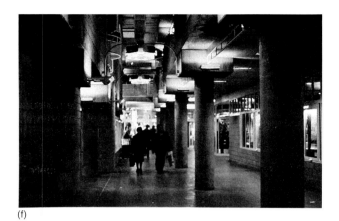

(f)

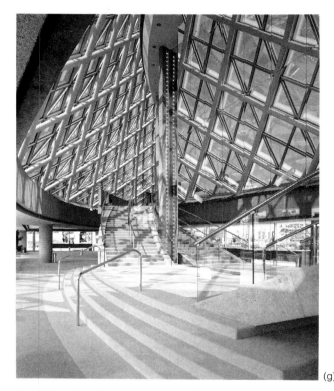

(g)

Fig. 13.4 continued *Approaches to the foyer design and layout. (f) Music Centre, Utrecht. The foyer spaces and circulation surround the auditorium with the predominant space being the internal covered pedestrian routes which connect with the adjacent shops, offices, library, places to eat and drink and exhibition areas. The social aim is the integration with the town centre activities. (g) Roy Thomson Hall, Toronto. Ambulatory circulation around auditorium, with a glazed curtain hung off the auditorium walls draped over the foyer, allowing daylight in and, in the evening, artificial light out*

counters should not impede circulation, nor should furniture. Movement along circulation routes should be easy and pleasant and perpetuate the sense of occasion.

If the public spaces are serving more than one auditorium operating at the same time then a multiplication of circulation routes is required: the

routes to, and into, the auditoria require to be clearly marked.

The minimum width of the circulation routes should allow for peak use – this will be the concentrated egress from the auditorium at the end of a performance. Except for a small auditorium, it is inevitable that vertical circulation will be necessary and staircases, ramps and lifts will be elements of the circulation design (Fig. 13.5). Staircases, for example, may be considered as a special feature within the public spaces. Changes of level for access to positions within the auditorium by disabled persons in wheelchairs will require ramps and/or lift access.

Access to other areas

Access to toilets, cloakrooms, foyer, places to eat and drink, sales areas and meeting rooms should all be off the main circulation routes to the auditorium.

Auditorium points of entry

Points of entry relate to the various levels and gangway positions within the auditorium and require space for:

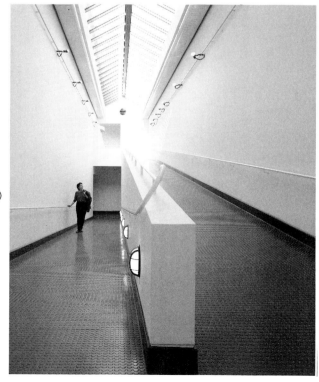

Fig. 13.5 *Vertical circulation. (a) Ramp. Processional use of ramp as only vertical circulation from entrance foyer to auditorium: Staatgallerie Theatre, Stuttgart.*

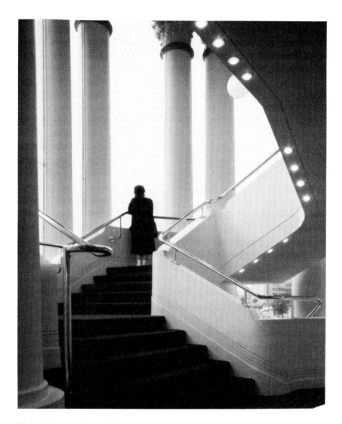

Fig. 13.5 continued *Vertical circulation. (b) Staircase. Movement from one level to another can be a visually important part of the theatre-going experience*

- the avoidance of noise and light penetration during a performance, with a sound lock – a vestibule between two lines of doors;
- the checking of tickets and selling of programmes by attendants.

Places to eat and drink

The extent of refreshment provision depends upon managerial policy and is influenced by the length and time of performances and intervals, and also the availability of other places to eat and drink in the locality. Provision may cover the sale of alcoholic and non-alcoholic drinks, coffee, ice-cream and food, including sandwiches, cold meals and hot meals. Licensed bars are a common provision as is the sale of coffee.

Restaurants may be in competition with commercial premises in dense city centre locations which may preclude their inclusion, while, for buildings in rural areas, the public would welcome places to eat associated with a visit.

Refreshment facilities are desirable not only as a service to the public but also as means of income-generation. If used outside performance hours, the service may assist in building up a public for

performances, and foster a more congenial atmosphere.

Consider the possible scale and type of refreshment facilities described in the following sections.

Licensed bars (Fig. 13.6)

- *Single bar or bars distributed about the circulation/ foyer spaces*: total length of bar(s). There are economic benefits in concentrating on a single bar but a large scale facility may suggest more than one bar, each close to the points of entry on various levels into the auditorium.
- *Types of alcoholic and non-alcoholic drinks*: bottled, draughts.
- *Hours of opening*: bar to serve public attending a performance only *or* generally open to the public; peak use is the concentration of demand during intervals; opening hours are constrained by the licensing laws.
- *Ancillary facilities*: bar stores including cellar, manager's office.
- *Delivery of barrels and bottles and refuse disposal*: lorry delivery will require ease of access to an unloading point adjacent to the bar store/cellar.
- *Licensing requirements*: bar facilities are subject to licensing permission and the local requirements and regulations should be ascertained. If necessary, obtain outline planning permission and a provisional licence.
- *Security*: closing off the bar area during non-opening hours to ensure compliance with security arrangements; secure storage of wines and spirits.

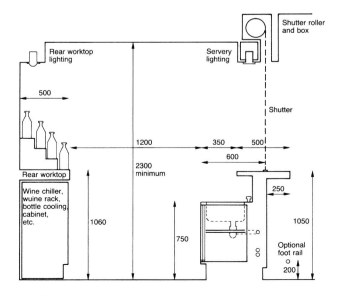

Fig. 13.6 *Section through bar servery: typical layout*

Coffee bar

- *Form of service*: table or counter self-service.
- *Number of seats and table size, type and layout*: individual, bench, banquet.
- *Hours of opening*: coffee bar to serve public attending a performance only *or* generally open to the public; peak use is the concentration of demand during the intervals.
- *Ancillary facilities*: beverage and food stores.
- *Delivery of goods and refuse disposal*: see note on bars above.

Food services

Facilities offering food can be many and varied. For example: coffee shop, snack bar, cafeteria, restaurant, private dining rooms, banquet facilities, food outlets. A number of points must be taken into consideration:

- *Form of service*: table or counter self-service.
- *Number of seats and table size, type and layout*: individual, bench, banquet.
- *Type of food and drink*: cold food, hot meals.
- *Management*: run internally or leased to another enterprise.
- *Hours of opening*: restaurant to serve public attending a performance only, *or* generally open to the public during lunch/dinner times; able to operate independently, when the building is closed.
- *Special requirements*: separate fire-escape, public toilets, cloakroom and entrance.
- *Ancillary facilities*: kitchen and/or other food preparation facilities, wash-up area, food storage, office(s) and rest room for staff, including toilets.
- *Delivery of goods and refuse disposal*: lorry delivery will require ease of access to an unloading point adjacent to stores.
- *Catering standards*: information on local requirements should be obtained from the local health department.
- *Furniture store*: space for tables and chairs if restaurant is to be cleared for other activities.

Exhibitions

Ascertain whether the displays of fine art, craft materials related to productions (or conferences), sponsors' materials and exhibitions of general interest are required.

Exhibitions and their requirements are grouped into five categories:

- A separate *art gallery* for the permanent and/or temporary display of fine art: paintings, prints, drawings, photographs, installations, sculpture and crafts. Security, fire protection, pattern of use, and possible conservation requirements suggest a separate space or series of spaces for works of historical, artistic or financial value. Security includes the detection of entry into the gallery spaces, including associated storage, during non-opening hours by visual or audible alarm, and may require attendants to be present when open. The enclosure must be fire protected, while adequate controls of the levels of lighting, heating, humidity and ventilation are necessary. The gallery spaces may be sub-divided by screens. The floor needs to be hard-wearing and able to receive heavy loads.

The gallery may be designed as a formal interior essentially for pictures, or less formal and specific, allowing exhibitions to be created for the space. Live Art should be considered, as should the use of gallery space for recitals, drama performances and so on, in which case the acoustic characteristics of the space would require particular attention. The whole of the gallery can be the foyer space to the auditorium, with refreshment areas, toilets, etc. off the gallery, thus making the gallery the focus of the public spheres.

- Ancillary accommodation may include: storage, with direct access off the gallery, for the depositing and packing of temporary exhibitions, and the screens and display units as well as being available for maintenance; an office for the custodian staff; access for the delivery of exhibitions, with doors and corridors of adequate size for the movement of the largest pieces. A lift or ramp will be required if there is a change of level.
- Permanent and/or temporary exhibitions of art works can be mounted on walls or screens within the foyer areas, or a distinct bay or separate space off the foyer, with items of modest artistic and financial value. Security can be covered by the general provision in the building, while pieces need to be firmly fixed to wall or screen. Pictures, photographs, posters and so on can be seen as part of the interior design approach of the foyer spaces.
- A display can be provided within the foyer associated with a performance or conference, exhibitions of local interest, sponsors' material and art-related displays, on walls or screens. Security can be covered by the general provision in the building.
- Objects, such as crafts, can be displayed in glazed cabinets with local lighting and sliding lockable sections for access. Such cabinets can be free-standing or set within walls or screens.

Walls and screens for the display of pictures, photographs and so on need to be flat and uninterrupted, with a plain textured finish which satisfies fire-spread requirements. Natural light, if considered necessary, should be from above but should be controlled, especially sun penetration. Display artificial lighting needs to be flexible and dimmable. Artificial and natural lighting should not come from an angle less than 45°, to avoid the shadow of the viewer falling across the display. Artificial lighting levels for display need to be tungsten, tungsten/halogen with fluorescent lighting restricted to general or working lights.

Security in relation to value of the exhibits may be a critical factor in the location and layout: lack of adequate security may restrict the type of exhibition to those of limited value. Discuss security with security consultants, the local police and the Area Museums Service.

Meeting rooms

Ascertain whether separate rooms are required for the following functions:

- Clubroom: a separate area for members of a club which is related to the company or main function of the building.
- Sponsors' rooms: for individuals and companies who are principal sponsors for entertaining.
- Entertainment room: for the entertaining of dignitaries, sponsors, members of the press, etc. by the staff in connection with a particular production.
- Meeting room for hire: a facility hired to groups and organizations for social and formal activities, not necessarily connected with the main functions of the building.
- Educational activities.

Consider, in each situation:

- The number and type of users.
- The uses to which the room is to be put: social activities, lectures, meetings, workshops, play reading, poetry reading, seminars.
- Refreshment facilities: a licensed bar, able to be closed off, with storage, wash-up and ease of delivery of bottles; food preparation areas, also able to be closed off, with storage, wash-up and ease of delivery of food.
- Period of use: available at all times public spaces are open (with exclusive use in the case of club members and sponsors) or restricted to specific times.
- Dual use: use of room for other activities such as conferences, board meetings, exhibitions.
- Ancillary accommodation: toilets and cloakroom, which may be necessary if rooms are to be used independently of the public spaces or if the general facilities are some distance away; storage of furniture, audio visual equipment, screens.
- Access requirements: off foyer and/or direct access from auditorium: direct access from outside.

Access to a meeting room may be through the entrance foyer or foyer only, or may also require direct access from the seating areas within the auditorium. Direct access from the auditorium is desirable for entertaining especially during the interval. Meeting rooms for hire not always connected to the performances, may require access directly from outside. So that a meeting room can be used independently of the rest of the public spaces then toilet and cloakroom, and possibly entrance lobby, may be necessary, to a suite of accommodation beyond the main public spaces. For conference or seminar use the meeting room should have an ante-room for registration and assembly as part of the suite.

Meeting rooms – clubroom, sponsors' room, entertainment room or room for hire – have similar requirements.

- Space standards per person, minimum area:
  - standing: 0.6 m^2
  - seated, with low tables and easy chairs 1.1 m^2
  - board meetings, with members seating around a table: 1.5 m^2
  - lectures: 1.0 m^2.
- Audio-visual equipment, pin boards, pictures, acknowledgement boards, television, closed-circuit television, chairs and tables: storage of equipment and furniture directly off the meeting room.
- Artificial lighting should be flexible: natural light capable of being closed off if projection (slide, film, video) is required. Artificial lighting should be directional towards wall display, speaker or performer, and general for lectures and board meetings, while being able to be lowered for social events and relaxation.
- It is desirable for meeting rooms to have a view and benefit from natural light, especially if used during the day.

Performance area

Consider a performance within the general foyer and/or places to eat and drink for informal shows: recitals, poetry reading, jazz performances, and so on. Provision includes stage, amplification, stage lighting and control, grand piano and so on: storage of stage units, furniture, seating, piano, and so on if area to be cleared for other activities. Performances may occur before, during and after performances in the auditorium.

The stage may be in a fixed position or flexible with its location in a variety of positions within the public spaces. It should be provided with stage lighting and sound and lighting systems as well as socket outlets for power to electrical instruments.

Outdoor areas

Consider outdoor areas related to public spaces: gathering area at entrance: areas associated with the foyers, places to eat and drink, and exhibitions and other forms of display. For places to eat and drink, consider whether tables and chairs are permanently provided or temporary, and have a store for when not in use. Areas for the consumption of alcoholic drinks will be subject to licensing laws.

Outdoor areas associated with public arrival can include:

- A threshold area between general public circulation and the entrance doors, under cover of a canopy; it will be essentially hard landscape of paving and other suitable material.
- A major civic open space serving more than one facility, able to accommodate large numbers of pedestrians and possible outdoor performances, with temporary roof structures and staging, signage,

seats, hard landscape and planting and lighting. An outdoor performance area should be served by socket outlets (for amplified musical instruments, stage lighting and sound equipment).

Pedestrian movement to the entrance must be clear with changes to level incorporating ramps.

Distinct outdoor areas associated with particular indoor activities, such as bar, coffee shop, restaurant and so on, could be incorporated into the design as a terrace at ground level or good use of roof space. Consider:

- Edges to the terrace as a barrier to contain users and discourage non-users: fences, walls, building form, levels, water, planting.
- Improvement of micro-climate: orientation towards sun, shading, protection from wind.

- External furniture: fixed *or* removable; storage of furniture when not in use.
- Landscaping: hard surfaces, planting, surface water, drainage.

The relationship between public spaces

The functional relationships between the various public spaces are shown in Fig. 13.7.

Performers' spaces

Performers require facilities to prepare for a performance and for relaxation and refreshment. Consider both the type – musicians, singers, dancers, actors – and the number of performers, including the

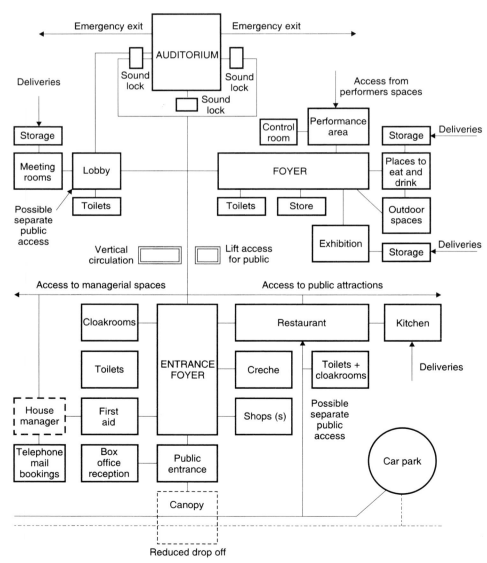

Fig. 13.7 *Relationship between public spaces*

number who may be children (children are subject to particular regulations) and the needs of disabled performers.

Facilities include: *changing rooms*, for musicians and choral singers who require provision only for the removal of outdoor clothes and, if necessary, changing into evening dress; *dressing rooms*, for singers, dancers, actors and other performers who require provision for supplying make-up and changing into costumes for, and during, a performance.

The number and type, and associated activities, depend on the type of production, and the scale and standard of the company. Changing rooms and dressing rooms can be single, shared (2–6) or communal (over 6): the number of occupants in each room is usually determined by the status of the performer. The larger professional companies tend to follow a traditional hierarchical structure with the principal performers in single rooms while the chorus, say, are in communal rooms. In contrast, small touring companies do not necessarily follow this pattern and can share one general room without gender and status division. Amateur companies accept lower standards than professionals and do not require single or shared rooms. Space standards vary, with the minimum subject to legislation.

Classical music: orchestral and choral

The number and type of changing rooms, with associated areas, for professional concerts and recitals are listed in Table 13.1. Members of a choir may consist of some or all who are amateur.

Table 13.1 Concerts: changing rooms: professional companies

Type of performer	Number	Occupancy
Conductors	2	Single
Soloists (instruments)	4	Single
Leader of orchestra	1	Single
Musicians	120	Communal
Soloists (singers)	4	Single
Choristers	250	Communal

For those soloists who are singers, provision for making-up may be required. Other associated areas include:

- *conductor's green room;*
- *pre-performance practice room(s);*
- *orchestra assembly area;*
- *choir assembly area;*
- *musicians' common-room;*
- *orchestra manager's office and other offices (e.g. tour manager) if touring orchestra.*

Further details on these areas will be found later in this chapter.

Facilities for changing will be required for recitals also, and occupancy levels are given in Table 13.2

Table 13.2 Recitals: changing rooms: professional companies

Type of performer	Number	Occupancy
Conductors	2	Single
Solosits (Instrumental)	2	Single
Musicians	40	Communal
Soloists (singers)	2	Single
Choristers	40	Communal

Associated areas are similar to those described under concerts.

Facilities for the use by *amateur* musicians only require communal spaces if they are exclusively without professional help. However allowance should be considered for visiting professional conductors and singers who will expect single rooms.

Pop/rock, jazz

Pop/rock and jazz performances fall into two categories:

- The classification of pop, rock and jazz musicians and singers in a manner similar to orchestral musicians and choral singers, with the provision of changing rooms, and associated areas, as described under concerts and recitals but with reduced numbers.
- Staged productions with performers requiring make-up and change of costumes, thereby needing dressing rooms, comparable to the provision described under musicals.

See Table 13.3 for type of accommodation.

Table 13.3 Pop/rock, jazz: changing/dressing rooms: professional companies

Type of performer	Number	Occupancy
Soloists	4	Single
Musicians	20	Communal
Singers	10	Shared
Dancers	20	Shared

Opera, dance, musicals and drama

For professional companies, the number and type of dressing rooms and changing rooms, with associated areas, are variously listed in Tables 13.4, 13.5, 13.6, 13.7, 13.8, 13.9 and 13.10.

The facilities apply generally to resident companies. Touring companies, especially for opera and dance, are likely to have fewer performers due to the cost and difficulties of transporting scenery and performers: such companies usually limit their repertoire and scale of production. For occasional productions with particularly large numbers of performers, temporary changing rooms and dressing room arrangements to supply accommodation can be considered with, for example, a rehearsal room able to be used.

Table 13.4 Opera: dressing rooms

Type of performer	Number	Occupancy
Male principals	3	Single
Female principals	3	Single
Male minor principals	20	Shared
Female minor principals	20	Shared
Male chorus	35	Communal
Female chorus	35	Communal
Extra chorus	40	Communal
Male dancers	10	Communal
Female dancers	10	Communal
Male supernumeraries	40	Communal
Female supernumeraries	12	Communal
Children	20	Communal

Associated areas include:

- *pre-performance practice-room for principals if a piano is not provided in their dressing room;*
- *waiting area for visitors and dressers adjacent to rooms for male and female principals;*
- *wig store and hairdressers' room;*
- *green room;*
- *specialist make up room, for use by chorus and supernumeraries if make-up is not self applied;*
- *pre-performance dance studio, for dancers to warm up;*
- *office for children's supervisor;*
- *company manager's office, and other offices (e.g. tour manager) if touring company.*

Table 13.5 Opera: changing rooms for the musicians

Type of performer	Number	Occupancy
Conductors	2	Single
Leader of orchestra	1	Single
Section leaders	6	Shared
Musicians	120	Communal

Conductors' rooms mentioned in Table 13.5 are for the use of performance conductors as distinct from facilities for the resident conductor, if applicable. One of the conductor's rooms should be large enough to accommodate an ensemble of six musicians for rehearsal. Associated areas include:

- *pre-performance practice room(s);*
- *orchestra assembly area;*
- *musicians' common-room;*
- *orchestra manager's office and other offices (e.g. tour manager) if touring company.*

Table 13.6 Dance: dressing rooms

Type of performer	Number	Occupancy
Male principals	3	Single
Female principals	3	Single
Soloists	24	Shared
Male *corps de ballet*	25	Communal
Female *corps de ballet*	35	Communal
Male supernumeraries	40	Communal
Female supernumeraries	20	Communal

Numbers of soloists and corps de ballet given in Table 13.6 depend on the scale of the dance and size of the stage. The number of performers relates to large-scale performance: smaller numbers would require accommodation especially for the touring contemporary dance companies. For contemporary dance generally the structure is not so formal and hierarchical. Associated areas include:

- *waiting areas for visitors and dressers adjacent to rooms for male and female principals;*
- *green room;*
- *rehearsal studio located near the stage for pre-performance practice by all performers;*
- *physiotherapy room;*
- *company manager's office, other offices (e.g. tour manager) if touring company.*

Table 13.7 Dance: changing rooms for musicians

Type of performance	Number	Occupancy
Conductors	2	Single
Leader of orchestra	1	Single
Section leaders	6	Shared
Musicians	100	Communal

The conductors' rooms mentioned in Table 13.7 are for the use of performance conductors, as distinct from facilities for the resident conductor. One of the conductor's rooms should be large enough to accommodate an ensemble of six musicians for rehearsal. Associated areas include:

- *pre-performance practice room;*
- *orchestra assembly area;*
- *musicians' common-room;*
- *orchestra manager's office, and other offices (e.g. tour manager) if touring company.*

Table 13.8 Musicals: dressing rooms

Type of performer	Number	Occupancy
Principals	4	Single
Minor principals	30	Shared
Chorus, dancers	60	Shared
Children	Variable	Communal

The number of performers depends on the production and the stage size. Figures given in Table 13.8 are for large-scale productions. Associated areas include:

- *waiting area for visitors and dressers adjacent to principals' rooms;*
- *green room;*
- *wigstore and hairdresser's room;*
- *specialist make-up room;*
- *office for children's supervisor;*
- *company manager's office, and other offices (e.g. tour manager) if touring company.*

Changing rooms for musicians are shown in Table 13.9.

Table 13.9 Musicals: changing rooms for musicians

Type of performer	Number	Occupancy
Conductors	1	Single
Musicians	30	Communal

Associated areas for musicals include:

- *pre-performance practice-room;*
- *musicians' common room;*
- *orchestra assembly area;*
- *orchestra manager's office, and other offices (e.g. tour manager) if touring company.*

Table 13.10 Drama: dressing rooms

Type of performer	Number	Occupancy
Principals	2 (6)	Single
Minor principals	16 (20)	Shared
Supporting cast	20 (40)	Communal

Figures in brackets in Table 13.10 are for large-scale drama productions. Associated areas are a green room and a company manager's office, if touring company, while specialist make-up room and supervisor's office for children may be necessary. Where drama only is performed it is not essential to provide changing rooms for musicians. However a drama production may include an orchestra and communal changing rooms (at least two) should be provided for a minimum of 30 musicians.

Medium- and small-scale opera, dance, musical or drama touring companies require less extensive performers' accommodation. For medium-scale companies, accommodation may include:

- *Opera, dance, musicals*: 2 single dressing rooms (each able to accommodate 2 performers, if necessary); 4 shared dressing rooms with 4 performers in each; 2 communal changing rooms for up to 20 musicians.
- *Drama*: 2 single dressing rooms (each able to accommodate 2 performers, if necessary): 3 shared dressing rooms with 4 performers in each.

For small-scale productions, accommodation could be limited to two communal rooms for not more than 10 performers, and a further room if there are musicians. Associated areas include an assembly/green room with provision for hot drinks.

For *amateur companies*, provide two communal rooms: one for 10 performers, the other for 20. A specialist make-up room will be required if performers are not likely to apply make-up themselves. Provide facilities for preparing hot drinks.

Multi-auditoria centres

If the building complex contains more than one auditorium with simultaneous performances then each requires its own set of dressing/changing rooms.

Multi-purpose auditorium

If the auditorium is to combine music and, say, drama then the most onerous requirements of each production type prevail. For buildings with a resident company, but where performances of different productions are staged in the same auditorium by different companies, then each company should have its own separate set of dressing rooms.

Changing room: requirements

Single room

The illustration in Fig. 13.8 shows the minimum practical dimensions and the relationship between items of furniture and fittings in single changing rooms. The following approximate areas may be taken as a guide to space requirements:

- single room with direct access to shower, wash hand basin and WC, 19 m^2;
- as above but with space for piano, 21.5 m^2;
- single room with space for an ensemble to practise or for auditioning and with direct access to shower, wash hand basin and WC, 40 m^2.

Shared room

The maximum number of performers in a shared room should be four. Provide space for hanging clothes, a chair for each occupant and a table or wide shelves for general use: lockers or cupboards and drawers for personal possessions, especially for resident companies; direct access to shower and wash hand basin and, preferably, WC in a bathroom; a long mirror and two small mirrors are required; minimum space for each occupant, excluding the bathroom, is 2 m^2.

Communal room

The numbers using communal rooms should not exceed 20. Provide space for hanging clothes, a chair for each occupant and a table for general use: the minimum space required for each occupant is 1.5 m^2.

Clothes should be accommodated on coat hooks at a minimum of 450 mm centres: lockers or cupboards should be provided for resident companies. The size of the tables should be 1500 mm × 600 mm with 750 mm minimum space all round. Provide a long mirror in each room near the door, and wash hand basins (1 between 4 occupants). Access is necessary to WCs and showers. Flexibility of use is increased if the larger communal rooms can be sub-divided into smaller spaces if required. Combining two communal rooms can provide an extra rehearsal space or committee room.

Dressing rooms: requirements

In each room consider the following:

- Provision for make-up, including mirror, lighting
(strong tungsten), worktop, pinboard, storage, towel
rail, shelf for wigs and hats, waste bin and socket
outlets for electric razors and hairdryers. The typical
arrangement for make-up facilities are illustrated in
Fig. 13.8.
- Hanging space for costumes and day clothes,
located near the door to the dressing room. Clothes
are normally hung on coat hangers. A shelf over the
hanging rails for storing luggage and hats is
desirable.
The lengths of hanging rails are: 1000 mm – usual
minimum; 1200 mm when numerous changes of
costume occur, or when costumes are retained in a
dressing room for a repertoire of productions; 750
mm in communal dressing rooms.
It is convenient to use wheeled racks for hanging •
costumes as they can be easily moved with
costumes to and from the wardrobe and/or repair
and maintenance room. Costumes may be delivered
in baskets, especially in touring venues, and the
means of transporting should be checked.

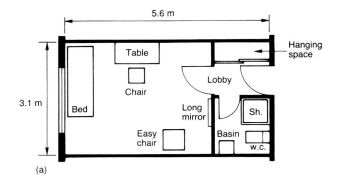

(a)

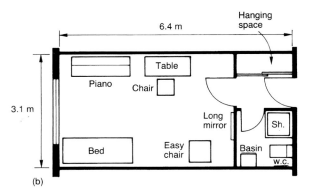

(b)

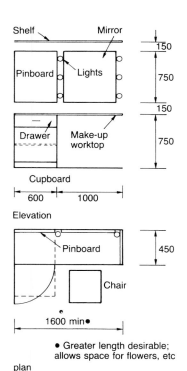

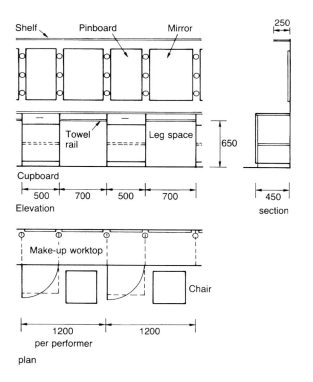

Fig. 13.8 *Changing rooms and dressing rooms: examples of changing rooms for single occupancy, i.e. conductor. (a) Plan of changing room with direct access to shower and WC. (b) Plan of changing room with piano and direct access to shower and WC. (c) Minimum space standard for making-up*

- Wash-hand basins with hot and cold water must be provided in all dressing rooms. Allow 900 mm minimum wall space and mirror over.
- A long mirror should be provided in single and shared room, located near the door, with one per eight performers in communal rooms: minimum size, 600 mm wide × 1200 mm high, mounted 750 mm above floor; the performer should be well lit with tungsten lighting.
- Day-bed, for resting in single and shared rooms.
- Windows are essential for daylight, ventilation and view.
- Toilets: provide an adequate number of toilets (WC and wash hand basin) on each floor for the performers: the minimum, as a guide (and laid down by legislation) is one toilet to 6, allocated male or female, according to the numbers in a particular production.
- Performers in wheelchairs: bathrooms and toilets to dressing rooms, at least those on stage level, to be suitable for use by wheelchair users; doors to be at least 850 mm wide.

Dancers in particular need to be warm as cold affects dancers' muscles and can result in injury: the temperature should be constant in all areas inhabited by the dancers, including the stage.

Single room

Single rooms should be able to accommodate two performers, if necessary. For opera, a piano is required in at least one room each for the male and female principals. Access to a bathroom with shower and WC off the room is necessary, with a wash hand basin within the room. Recommended dimensions are:

- room with a bathroom: 15 m^2;
- room with a piano and bathroom: 19 m^2

For pop/rock concerts and musicals there may be a requirement for a 'star' dressing room, with spaces for relaxation, entertaining, and television as well as bathroom, storage and make-up facilities.

Shared room

Usually there should be not more than four performers in a shared room. Direct access to a shower is necessary, with a wash hand basin within the room. Access to toilets is required, but not necessarily in the room. A room for four, with shower requires 18 m^2.

Communal room

Usually there should be not more than 16 performers. Direct access to showers (1 per 4 performers) is desirable: wash hand basins in the room (1 per 4 performers). Allow 3 m^2 per occupant. Communal rooms used by children require direct access to toilets.

Communal rooms should be planned so that they can be sub-divided into smaller spaces, with storey-height partitions and door access into each sub-division. Combining two communal rooms allows a larger space for rehearsal and committee meetings.

Associated areas

Green room

A green room is the term for the general area for performers for social activities, rest, refreshment and entertainment. Its size is determined by the number of performers (allow 1.4 m^2 per occupant), unless there are other special uses (e.g. meetings, rehearsals, extra dressing room) of the room which might dictate its size. Storage will be required to accommodate equipment for the additional uses. The extent and type of refreshment can vary from self service by the performers to meals prepared by separate staff, which will in turn require kitchen facilities, food delivery and refuse collection. The green room for dancers, singers and actors can function as an assembly area.

In addition to a green room, especially with multi-auditoria complexes for resident companies, a *canteen* providing full-scale meals may be appropriate, able to be used by all the staff of the building.

Musicians' common-room, and conductor's green room

Further rooms suitable for resting and refreshment should be provided for musicians and conductors; details as for the Green Room.

Pre-performance practice room

Space is required for musicians, singers or dancers to practise before a performance. Musicians and singers will need a 15 m^2 room with piano which is acoustically isolated. A 'warm-up' and practice studio for dancers is critical; it will need a minimum size of 100 m^2, with barres and mirrors, and a wooden sprung floor.

Orchestra assembly area

An area large enough for an orchestra to assemble before entry onto the platform or into the orchestra pit: the orchestra assembly area should contain bench seating and wide shelves for instruments; a lobby needs to be formed as a sound and light lock at points of entry onto the platform or into the orchestra pit: allow 1.0 sqm per occupant.

Choir assembly area

An area, or areas, large enough for a choir to assemble before entry into choir stalls: allow 0.6 m^2 per occupant.

Waiting area for visitors and dressers

Adjacent to the entry to each of the principal dressing rooms an area should be set aside with lounge seats and a coffee table, and with provision for making refreshments.

Specialist make-up room

When performers are unskilled at making up (as may be the case with amateur companies), an area is necessary for the application of make-up by another person. The area should be separate and contain a table for make-up equipment and chair(s) for performers being made up. The performer should be illuminated by a strong general light. 10 m^2 per person should be provided.

Wig store and hairdresser's room

For productions with an extensive use of wigs then a store near the dressing room, with shelves, will be required: room size 5 m^2. Where performers use their own hair, but it requires styling, then a separate room associated with the dressing rooms may be required, fitted out with appropriate equipment: a minimum size is 10 m^2.

Child supervisor's office

The person acting as chaperon for child performers requires an office containing chair, desk and storage.

Company manager's office/orchestra manager's office

A separate office or offices for the management of the company may be necessary in those buildings receiving touring companies. Similarly facilities for a touring orchestra and its management will be needed.

For touring companies, especially pop and rock concerts, the office(s) may be required for a tour manager, promoter and assistants: such an office should be equipped with telephones, fax machines and reproduction machines.

Physical therapy room

For large dance companies, a room for massage and physiotherapy will be required: minimum size 15 m^2.

Location and access

Changing/dressing rooms should be positioned at or near the platform/stage level so that performers have ease of access to the platform/stage. The performers' spaces should be grouped together on one side of the platform/stage adjacent to the main entry to the platform/stage and planned to be close both in section and on plan, with staircase access to upper and, possibly, lower floors. Rooms should be not more than three storeys above (below) platform/stage level. Staircase access needs to be near the entry point to

platform/stage. Lift access should be included for general use and costume distribution, if applicable, but performers should not rely on a lift. Principal changing/ dressing rooms, green room and assembly area require to be located at platform/stage level. For productions which include a large number of performers, especially with a chorus and supernumeraries, principals' rooms should be separate from those of other performers.

For music, the musicians' spaces should be grouped around the orchestra assembly area with direct access to the platform/stage. Members of a choir must have direct access to the choir assembly area and choir stalls.

For orchestras with opera, dance, musical and, perhaps, drama productions, changing facilities need to be grouped around the orchestra assembly area with direct access to the orchestra pit. For curtain calls – traditional with opera and ballet – the conductor has to travel quickly from orchestra pit to stage. A convenient location for the musicians' spaces is at the level of the orchestra pit.

Access is also required by musicians to the instrument store.

The minimum width of corridors serving changing and dressing rooms should be 1500 mm: corridors should avoid sharp turns.

Stage door or performers' entry

An external access to the performers' spaces will be required, with the following:

- Entrance door, which should be protected from the elements by a canopy and include a lobby as a sound and thermal barrier.
- Direct access between the entrance door and the platform/stage without passing through other functions: direct access to rehearsal room/studio and green room.
- Vestibule with circulation and waiting area, including easy chairs, notice board and public telephone.
- Space for a doorman, either as an office with a glazed panel or an open desk, to control and supervise entry: access to toilet and provision for storing outdoor clothing.
- Doorman's desk to include key boards, pigeon holes, letter rack, provision for flowers and parcels, telephone and directories.
- Entrance can be a control point for the security, fire alarm, paging and internal telephone network, and smoke vent release to flytower.

Relationship between performer's spaces

The functional relationships are shown in Fig. 13.9.

Performance organization

The work of the performers requires to be complemented by work beyond the performance area unseen by the audience. Also the platform/stage

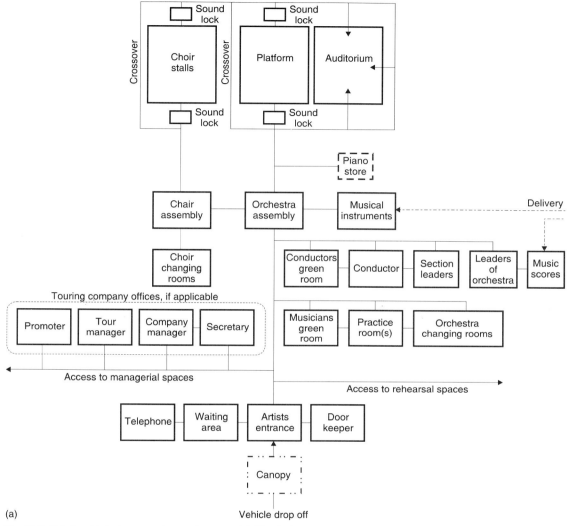

(a)

Fig. 13.9 *Relationship between performers' spaces. (a) Classical music*

requires to be set up for a performance as well as, where applicable, scenery and costumes repaired and maintained. A resident company has a full complement of staff to carry out these functions while a building receiving touring companies would have a core resident set of staff supplemented by the incoming company. One-off events or those running for a limited period would require the construction of the staging, seating areas, lighting and sound control and so on as well as the setting for the performance, with their removal after the event.

Orchestral and choral music

Supplementary functions for orchestral choral performances and include:

- Organization of the platform for, and during, a performance: setting up of the rostra, music stands, piano, etc. and settings: *platform management*.
- Operation of the performance lighting, sound and, possibly, machinery during the performance, and for the repair and maintenance of equipment: *electricians*.
- Delivery of musical instruments and their storage for the current performance(s): *platform hands*.
- Change of auditorium/platform configurations in multi-purpose facilities: *platform hands*.

Supplementary facilities will include:

- offices and associated areas including changing and resting facilities;
- lighting control room;
- dimmers;

Fig. 13.9 continued *Relationship between performers' spaces. (b) Pop/rock music, touring company; (c) Jazz*

- television and radio transmission and recording: control room;
- follow spot;
- observation room;
- piano store;
- storage of musical instruments;
- delivery of musical instruments;
- access for deliveries;
- parking provision for touring vans and performers' coaches.

Opera, musical, dance and drama

The supplementary functions required for opera, musicals, dance and drama include:

- Organization of the stage for, and during, a performance: *stage management*.
- Movement of scenery during a performance: *stage hands and flymen* (if there is a flytower).

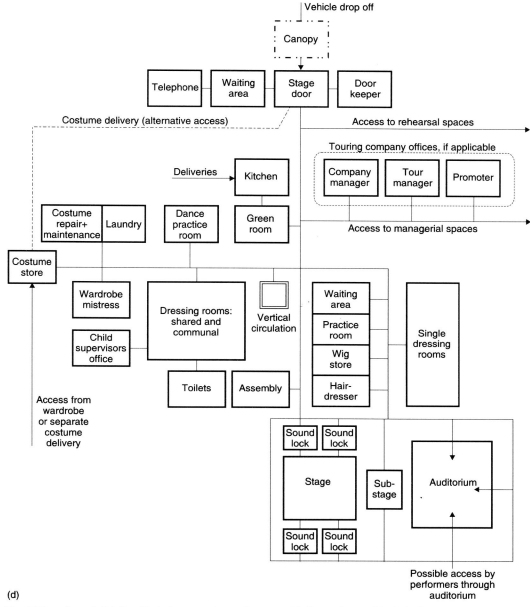

Fig. 13.9 continued *Relationship between performers' spaces. (d) Opera, Dance, Musicals, Drama*

- Repair and maintenance of the scenery being used for a particular performance: *master carpenter.*
- Provision of performance properties for use on the stage, and for their repair and maintenance: *property master.*
- Provision of performance costumes for the performers, and for their cleaning, repair and maintenance: *wardrobe mistress.*
- Operation of the stage lighting, sound, special effects, and machinery during the performance, and for the repair and maintenance of equipment: *electricians, machinists and specialist technicians.*

- Delivery of scenery, costumes, stage lighting and sound equipment and musical instruments (if applicable) and their storage for the current performance(s): *stage hands.*
- Change of auditorium/stage configurations in multi-purpose facilities: *stage hands.*

If production spaces are included in the building complex then certain responsibilities may be combined and carried out by one person, e.g. the property master may be responsible for both performance and production organization. Touring companies, especially

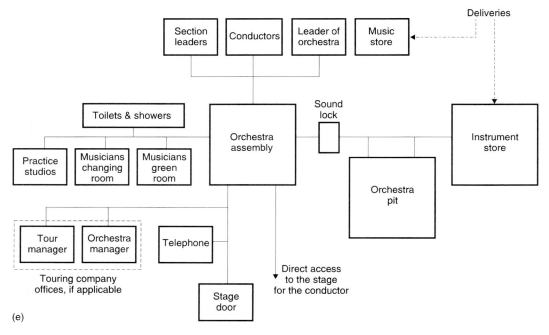

Fig. 13.9 continued *Relationship between performers' spaces. (e) Musicians' spaces: orchestra pit*

for opera, dance and musicals, may travel with their own piano tuner and catering staff serving technicians during the setting of the stage: extra space for temporary use as catering facilities will be required.
   Facilities include:

- offices and associated areas including changing and resting facilities;
- lighting control room;
- dimmers;
- follow spot;
- scenic projectors;
- sound control room;
- observation room;
- TV and radio transmission: control room;
- stage manager performance control;
- quick change;
- scenery and properties: repair and maintenance;
- storage of scenery: scene dock;
- delivery of scenery;
- refuse: performance organization;
- properties store;
- piano store;
- costumes: repair, maintenance and laundry;
- delivery of costumes;
- lighting equipment: repair and maintenance, storage;
- sound equipment: repair and maintenance, storage;
- musical instruments: storage and delivery, if applicable;
- access for deliveries;
- parking provision for touring vans and performers' coaches.

Those involved in performance organization also closely follow the rehearsal and production developments: stage management, technicians (lighting, sound and stage machinery) and others need to be in close proximity to the stage and also the rehearsal room/studio and production workshops.

Pop/rock, jazz

The functions and facilities required for pop/rock and jazz events can be similar to orchestral and choral music, with the addition of the delivery of amplification equipment and the provision of an auditorium sound mixing position, as well as lighting rig over the stage. However for the more theatrical pop and rock concerts, the functions and facilities are similar to those listed under opera, musicals, dance and drama.
   For temporary stadium concerts, the organization of the stage and provision for the audience require toilets, first aid facilities, relay towers, ground protection, safety barriers, lighting positions, raked seating, sound and lighting control locations and control points as well as the staging and performers' spaces. A temporary auditorium in an open area may also require perimeter fencing.

Offices and associated areas

The following staff may require individual offices; with each office being 12–15 m^2:

- Platform/stage manager;
- Assistant platform/stage manager;

- Secretary;
- Chief technician;
- Master carpenter;
- Property master;
- Wardrobe mistress/master.

In addition electricians, and platform/stage hands and including flymen (if appropriate) require changing rooms: allow 3 m² per person. Stage hands for opera, musicals, dance and drama productions, if seen within a performance will require make-up provision and to change into costumes. Showers should be available to stage hands and flymen, off their changing rooms. A separate toilet can be located at platform/stage level, suitable for wheelchair users.

Lighting control room (Fig. 13.10)

This room is usually positioned centrally at the rear of the auditorium where the operator has an unrestricted view of the platform/stage. It should be an enclosed sound proofed room, with an observation window; it needs space for a lighting control console and the operator who is required to sit by the console and view the performance through the observation window. Additional space is required for an assistant, worktop for lighting plans and script. The room's size and shape should be: minimum 3 m wide, 2.5 m deep and 2.4 m high, with separate mechanical ventilation.

For temporary, multi-use and possibly small scale auditoria, control may be by a remote console located

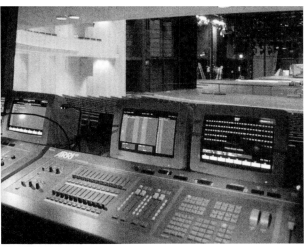

(a)

Fig. 13.10 *Lighting control room. (a) Viewing requirements through control room window or opening. Clear view of performance by seated operator is essential with a clear view by standing operator desirable. The window needs to be sound-proof and it may have to be possible to open it in part or in whole to allow the technical staff to communicate directly with the director during rehearsals. The window may slide horizontally, concertina or (as illustrated) slide vertically into the panel below. The glazing to the window may have to slope to avoid reflection of operator and/or performance, as the angle illustrated. The sound control room may need to be within the acoustic volume of the auditorium, with a simple opening and no window or with a retractable window. (b) An example of a control room showing view of the stage over the control desk through the window. The control desk includes computer screens showing cues during a performance, dimmer controls for stage lighting, discrete artificial lighting illuminating the desk top with no glare of spillage into the auditorium during a performance*

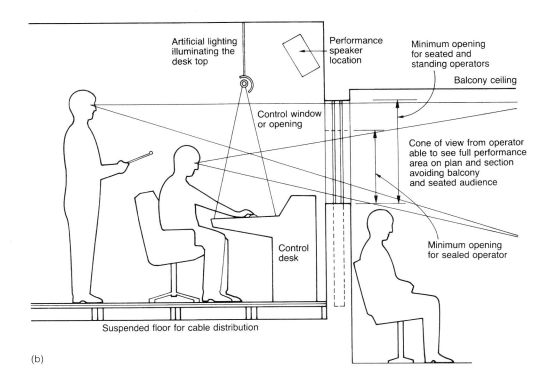

(b)

at the rear of the seating within a distinct area but not enclosed.

Equipment for the control of the lighting will depend on the standard of the company and the level of skills of the technicians: an amateur drama company will require a modest level while the equipment for a professional opera company will be more sophisticated. The design of the console, for example, is constantly evolving while the requirements of the lighting designer are developing: these suggest that the design of the control room requires to accept change. The tendency in recent years, however, has been that, while becoming technically more sophisticated (with memory control the main advance), lighting control consoles have become smaller.

Consideration should be given to the operator being in a wheelchair, by allowing sufficient space within the control room (allow 1500 mm turning circle), and having the console and other equipment conveniently located and access into the control room on the level. In the case of positioning and focusing stage lighting within the stage and auditorium, then developments in computer-programmed, mechanically adjusted positions allow the operator to be virtually static and not have to use lighting bridges and ladders.

Entry into the lighting control room should not be directly from the auditorium and public circulation. The location should give easy access to the stage, dimmer room, stage lighting bridges and vertical slots. There should be a direct link with the sound control room, especially if the same operator is required at times to operate both lighting and sound equipment. Similarly there should be direct access to follow spots, and projectors.

For access to performance lighting positions, see Fig. 13.11.

Dimmers

A dimmer is a unit of electrical apparatus inserted in a lighting circuit to permit platform/stage performance lights to be faded smoothly from zero to full intensity. Dimmers require a separate room away from the auditorium and platform/stage, but economy of cable run should be considered, as cables from platform/ stage and auditorium lighting are concentrated on the dimmers. The dimmer room should be easily accessible from the lighting control room.

Follow spot (Fig. 13.12)

Follow spot positions are located at the rear and side of the auditorium. Each position accommodates a spotlight on its stand, with an operator. The location of

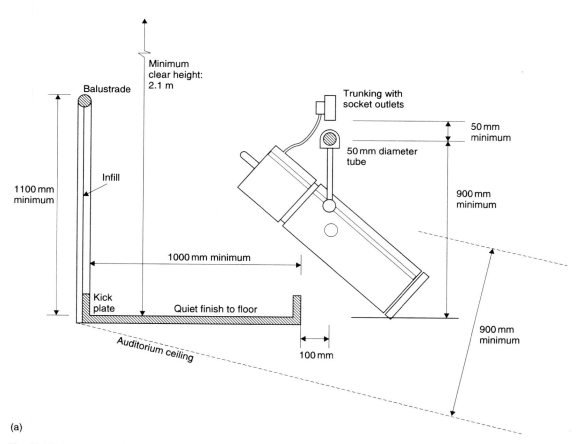

(a)

Fig. 13.11 *Access to performance lighting. (a) Auditorium lighting bridge at ceiling level with lighting directed towards platform/stage.*

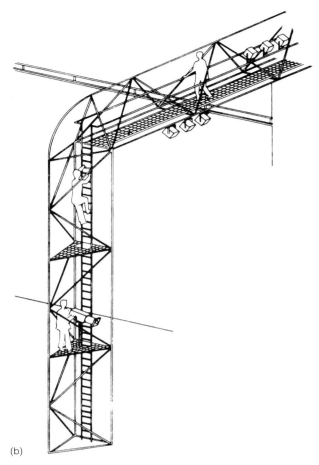

Fig. 13.11 continued *Access to performance lighting. (b) Example of vertical and horizontal access to lighting position, in this case, integrated into the structure*

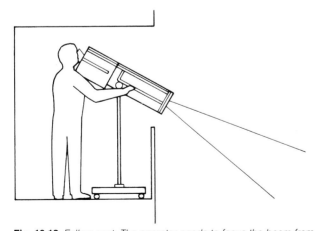

Fig. 13.12 *Follow spot. The operator needs to focus the beam from the follow spot on a moving performer or performers, with the follow spot located at the rear of the auditorium, usually at a high level, and/or on a lighting bridge at ceiling level. The beam requires an uninterrupted cone to any part of the performance area on plan and section, avoiding illumination of, and spillage onto, the seated audience. The minimum area for follow spot and operator is 1.5 m × 2 m*

a follow spot position should be behind or over the seating in the auditorium, with a direct projection of the lighting onto moving performers within the platform/stage area. Follow spots may be operated by the stage lighting operator and it is convenient if the positions are adjacent to the lighting control room. The minimum area is 2 m × 2 m.

Scenic projectors

Film, video and slide projection can be part of the stage scenery as a visual effect (as opposed to an exclusive use of film projection) requires space at the rear of the auditorium and can be within the lighting control room. Projection must be central to the performance area.

Sound control room

Accurate control of sound equipment depends on the operator hearing the sound the audience hears. The control room should be an enclosure with an open observation window in a representative position within the auditorium. The operator requires an uninterrupted view of the performance area as well as being able to hear the performance.

The sound control room contains: a control desk, with the operator sitting viewing the performance area, while seated at the desk; space for the desk operator including a seat; tape decks; equipment racks; monitor loudspeakers; worktop for scripts; observation window with an opening size determined by the sightlines (seated operator seeing the performance area) and sound quality. The opening should be capable of being closed off by a glazed panel. Wall and ceiling finishes should not distort the sound as experienced by the audience. The minimum size of a sound control room is 3 m wide × 2.4 m deep × 2.4 m high.

Auditorium sound mixing position

For amplified concerts, musicals and music within other types of production, a central position within the seating areas of an auditorium for the mixing of amplified sound from the stage may be necessary. The aim is for the operator to hear adequately the sound the audience hears.

The area needs to be flat, and set in to the seating tiers to minimize distraction. The area required is a minimum of 2 m × 2 m, with a protective barrier all round and equipment securely located. Equipment will include a mixer and sound control desk.

Television and radio transmission and recording: control room

Television and radio companies bring their own equipment and the camera and microphone positions are considered under the section entitled Auditorium. A separate enclosed soundproof control room, with observation window, may be required, for announcers, balancing and directing, or a position within the lighting control room to monitor and direct the television and radio transmission of a performance. Similarly the recording of a performance may require a separate room or position in the lighting control room for monitoring. The minimum required area is 2 m × 2 m.

Observation room

The director/choreographer/designer and others associated with a particular production may wish to check and view a performance without necessarily entering the auditorium during a performance. An observation room at the rear of the auditorium with a clear view of the performance area allows for such activities. The minimum required area is 2 m × 2 m.

Stage manager's performance control

The concentration of the control of a performance is with the stage manager (or assistant stage manager) in the prompt corner. If a proscenium format then the prompt corner is situated in the stage behind the proscenium way on stage left – facing the audience. Control equipment includes communications and public address systems. The stage manager requires a clear view of the performance area to direct the performance, and, if necessary, the release of the safety curtain and/or drencher and release of the vents at the head of the flytower (if applicable). The stage manager should also be in telephone communication with lighting and sound technicians, fly gallery, conductor, etc. and may be responsible for prompting those on the performance area.

Quick-change

For the application of make-up and rapid changes of costume, quick-change rooms or mobile units need to be available within easy access of the performance area. They can be separate rooms, preferably near the prompt corner, or mobile units which can be placed in the rear and side stages at strategic points of egress from a stage setting. The shorter the distance from the performance area to the quick-change the better.

The area should contain two make-up positions and hanging rails for costumes (see under Dressing Rooms for details, p. 171).

Scenery and properties: repair and maintenance

An area should be designated at the side of the stage for the repair and maintenance of scenery and properties currently in use on stage for a performance; it should be an enclosed area so that the work can be carried out without disturbing activities on the stage. The area needs to be large enough to accommodate the maximum height and width of scenery, with working space for the staff including a carpenter's bench. These facilities are additional to those provided under the Production Spaces.

Storage of scenery: scene dock

An area at the same level of the stage should be provided for the storage of scenery. Direct access will be needed to the stage and unloading bay. The scene dock should be an enclosed area adjacent to, but separate from, the stage.

The opening between scene dock and stage should be at least 3 m wide and sufficiently high to allow for the maximum height of scenery. The door may require to be fire-proof and to insulate the scene dock acoustically from the stage. The height of the scene dock needs to be the same as the side and rear stages.

Delivery of scenery

An unloading bay for the delivery of scenery, including backcloths, will be required, with the delivery vehicles able to reverse close to the unloading bay. For a large touring company allow for more than one vehicle delivering at a time. Allow 3 m of opening per vehicle. Provide overhead cover from rain and screening of the opening from the wind.

Refuse: performance organization

The extent of refuse from the stage will vary and will relate to the extent of re-use of scenery. If scenery is mainly dismantled and thrown away after a production is complete, then consider using a skip.

Properties store

Provision should be made for a store room with a fire-resistant enclosure, opening directly to a side stage for

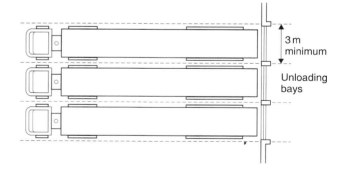

Fig. 13.13 *Delivery of scenery, properties and costumes as well as staging and lighting and sound equipment. Vehicle loading bays for off-street unloading can be head on (as shown in the diagram) or finger docks where depth for manoeuvring is limited. Vehicles can be vans (for the smaller productions), or lorries, with articulated lorries having either 12 m or 14 m trailers, for the larger productions. Unloading should be directly into a scene dock with at least two bays for touring companies. The opening can be 2.4 m wide and 4.5 m high for each bay, with a raised platform at the level of the trailer tail. The turning circle for the larger lorries is 25 m. A trailer park within, or beyond, the curtilage of the site, which may have to accommodate 1 to 30 plus trailers, with musicals and pop/rock concerts competing for the record of the larger numbers*

properties in use during a performance. A sink, worktop storage, refrigerator and cooking rings (for preparation of food used on the stage) need to be provided.

Piano store

A grand piano or baby grand will require storage when not in use. The movement of the piano from platform/ stage to store should be on the flat with openings wide enough for a grand piano. A change of level will require a lift: in a concert hall a lift on the platform, preferably at or near the location of the piano on the stage, can take the piano to a store below the stage. The space must be ventilated and kept at a temperature similar to the stage conditions. The minimum area for a store is 2.5 m × 3.5 m.

Costumes: repair and maintenance

An area should be provided within easy access of the dressing rooms for the repair and cleaning of costumes and associated items. There should be sewing machines and storage space for smaller items; a laundry with sinks, draining boards and washing machines, as well as drying cupboards, ironing boards and storage. The minimum space required is 20 m².

Delivery of costumes

Costumes may be delivered through the unloading bay, through the stage door or through a separate unloading access for costumes only.

Storage of costumes

Touring companies may deliver costumes in a skip and/or on rails. Costumes can be delivered directly to the dressing rooms or, if the programme is a repertoire of productions, stored: space will be required for the skips and/or rails. Empty skips and/or rails may be required to be stored if they cannot be accommodated in the dressing rooms.

Lighting equipment: repair and maintenance

A separate workshop will be needed for the assembly, storage, maintenance and repair of lighting equipment. It should be at least 3 m × 3 m with worktops, a metalwork vice and storage. Location can be at stage level or at the upper level of the lighting bridges: in either location the noise from the workshop should not penetrate to the stage and auditorium.

Lighting equipment: storage

Storage of lighting equipment – covering small supplies, lanterns, stands, cables, groundrows and colour filters – can be located at stage level and/or at an upper level adjacent to the lighting bridges.

Lighting equipment: use on stage during a performance

Storage will be required for items ranging from chandeliers to hand properties. A suitable area will contain shelves on the wall, some clear floor space and bars overhead, for storing such light fittings. This store should be located at stage level with ease of access onto the stage.

Sound equipment: storage and workshop

An area will be needed close to the stage or electricians' workshop for the storage and maintenance of sound equipment, such as microphones, speakers, stands and so on.

Musical instruments: storage

Smaller musical instruments can be carried and looked after by their owning musicians: the large instruments and their cases need to be securely stored near to the concert platform or orchestra pit and at the same level of the platform or pit.

The size will depend on the number of instruments determined by the scale of the orchestra/group. Provide shelves 1.2 m deep, at 600 mm centres vertically.

Musical instruments: delivery

Larger instruments in their cases travel by lorry or van for touring companies. For pop/rock groups this may also mean the transportation and delivery of loudspeakers and sound control desks. In a concert hall delivery should be directly to the platform and instrument store. In buildings for opera, musicals, dance and drama delivery can be through the unloading bay to the scene dock, or via a separate entrance.

Access for deliveries (musical instruments, scenery and costumes)

Lorry and van access should be off-street, with space to turn or exit conveniently. With large touring companies, vehicles are usually articulated lorries with 12 m containers: the small touring company may have only a transit van.

A service yard for access and parking may require a secure enclosure or security barrier to restrict entry, and an intercom to reception.

Parking for touring vehicles and performers' coaches

Vehicles for transporting musical instruments, amplification equipment, scenery and properties by touring companies can be parked within the curtilage of the building complex. Performers may travel in vans and coaches which may also require parking facilities.

Location and access

For orchestral and choral music, direct access is required to all performance lighting and sound positions in the auditorium and about the platform out of sight of the audience and linked to the control rooms at the rear of the auditorium. Access is required for the delivery of musical instruments in buildings receiving touring companies. A separate entrance is preferable. Music scores for classical and choral music may be transported with the instruments and stored near the orchestra ladder.

For opera, dance, musicals and drama direct access is required to all performance lighting and sound positions in the flytower, on stage, auditorium bridges and lighting slots, follow spot positions and projection at the rear of the auditorium. Access is necessary from the stage to the lighting positions and also the control rooms at the rear of the auditorium, out of sight of the audience. Vertical access is required into the flytower for loading scenery at grid level and operating the movement of scenery from the fly gallery, if applicable. In a proscenium format the stage manager's control should be at the side of the proscenium opening: in an open stage format a more usual location is at the rear of the auditorium. Scenery, property and lighting stores should be directly associated with the stage. The permanent storage of lighting and sound equipment needs to be off-stage and associated with workshops, chief electrician's office and staff room. It should be possible for a touring company to deliver scenery easily and directly from an unloading bay into a scene dock and onto the stage, with egress following the reverse route. Access needs to be at street level with the scene dock and stage at the same level. A change of level would require a lift: the inconvenience of which does not suggest incorporation. For touring companies the delivery point for costumes can be either through the scene dock stage door or a separate access point. When the wardrobe department is within the building complex, access is required from costume storage to the dressing rooms. Ease of distribution of costumes to all levels of dressing rooms is required. Provision for maintenance of costumes and an office for the wardrobe mistress should be grouped with the costume storage and have easy access to all dressing rooms. Access is required for the delivery of musical instruments in buildings which receive touring companies. A separate entrance is preferable but it may be combined with the scenery entry or stage door. Lift access to the level of the instrument store may be necessary. A piano is usually permanent but, if not, delivery can be across the stage and into the pit via a fore-stage lift. Music scores may be carried in bulk by touring companies with the instruments: they need to be stored near the orchestra leader who will be responsible for their distribution. The relationship between the main activities is shown in Fig. 13.14.

Managerial spaces

Managerial spaces refer to the accommodation for the administrative staff: the pattern of provision reflects the management structure of the client's organization, size of the company, and whether all functions are carried out within the building complex. These functions are common to both buildings receiving touring companies and those hosting resident companies: the requirements of the resident company and its organizations are considered under Production Spaces, p. 190.

Provision includes offices, box office, rest rooms, storage, workshops and storage. The relationship between the activities is shown in Fig. 13.15.

Administrative offices

Identify the management structure, number and type of staff requiring office space, and whether individual, shared or general offices are needed. The following functions are listed as a briefing guideline.

- *Policy*: Provision for General Manager or Administrator and Assistant General Manager or Administrator.
- *House management*: Supervision and welfare of the pubic, organization of staff, daily maintenance of the building and its security, which may consist of House Manager, Assistant House Manager and Catering Manager. The House Manager usually needs to ensure compliance with the licensing requirements that control places of assembly and public entertainment.
- *Accounts*: Responsible for the financial records, payments and control of expenditure: Finance Officer.
- *Personnel*: Staff relations and development: legal and contractual functions.
- *Lettings for functions*: Responsible for letting facilities to outside bodies and control of the arrangements.
- *Press, publicity and marketing*: Public relations and information to the media: dealing with mailing lists, subscriptions, audience development, general publicity, interviewing journalists, entertaining, displays in public spaces and elsewhere (posters, leaflets and so on), promotion direction: Publicity Manager.
- *Graphic design*: There is printed material – posters, leaflets, programmes and so on – which may be of a sufficient volume for the design, production and distribution to be carried out in the building.
- *Development Programme*: Responsible for raising capital and revenue funds, including sponsorship: functions include entertaining existing and potential funders and sponsors: Development Officer.
- *Community Programme*: Responsible for exhibitions, foyer activities, conferences and seminars, festivals, tours of building, events beyond the building: Community Officer.

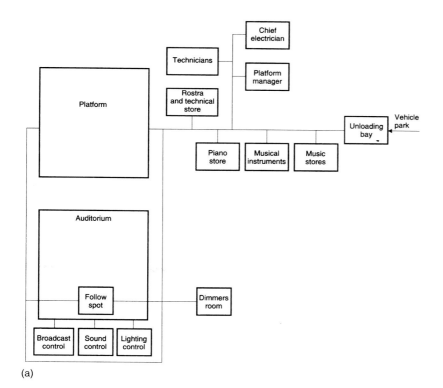

(a)

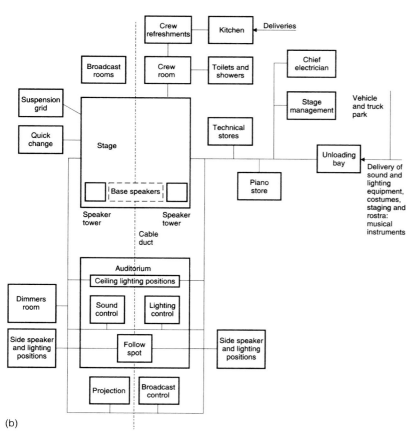

(b)

Fig. 13.14 *Relationship between activities: performance organization. (a) Classical music. (b) Pop/rock music*

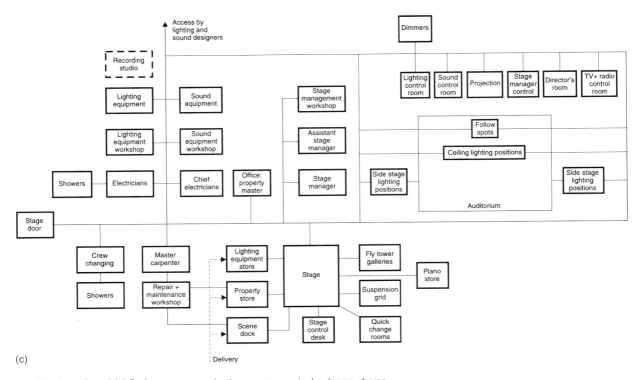

Fig. 13.14 continued (c) Performance organization: opera, musicals, dance, drama

- *Clerical*: Assistants and secretaries.
- *Storage*: Central or local storage of records, accounts, pamphlets, posters, programmes, video material, production records, press material, office consumables and so on.
- *Conference*: Separate conference room for board, staff and visitors meetings as well as entertaining sponsors and others: conference provision within offices.
- *Reception*: Separate area with receptionist, telephone operator, information and waiting area: delivery point for small items.
- *Office services*: Copying and printing, mailing facilities, telephone and other communications, refreshment areas.
- *Special Requirements*: Safe/strong room, equipment and machinery including computerized operations: acoustic privacy from noise.
- *Toilets*: Provision laid down by legislation including facilities for disabled persons.

The types, sizes and number of offices depend upon management policy and organization, and the scale and category of building: in the smaller categories more than one function may be combined in a single member of staff, while the larger complexes will encourage extensive office requirements and a departmentally-based structure.

The offices should be grouped together with access from both the public spaces and backstage, with either a separate entrance for staff or through the public spaces. Offices should be located on an external wall to benefit from natural light and ventilation, and views. For the relationship between managerial spaces see Fig. 13.15.

Box office

If seats in the auditorium are bookable, then a separate area is required for booking, and issuing, tickets to the public. Consider:

- The number of positions of box offices, which could be:
  - a single box office serving one or more auditorium;
  - separate box offices serving individual auditoria in a complex with more than one auditorium.
- Times of opening. The box office may be open when the rest of the building is closed to the public.
- Counter requirements, including number of positions (current, advanced and other bookings), open or kiosk, computer booking system, public information and cash arrangements. The assistants must be able to see and hear the person buying the tickets – including persons in wheelchairs and those with impaired hearing – and receive money and issue tickets easily (Fig. 13.16).

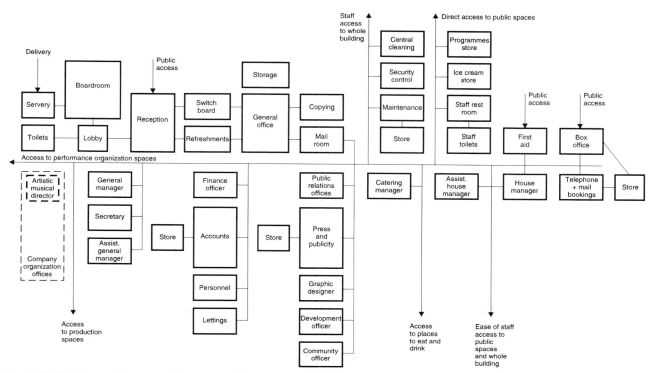

Fig. 13.15 *Relationship between activities: managerial spaces*

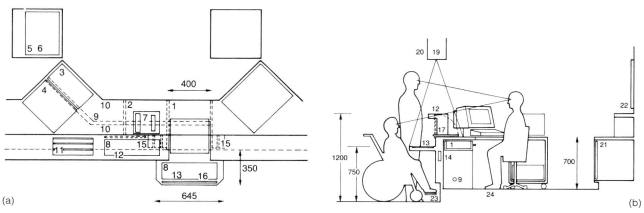

Fig. 13.16 *Box office. (a) Plan and (b) section through a box office position showing counter levels for standing customer and customer in a wheelchair. An alternative is a single low level counter for both users with customers seated. 1 Drawer for stationery, 2 till drawer, 3 keyboard, 4 VDU, 5 printer of tickets on mobile unit, 6 controller in mobile unit, 7 telephone, 8 display plans of seating layouts, 9 foot rest, 10 writing space, 11 leaflet dispenser, 12 upper customer counter, 13 lower customer counter, 14 three section trunking, 15 pigeon holes for messages and tickets booked in advance, 16 upstand to ease cheque writing, 17 gate: counter in lower position, barrier in vertical, 18 message clip and local light under upper counter, 19 lighting to illuminate counters, 20 display: performance information, function of box office position (current performance, advance booking), 21 storage, 22 display: posters, ticket prices, performance information, 23 foot recess, 24 raised floor*

- Postal and telephone bookings, and counting and checking money. These activities may be incorporated into the box office counter, or located in a separate adjacent area or office.
- Storage of tickets, seating records, accounts and so on.
- Staff requirements including numbers and access to changing facilities, rest area and toilets.

Access is required to the box office from the entrance foyer by the public and possibly directly from outside, with the box office area capable of being closed off from the public spaces. The box office should be adjacent to the House Manager's office.

Other accommodation

Rest rooms

Facilities for changing (lockers), resting (lounge chairs) and refreshment (sink, provision for making hot drinks) are required for sales staff, usherettes, stewards, cloakroom staff, commissionaires, doormen and other staff serving the public; fire officers and first aid staff (including nurses); security staff, and cleaners. Rest rooms should be capable of accommodating the maximum numbers using the building at one time. Access is necessary to staff toilets. The rest rooms require direct access off the public spaces.

Storage

Provision must be made for the secure storage of ice cream, confectionery, programmes and other items for sale or distribution to the public. Such storage areas should be located with direct access off the public spaces.

Maintenance

Building maintenance, including fabric, equipment and engineering services (heating, cooling, ventilation, water, waste, electrics and control systems) will require workshops, office(s) and storage for maintenance items. External maintenance, including landscaped areas, pedestrian routes and access roads, will also require storage space for maintenance equipment.

Cleaning

Central storage of materials and equipment will be required plus offices and arrangements for refuse collection. Provide cupboards, with sinks for cleaning materials and equipment distributed throughout the building.

Security

Security for the building will require a central control room with surveillance monitors, fire-detection systems, alarms, services monitors, paging system and locking devices.

Production spaces

For those companies which *initiate* their own productions, spaces are required for the company organization, rehearsal and, if for opera, dance, musicals, and drama, the organization and preparation of scenery, properties and costumes. Buildings hosting touring companies only would *not* require production spaces as such companies would have rehearsed and prepared scenery, properties and costumes elsewhere. Production spaces for rehearsal and for the preparation of scenery, properties and costumes, however may not be included in the building complex and inclusion will depend on their extent and type:

pattern of use and frequency of change of productions; land and labour cost; availability of facilities and services elsewhere.

For buildings with a pattern of use of long runs and one-off events, inclusion of production facilities would not be justified and commercial firms can make the scenery, rehearsal spaces can be hired and so on. High land costs, for example in a city centre, may discourage the building of production spaces, especially the scenery and properties workshops, within the complex. It might be preferable to erect such facilities on land of lower value not in the city centre.

Production spaces may be also seen as a separate complex providing a service to a range of companies who hire the rehearsal spaces and the scenery, properties and costumes.

Company organization

Spaces for the organization of a *resident* company and the extent of accommodation will vary from company to company, according to its size and type, and type of production. A small resident company with a permanent group of performers may be able to organize themselves without additional assistance, while the larger companies, such as a national opera company, will require an extensive organization. For the relationship between activities see Figs. 13.17 and 13.18.

Consider the number and type of staff requiring single, shared or general office space, and associated area, for the following functions:

- *Artistic policy*: General production aims and their implementation: Artistic Director, Musical Director.
- *Direction*: Responsible for the directing of a production: resident, visiting, assistant and associate conductor(s), director(s) and choreographer(s). Opera and musical productions, as examples, can involve a director, conductor and choreographer, while a drama production usually requires only a director.
- *Production development and instruction*: Resident composer, playwright, or lyricist; instructors, *répétiteurs*, coaches, prompters, choir masters, ballet masters, rehearsal pianists, dance staff, dance medical staff, and so on, according to the type of production.
- *Design*: For pop/rock concerts and opera, musicals, dance and drama productions, the design of scenery, properties, costumes, and stage lighting and sound: resident and visiting scenic designer, costume designer, lighting designer and sound designer as distinct or combined functions. Designers may not work within the building complex except for the initial coordination and supervision of the execution of their designs.
- *Production organization*: For pop/rock concerts and opera, musical, dance and drama productions, the technical planning of the stage and coordination of the production staff including administration and

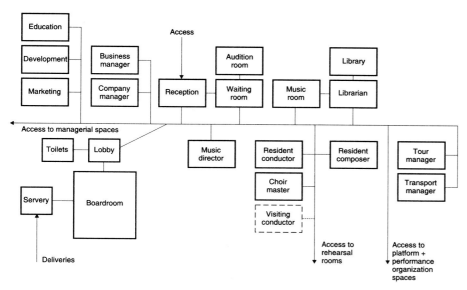

Fig. 13.17 *Relationship between activities: company organization – orchestral music with professional company*

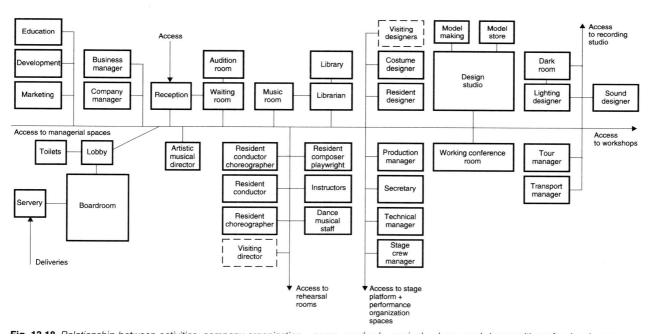

Fig. 13.18 *Relationship between activities: company organization – opera, pop/rock, musicals, dance and drama with professional company*

interviewing: production manager, technical manager, stage crew manager.
- *Business management*: Financial, legal and contractual management of the company: company manager, orchestra manager, business manager.
- *Development and education programme*: Sponsorship of company and productions; promoting company and productions; press,

publicity and marketing of tours; educational function – company tours of schools, places of higher education, lectures and exhibitions. Friends of company: development officer, sponsorship officer, press officer, marketing officer, merchandizing officer, education office, theatre-in-education staff; the extent of printed material may suggest a graphic design department.
- *Clerical*: Assistants and secretaries, local storage.

Associated areas may include:

- board room, with lobby, toilets and severy;
- library and facilities for a librarian;
- music room, with piano and provision for recorded music, for selection of orchestral music, opera or dance;
- audition room, with adjacent waiting area;
- working conference room: for direction and design meetings;
- model-making facilities for the preparation of models of sets and model store;
- photographic dark room, for lighting designer;
- general storage;
- toilets;
- office services: copying and printing, mailing facilities, telephone and other communications, refreshment areas; separate entrance and reception.

Provision may be necessary for the organization of a *touring* company without a 'home' concert hall or theatre, or a resident company which also tours, within and beyond its region, who initiate their own productions. For such companies they may require:

- *Tour management:* Tour planning and promotion: tour manager, promotion manager.
- *Transport:* Either by owning, leasing or hiring vehicles. If owned, provision for parking must be considered. Organization of the transportation of personnel, equipment, staging, musical instruments and other items, as appropriate: touring may be local, regional, country-wide, continent-wide or world-wide. This is an important aspect of organization for national companies – opera, dance, drama, symphonic music – as well as musicals, and pop/rock concerts in particular. Such planning of tours and transport arrangements become a major function of the organization: transport manager.

Offices, and associated areas, for the organization of a resident company should be grouped together and located within easy access of rehearsal spaces, the auditorium and platform/stage, managerial offices and, for the designers and production manager, other production departments. Certain functions may be shared with the managerial offices such as board room, copying equipment, library, archives and so on, which suggest that grouping of the offices for company organization and management would be beneficial. The juxtaposition of, say, the artistic/music director and general manager/executive would have operational benefits.

Catering

The scale of the company organization, along with the management organization requirements, may justify the inclusion of catering facilities as the common social and refreshment area. Such a facility could be also used by the performers and technicians if within the same building.

Within the production organization the catering facilities can act as a lounge for performers awaiting rehearsals, a venue for social occasions and business lunches, and a general point of contact. Consider

- hot meals, beverages, alcoholic drinks;
- size and shape;
- kitchen layout;
- method of service (e.g. self-service);
- method of supplying goods to, and removing refuse from, the kitchen;
- catering staff facilities including office, rest room and toilets;
- users' toilets and cloakroom, especially if used by invited visitors.

Rehearsal spaces

Rehearsal spaces – rehearsal room, rehearsal studio and practice studio – are used for the development of a production by the conductor, director, choreographer or instructor.

Rehearsal room and rehearsal studio

Consider the number, type and size required:

- For orchestra, choir and opera chorus: a *rehearsal room* with a tiered floor, able to accommodate the total numbers in the orchestra, choir or chorus.
- For chamber orchestra and jazz groups: a *rehearsal room* with a flat floor able to accommodate total numbers in orchestra or group.
- For opera, musical and drama, and also rock/pop: a *rehearsal room* with a flat floor, able to accommodate the largest performing area on the stage. These rehearsals may require partial or complete use of the performance scenery or staging arrangements (Fig. 13.19).
- For dance: a *rehearsal studio* with a wooden sprung flat floor, able to accommodate the largest performing area on the stage; may also be used for exercise and practice before a performance by the resident company; practice barres and wall mirrors are necessary (Fig. 13.20).

Other aspects of rehearsal spaces to be borne in mind include:

- Other users: rehearsal spaces could be hired out to other companies, if not fully used by the resident company.
- Other uses: rehearsal spaces could be used as a recital room or drama studio theatre with public access, especially if there is temporary or permanent seating, performance lighting and sound their control, access from changing/dressing rooms. Further uses could be as temporary changing/dressing room; for recording music;

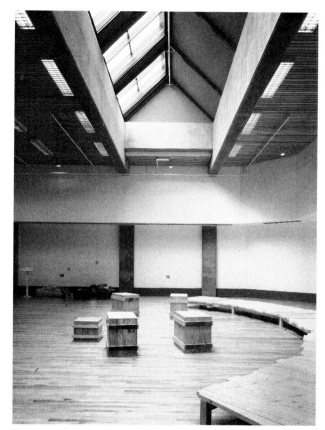

Fig. 13.19 *Rehearsal room. An example of a rehearsal room with top daylight (able to be blanked off) and sprung floor: The West Yorkshire Playhouse, Leeds*

holding fitness classes or drama and music workshops.

- Changing rooms, toilets, lounge: these will be necessary if the rehearsal room or studio is separate from the building complex, if changing or dressing rooms are not available during rehearsal hours, or if other companies are rehearsing.
- Storage: directly off rehearsal room or studio, a store will be needed for accommodating furniture, equipment, rostra and so on when not in use.
- Public entrance: if the public are to be admitted for performances and other uses then separate access is necessary with a sound lobby and access to toilets.
- Location: rehearsal spaces should be at the same level as the platform/stage and workshops for the convenience of movement of, as applicable, scenery, properties and musical instruments, with ease of access from stage door/performance entrance and changing or dressing rooms.

The relationship between activities is shown in Fig. 13.21.

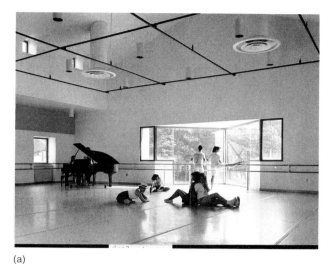

(a)

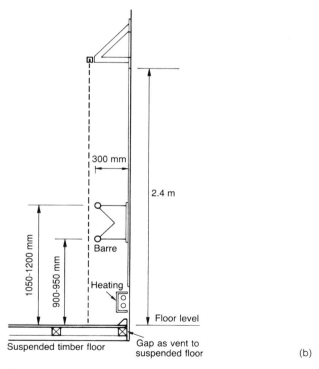

(b)

Fig. 13.20 *Rehearsal Studio. (a) An example of a rehearsal studio: Performing Arts Centre, Cornell University, Ithaca, New York State. (b) Section through wall barres in rehearsal studio for dance practice showing heights of barres and mirror: continuous heating below the barres is necessary as is the suspended timber floor*

Practice studios

For the development of performers or students it may be necessary to provide studios for individual or group practice, tuition or rehearsal. Consider the number and type required for speech, movement, singing, instrumental music, whether for individuals or groups; other uses such as changing or dressing rooms,

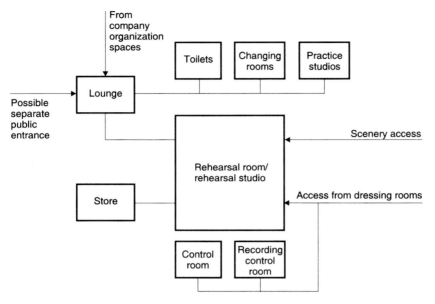

Fig. 13.21 *Rehearsal room/rehearsal studio: relationship between activities*

sound recording room; equipment requirements which may include piano, music stands, gramophone and tape recorder, according to the function of the studio. The studios may be located as part of a rehearsal complex with ease of access for the performers and instructors. Practice studios may be associated with educational institutions: music schools, drama schools, music departments in schools and places of higher education.

Scenery workshops

The mounting of any opera, dance, musical or drama production and also rock/pop concert requires spaces for the preparation of scenery and properties. Consider the facilities described in the following sections.

Offices

Those requiring office space can include head of carpentry workshop, head of paint shop, and head of property department, i.e. those in supervisory positions in each of the main working areas.

Carpentry workshop

For the construction of scenery, power-operated tools (such as wood working machine, mortise, lathes, circular and bandsaws); benches for carpentry, assembly and canvassing; storage of raw materials such as timber, sheet materials, rolls of materials, nails, and screws and so on, including polystyrene sheets which may require a separate fire resistant enclosure (Fig. 13.22).

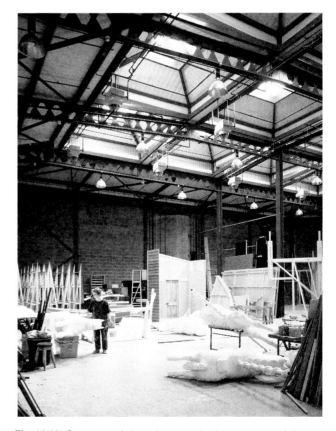

Fig. 13.22 *Scenery workshop. An example of a scenery workshop with a trail assembly area and carpentry shop beyond: The West Yorkshire Playhouse, Leeds*

Paint shop

The paint shop is for the painting of scenery, backcloths and flats (painted flat on the floor or on a paint frame) and three dimensional pieces. Benches will be needed for mixing paints and for other preparation and cleaning brushes. Storage will be required for raw materials such as paints and equipment such as brushes and spray equipment. Paints may need to be stored in a fire-proof enclosure.

For details of a paint frame, see Fig. 13.23.

Metalwork shop

The use of metal in the preparation of scenery is increasing. Provision for welding, cutting and fabricating metalwork items includes benches, welding screens and bending machinery and storage arrangements for raw materials such as sheets, tubes and bars, and bolts, nuts and screws.

Trial assembly area

An area should be provided for the erection of a trial assembly of the set under construction, at least the size of the performing area of the stage.

Property department

For the preparation of properties, worktops and storage areas for raw materials will be required. Two separate workshops may be required: one for polystyrene and fibreglass work with associated fire-resistant requirements and extraction of toxic gases; the other for work with other materials.

Delivery of raw materials

Provision should be made for the delivery and storage of raw materials to the carpentry workshop, paint shop, metalwork shop and property department, including arrangements at the unloading bay and for parking of delivery vans and lorries.

Storage

Storage facilities are needed for scenery and properties, including armoury, for re-use.

Sequence of operations

The main activities in the preparation of *scenery* are carpentry and painting. The sequence of operations include:

1. Delivery by van and lorry and subsequent storage of the raw materials.
2. Cutting and making up of scenery in the carpentry shop.
3. Trial assembly of the set: the trial assembly area should be the focal point of the workshop.
4. Painting of the backcloths and flats on a paint frame in a separate area, and of the three-dimensional pieces in the trial assembly area.
5. Storage before movement onto the stage.
6. Return of scenery for re-use or to permanent storage in the building or elsewhere.

The following points must be considered:

- The floor should be at the same level for workshops, unloading bays, scenery store and stage, with a clear broad passage of movement of scenery to the stage. If change of level is inevitable then a lift will be necessary but is not recommended.
- The paint frame and backcloth storage should be positioned so that the rolled backcloths can be moved horizontally into position under the flytower (if applicable) or grid and, when flown, the painted surface faces the audience.
- It must be possible for people to pass from area to area and to the stage without having to use the large doors or roller shutters required for the movement of scenery.
- The carpentry shop should be separate from the paint shop because of noise and possible sawdust penetration.
- The carpentry shop and paint shop should be so planned that noise from them does not penetrate the stage. Scenery storage located between workshops and stage will act as a sound barrier.
- If touring companies are anticipated, the unloading bay should be provided directly onto the stage without interfering with the workshops.
- Openings between spaces and the relationship between spaces should be designed to facilitate the easy movement of scenery. Minimum dimensions of openings are determined by the maximum height and width of scenery.

The preparation of *properties* follows a similar sequence: delivery and storage of raw materials,

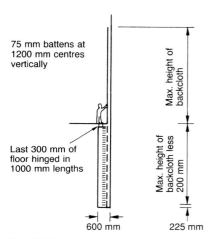

75 mm battens at 1200 mm centres vertically

Last 300 mm of floor hinged in 1000 mm lengths

Max. height of backcloth

Max. height of backcloth less 200 mm

600 mm   225 mm

Fig. 13.23 *Paint frame. Section through vertically movable paint frame in slot in floor*

making-up, storage before use on the stage, re-use or stored. For the relationship between activities see Fig. 13.24.

Wardrobe (Fig. 13.25)

Space will be required for the making and fitting of performers' costumes and associated items such as wigs, as well as facilities for storing, repairing and cleaning the costumes for a performance. Consider the amount, type and size of equipment and benches

required for cutting and making-up costumes, and the number and type of fitting rooms for performers to try on their costumes. Separate spaces will be needed for wig making and millinery accessories; dyeing cloth and spraying materials; storage of raw materials (rolls of cloth, pattern paper) and small items (sewing materials, dye stuffs and so on). Arrangements should be made for taking delivery of raw materials including at the unloading bay and for the parking of delivery vans and subsequently for the method of moving finished costumes to the dressing rooms. An office will

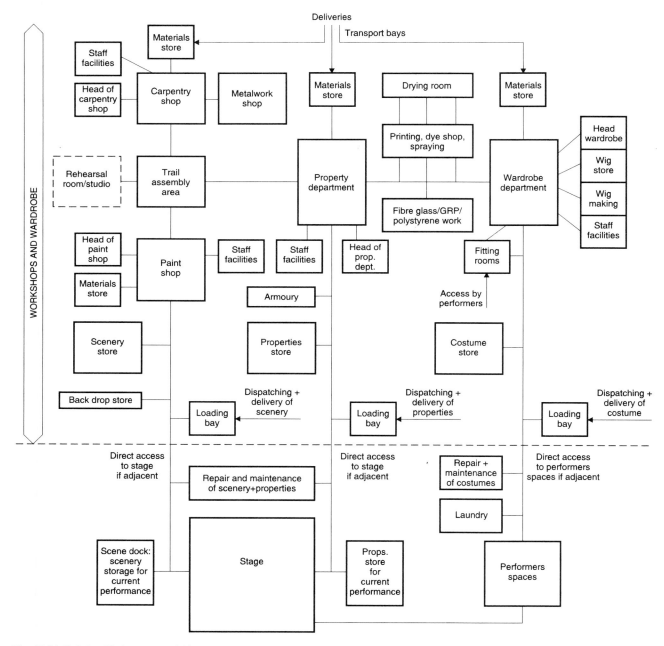

Fig. 13.24 *Relationship between activities: scenery workshop and wardrobe*

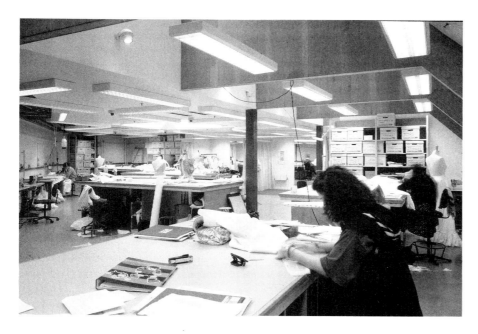

Fig. 13.25 *Wardrobe. An example of a wardrobe showing work room and office beyond: The West Yorkshire Playhouse, Leeds*

be needed for the costume supervisor, located in a supervisory position.

The sequence of operations for preparing *costumes* is

1 Delivery of materials e.g. rolls of cloth by van and lorry and the storage of the materials.
2 Cutting and making up.
3 Fitting costumes on performers in fitting rooms.
4 Finishing off and adjustment.
5 Storage before delivery to dressing rooms.
6 Re-use or put into storage within the building or elsewhere.

Wig making should relate to the main working area: printing, spraying and dyeing and glassfibre work should be carried out in separate areas with access to both property and wardrobe departments.

Performers require ease of access to the wardrobe for fitting costumes, while the distribution of finished costumes for, and their cleaning during, a production suggests a location close to the dressing rooms. For the relationship between activities see Fig. 13.24.

Recording studio (Fig. 13.26)

Sound effects and music

An isolated space, with a control room, will be required for the recording of sound effects and music associated with a production. It will be used by the sound designer working with the director or choreographer. Consider the size and shape of the recording studio – the number of musicians is a critical

aspect – and the control room, including its equipment and play-back facilities. Associated areas include a library of tapes and discs.

Facilities for recording within the building complex can be grouped with the electrician's workshop, office and sound equipment store as well as the control rooms to the auditorium to form a 'suite' of accommodation centred around the electricians. A sound lock is required between the circulation and control room, and between the control room and the recording studio. The first could be expanded to form a small lounge for visitors, with a sound lobby into the control room. A viewing panel is required between

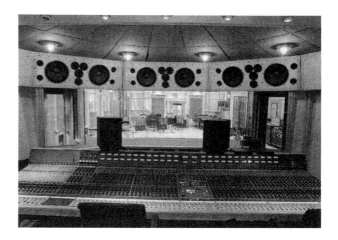

Fig. 13.26 *Recording studio. (a) An example of a recording studio with the control room, observation window and studio beyond.*

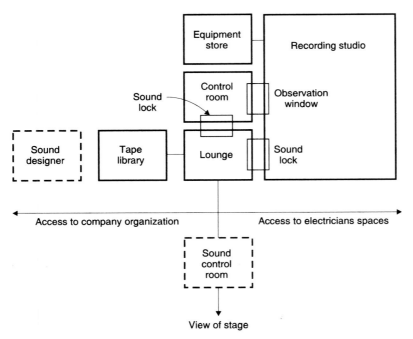

Fig. 13.26 *Recording studio. (b) Relationship between functions*

control room and studio. The area needs to be acoustically isolated.

Subsequent sound facilities include:

- *Library*: Storage of tapes and discs, requiring cupboard or room, with shelves, 300 mm wide, and catalogue system.
- *Studio*: If it is only to be used for sound effects the studio can be small: for the recording of live music then the space needs to allow for the number of musicians (though this would be restricted). If a large number of musicians were required then hiring commercial facilities, especially if an infrequent occurrence, would be economically beneficial.
- *Control room*: For the operators, recording equipment and play-back facilities. The control room requires a double-glazed sound-insulated window to the studio and a double door/lobby access. The mixing and editing of recorded music and sound effects can be carried out in the control room: if so, then the quality of the sound reproduction and internal acoustics need to satisfy the needs of the listener. As with the studio, the control room needs to be insulated from sound from adjacent areas and the ventilation should be silent.
- *Lounge*: If the recording studio is to be used by others, or on behalf of others, then it is desirable to include a lounge for visitors with a sound lobby into the control room.

- *Lobby*: A sound lobby from the access corridor is necessary to ensure isolation from adjacent areas.

Electronic music

For composers of electronic music, facilities are necessary for the production, recording and editing of sounds. Briefing requirements are similar to those listed under recording studios above. The recording studio for electronic music can be located with ease of access by the resident or visiting composer from their offices and entrance.

Electronic music can be composed using a computer where the facilities for the composer include such equipment – a processor unit and a VDU.

Common facilities

Consider the number and type of staff for each section of the production spaces, and the facilities required for resting, changing, refreshment and other provisions such as toilets and showers.

Transport

For those buildings for the performing arts initiating their own productions, a van or vans for the collection and delivery of goods may be justified. Parking space will be necessary within the curtilage of the site.

14

14 Building design

The initial brief will have produced a schedule of accommodation as a list of functions, their spatial requirements and their floor areas. The schedule should be checked against known comparable examples. Relevant current literature should be surveyed and appropriate existing buildings visited to extract experience of the building type.

Layouts should be considered which satisfy site, circulation, construction, environmental, statutory, economic and other requirements.

General considerations effecting the building design include the following:

Relationships between functions
External access
Internal circulation
Means of escape
Sub-divisions
Phasing and flexibility
Acoustic strategy
Energy strategy
Fire protection
Security
Ventilation
Heating
Lighting
Communications

Plumbing and drainage
Cleaning and refuse
Plant rooms
Integration and distribution of services
Structure
Internal finishes, windows, doors, fittings and equipment
Signage and works of art
External works
Form
Approvals

Relationships between functions (Fig. 14.1)

The operational patterns and relationships between functions are common to each of the broad categories of buildings for the performing arts, covering:

- buildings for music, with or without rehearsal facilities;
- buildings for opera, musicals and drama, with or without production facilities.

External access

External pedestrian and/or vehicular access is required for the following where applicable:

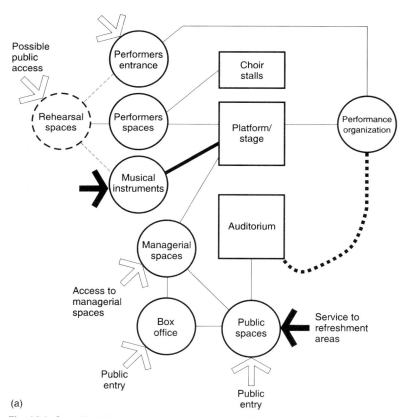

(a)

Fig. 14.1 *Overall relationships between functions. (a) Buildings for orchestral and choral classical music (with choir stalls), jazz and pop/rock music (without choir stalls).*

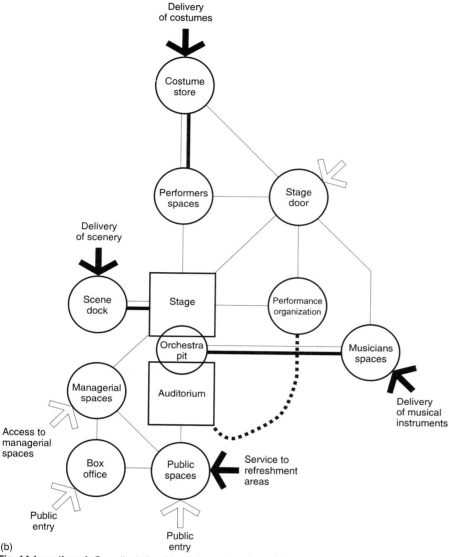

Delivery
of costumes

Costume
store

Performers
spaces

Stage
door

Delivery
of scenery

Scene
dock

Stage

Performance
organization

Orchestra
pit

Musicians
spaces

Managerial
spaces

Auditorium

Delivery
of musical
instruments

Access to
managerial
spaces

Box
office

Public
spaces

Service to
refreshment
areas

Public
entry

Public
entry

(b)

Fig. 14.1 continued *Overall relationships between functions. (b) Buildings for opera, musicals, dance and drama, which receive touring companies only, or with a resident company whose production facilities are located elsewhere. The orchestra pit and musicians' spaces may not be applicable if for drama only.*

- public, with general and special needs, to the entrance foyer, box office, restaurant and other facilities; orientation towards principal pedestrian and vehicular routes;
- staff: combined or separate access for performers, management, technicians and workshop staff;
- goods delivery and collection: food and drink, empties and refuse collection, scenery, properties, costumes, musical instruments, raw materials, small goods, workshop refuse; separate entrance, road access and off-street lay-bys are necessary for vehicles delivering and collecting;
- fire engines, ambulances, TV and radio transmission vans, disabled persons' cars, external maintenance and access to replace equipment;

- replacement of boilers, chillers, air-conditioning units and other equipment.

Internal circulation

Routes taken by the public and by the various categories of staff are specific and mainly follow a sequential functional pattern through the different sections of the building complex. The layout and planning of each section should allow for ease of movement within and between each section to ensure efficient and effective use. The following should be considered:

- food and drink delivery, and empties and refuse collection: vertical movement, if necessary, requires

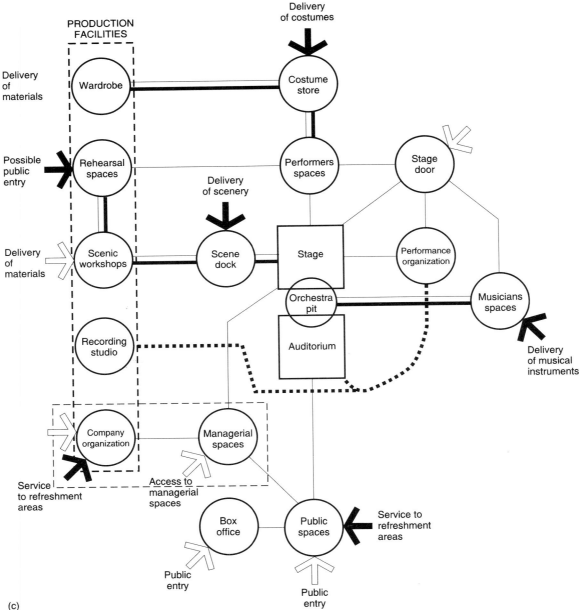

PRODUCTION
FACILITIES

Delivery
of costumes

Delivery
of
materials

Wardrobe

Costume
store

Possible
public
entry

Rehearsal
spaces

Performers
spaces

Stage
door

Delivery
of scenery

Delivery
of
materials

Scenic
workshops

Scene
dock

Stage

Performance
organization

Musicians
spaces

Orchestra
pit

Recording
studio

Auditorium

Delivery
of musical
instruments

Company
organization

Managerial
spaces

Service
to refreshment
areas

Access to
managerial
spaces

Box
office

Public
spaces

Service to
refreshment
areas

Public
entry

Public
entry

(c)

Fig. 14.1 continued *Overall relationships between functions. (c) Buildings for opera, musicals, dance and drama, with their own production facilities. The orchestra pit and musicians' spaces may not be applicable if for drama only*

a lift to serve the bars, cellars, kitchen and stores from delivery and collection points;

- public areas: vertical circulation requires stairs and lifts with ramps and escalators also possible; horizontal circulation requires access to all points of entry into the auditorium and to all amenities;
- changing/dressing rooms: staircase access only from upper and lower floors to the stage level; lift primarily for costume distribution;
- scenery and properties: the scene dock, stage and workshops should be at the same level, and the

width of openings able to accommodate the size of the scenery (minimum width of 2.4 m); change of level should be avoided but, if inevitable, then a large goods lift will be required;

- wardrobe: lift access is necessary for delivery of raw materials, and distribution of costumes, if the wardrobe is at an upper level;
- performance lighting and sound: horizontal and vertical access needs to be out of sight of the audience; lift access is desirable for the transport of lighting and sound equipment to the upper levels

serving the control rooms and lighting bridges, and the electrical store(s).

- flytower: if included in the brief, the flytower, could be served by a small lift as well as an access staircase.

Principal aspects of internal circulation are dependent on regulations and controls arising from fire safety considerations. Stairwells and corridors need to be wide enough and free of obstruction (fixtures recessed) to provide safe movement. Congestion and conflict of movements can be avoided by the incorporation of threshold spaces at access points, where people will change direction and particularly in the area of staircases.

Lifts, other than the one serving the flytower, should accommodate a wheelchair user.

Means of escape

Escape routes are required from each level within the auditorium: the number and width are governed by legislation. Separate escape routes will be necessary from each level and for persons in wheelchairs through protected areas directly to the outside as places of safety. Legislation is applied by the local government and fire authority to whom formal applications for approval are required: layouts should be discussed before application. The local fire authority is required to inspect and approve the escape routes (and other conditions) before issuing a certificate and licence.

Escape routes are also needed from the technical areas, platform/stage, performers' spaces and public areas as well as, if applicable, the various workshop spaces. An alternative escape route will be required in most instances from each of the functional areas and from each of the floors. Staircases, as a means of escape, may have to be enclosed with fire-resistant walls to form protected areas. The maximum travel distance from the furthest point in a space to a protected area is defined by legislation.

Sub-divisions

Certain areas may need to be closed off for security or operational reasons. The workshops may be in use during times when the rest of the building complex can be closed off. With multi-auditoria complexes, one auditorium and its back-stage facilities, should be capable of being closed off if not in use.

Phasing and flexibility

The building complex may need to be divided into phases to be developed over time or constructed in a single operation. However it should be recognized that an auditorium and its performance support facilities is an autonomous unit and cannot be so sub-divided. Production facilities, if applicable, can be considered for construction during a later phase, as can storage, Theatre-in-Education, and other similar discrete facilities. Similarly with multi-auditoria complexes and

when part of a large building such as an educational establishment, phasing is more easily achieved. The implication of noise penetration from construction of the subsequent phases on the built auditorium should be carefully considered. Areas need to be allocated on the site for the future expansion.

Allowance needs to be made for changes internally to the technology – performance and sound equipment, platform/stage machinery, information and communication technology, security systems – and to the organization requiring, say, changes to the layout of the offices, dressing/changing rooms, workshops and similar spaces.

Acoustic strategy

Acoustic control is required between potentially conflicting internal activities and external noise sources, while also considering the acoustic performance of those spaces with particular characteristics such as the auditorium. These cover:

- isolation of noise sources within the building. These include: use of foyer and public places to eat and drink during performance times; washing up noises in bar and kitchen areas; workshop and wardrobe; toilets; talking in green room and other performers' spaces; plant rooms.
- exclusion of external noise, from acoustically sensitive areas such as the auditorium and platform/stage, and the rehearsal room/studio, with transport (vehicles, trains, aeroplanes) usually the main source of external noise. Support accommodation can be located as an acoustic buffer between the external sources and, say, the auditorium. The method of construction can increase the sound reduction, while the layout can position the more sensitive areas away from the external sources of noise.
- isolation of the auditorium, including structural separation from support accommodation and pad foundation separating structure from ground-borne sound; auditorium surrounded by a corridor as acoustic buffer which has the added benefit of providing a circulation route.
- restrictions on the noise level generated by the activities in the building affecting adjacent properties such as rock music from the auditorium, delivery and removal of scenery by lorry and van and the public arriving and leaving before, and especially after, a performance. These aspects should be evaluated under site considerations as to the acoustic sensitivity of the surrounding areas: the design though can assist in reducing or avoiding interference.
- sound locks at points of entry into acoustically sensitive areas, such as public access into the auditorium, performers entry onto the platform/stage, and rehearsal room/studio, technicians entry into control room, flytower and lighting bridges.
- local acoustic treatment, e.g. acoustic insulation to pipework through sensitive areas.

- acoustic design of the auditorium and platform/stage and also the rehearsal room/studio, foyer (especially if used for performances) and recording studio, including ventilation system and air-conditioning which require to serve each space only.

Energy strategy

Consider sources of energy and the need for energy efficiency as well as computation of energy demand from cooling, heating, ventilation and electricity. Analyse the pattern of use and possible need for zoning to allow independent use of separate areas. Such calculations will indicate loadings, equipment type and size of plant rooms.

Measures to *conserve* energy which may affect the layout and fabric of the building include:

- compact form to reduce internal volume and external surface;
- orientation of those areas that would benefit thermally from controlled solar gain;
- active solar devices and heat storage;
- protection from prevailing winds, including landscape;
- reduction of openings, especially on north side in the northern hemisphere;
- air locks at external doors, to avoid escape of warm air, including scene dock and other unloading points;
- heat recovery systems and heat pumps;
- insulation levels within external walls and roof;
- selection of building materials to include renewable resources;
- fuel selection, in the light of a national energy policy, costs and future predictions; inclusion in district heating system;
- use of excess heat from cooling and extraction with the air-conditioning system to the auditorium in the rest of the building or adjacent buildings;
- avoidance of air-conditioning by including natural ventilation and cooling.

Buildings for the performing arts are relatively high-energy with especially high electrical loadings due to the performance lighting and sound, and air-conditioning. This affects the cost-in-use with heating, ventilation and electricity the main contributors.

Fire protection

The following precautions need to be considered:

- building divided into fire resistant compartments;
- enclosing staircases if part of the escape route with fire resisting material;
- automatic fire dampers, with access, in ducts at all points where they pass through compartment walls and floors;
- smoke exhaust/extract system: possible requirements in scene dock and other storage areas;

- detector system: heat and smoke activated sensors;
- automatic sprinkler system: most areas, except the auditorium and circulation routes, will require sprinkler coverage; consider routes, horizontal and vertical distribution and possible water tank requirement;
- alarms: connected to automatic detector systems and central indicator panel, with possible link to local fire station;
- extinguishers and hose reels: location and type, distributed through the building;
- fire resistance of walls and doors, and also services;
- fire fighting access point for local fire brigade and equipment.

Fire precautions need to be discussed with the local fire authority, fire insurers and building control inspectors.

Security

Buildings for the performing arts, as with other building types, are susceptible to theft and vandalism. Consideration should be given to the surveillance of public areas during opening hours, detection of trespassers on site out of opening hours, protection of the building from possible break-ins and the detection of break-ins as well as special protection of valuable items. Methods include:

- visual surveillance by staff of public at entrance, within places to eat and drink, and along circulation routes; control at entry doors into the auditorium;
- burglar alarms to openings – doors and windows – and within internal areas, activated at times of break-in;
- surveillance systems (closed-circuit television) at fire exit doors and other external doors, service yard, open spaces and 'blind' external walls;
- external lights, operating during hours of darkness;
- security guards in building when closed;
- selection of materials to discourage break-ins: such as door construction, glass thickness, shutters to windows and other materials selected to be anti-vandal;
- locking off sections of the building when not in use;
- door locks with key or card control to dressing rooms, pass door to offices from public areas or to back stage areas, and so on;
- checking of vehicles entering and leaving service yard with automatic barrier at entrance;
- staff entry control: stage door, management reception;
- special protection: money, computer data, records and so on able to be locked away in safes.

A central control point for the security and surveillance systems needs to be identified, associated with, say, entrance reception desk or stage door.

Discuss proposals with local police advisory service and insurance company.

Ventilation

Areas possibly requiring *air-conditioning*, as separate systems for reasons of noise control, include the auditorium, recording studio, meeting rooms, public areas, particularly bar and kitchen servery, and rehearsal room/studio. *Mechanical* ventilation will be necessary where rooms are internal, such as toilets, showers, stores and circulation as well as meeting rooms, public areas and rehearsal room/studio if air-conditioning is not required. *Natural* ventilation will be appropriate to perimeter offices, dressing/changing rooms and other rooms, and rooms at roof level which can benefit from top light.

Heating

Consider the methods of heating:

- in the auditorium and other spaces which have air-conditioning there will be heating and also cooling included within the system.
- other areas can have warm air heating, radiators, convectors or radiant panels. A simple radiator system should be adequate for offices, dressing rooms and other small rooms: space heaters and radiant panels, for the workshops; radiant panels for stage areas and scenery storage.

Lighting

Consider the following general issues: particular requirements are discussed within the description of each space:

- *Natural lighting*: Glazing to be positioned to avoid glare, reflections and unwanted solar gain and heat loss.
- *Artificial lighting*: General considerations include quality and quantity of light, efficiency and initial and on-going costs as well as type (fluorescent, low voltage, tungsten, tungsten/halogen, sodium), location (ceiling, wall or track-mounted, uplighters), shielding of fittings (for protection, say, in workshops), if dimmer switching and location of lighting control (locally in dressing rooms, centrally in public areas).

Lighting installation should consider:

- task lighting: intensity of light on the working plane;
- amenity lighting: general lighting within a room or circulation area;
- special lighting effects, including performance lighting in auditorium;
- safety;
- security;
- emergency: automatic alternative system if power fails;
- external: floodlighting to emphasize and model architectural features, and assist awareness of building; screened floodlighting of trees, works of art, display; lighting of access routes, down lighting at entrance canopies; lighting of emergency exit doors and routes.
- warning lights: at points of entry to the stage/platform, rehearsal spaces, recording studios and possibly to the auditorium, indicating that the space is in use.

Communications

Consider the following:

- telephone systems: one or more exchange lines with either a small switching system or switchboard (e.g. PABX); external and/or internal systems and number of outlets for staff and public;
- provision of multi-core cable installation and outlets for computer consoles and closed-circuit television;
- public address, tannoy system, paging;
- facsimile transmission;
- video transmission of performance, television;
- postal services.

Power

Consider the number and distribution of power points for specialist equipment, cleaning and local lighting, and the size and location of distribution trunking.

Plumbing and drainage

Consider requirements, including:

- position and space for water tank(s) including mains water supply, overflow necessities and insulation as well as access and maintenance.
- position and size of water pipes and distribution around the building.
- position and size of soil-vent pipes in relation to sanitary installations and floor gulleys.
- position and size of internal and external manholes, including connections to existing foul and surface-water sewers.
- position and size of rain water down pipes and gulleys, and surface water gulleys to outdoor areas.
- water supply for sprinkler system and hose reels.
- number and location of interception, e.g. kitchen.

Cleaning and refuse

Consider when the cleaning of the building will be done and the method: provision should be made for cleaners' stores and sinks within each functional area; socket outlets as power supply to cleaning equipment within each space; selection of floor and other surfaces for ease of cleaning.

Consider the method and frequency of refuse disposal: position and number of containers and skips, and method of enclosure, full enclosure will need to be ventilated.

Plant rooms

Spaces are required to accommodate plant and include:

- water storage tank(s);
- electrical sub-station;
- emergency installation;
- boilers and other space heating;
- ventilation/air treatment plant, including cooling;
- gas meter;
- fuel storage: oil tank, coal bunker;
- control and monitoring equipment;
- electrical meters.

Consider internal and external access to plant rooms, maintenance requirements and location and size of air supply and extract grilles, as well as provision and location of services: gas, electricity, water, drainage and telephone and cable television. Local suppliers of services have to be consulted: check capacity and ability to accept increased loading, connection charges and ability to meet building programme if supply is to be changed. Ensure that adequate supply services are available: note that very heavy electrical loads will be involved.

Integration and distribution of services

Consider size and location of horizontal and vertical ducts to receive services: position of distribution boards; access to ducts and trunking; flexibility with the future addition of cabling; separation of power, telephone, co-axial, performance lighting and performance sound cables. The location of plant rooms and main distribution runs must be considered together with the structure at an early stage in the design and development, if the services are to be satisfactorily integrated. An aim is to keep service runs to a minimum.

The use of the ceiling zone to the corridor about the auditorium can be the principal horizontal distribution for circulation and noise control services.

Structure

Investigate structural options for various layouts as either frame structure or load bearing walls, as well as establishing floor loads, storey heights and distribution of services. The structure to the auditorium is discussed on p. 131 and the platform/stage and flytower on p. 144. Workshops are basically industrial spaces but note the height requirements for large items of scenery. Most other spaces are cellular in character and have requirements similar to those for offices and domestic work.

Selection of external material – brickwork, blockwork, natural or cast stone, metal cladding, concrete, timber – will depend on context, cost and buildability: context includes attitude towards general character of the immediate area, the image being considered for the

building and the type of building for the performing arts.

Internal finishes, windows, doors, fittings and equipment

Public buildings are heavily used, not only all the areas used by the public but also the platform/stage, support facilities and workshops are subject to heavy treatment. Materials need to be robust to counter abuse, easy to clean, offer minimum maintenance, and be suitable for various functions within the building. The choice of finishes and components should respond to the general theme of the interior design in all functional areas, and respond to the requirements of disabled persons.

Signage and works of art

Both signage and works of art will need to be incorporated into the interior and exterior design. Signage needs to cover directional information for different users, instructions, statutory requirements covering means of escape, and information for people in wheelchairs at their eye level. Signage in braille should be considered. Signage is an important component in all areas and should be considered at an early stage in the design process. Direction signage in complexes with more than one auditorium within the public spaces needs particular attention to ensure clear instructions to direct the public to the correct level in each auditorium.

Works of art can be 'built in' or applied: a percentage of the capital cost of building should be allowed, and discussions with artists or arts promotion organizations should occur early in the design process.

External works

Landscape and siting proposals associated with the building design include:

- access requirement: roadways, pathways, links to adjacent buildings;
- planting and other landscape features, including improving micro-climate conditions, scale and protection;
- outdoor performance areas: informal and formal;
- terraces and outdoor seating areas, associated with public entrance and other spaces;
- artificial lighting: general access, landscape features, security, fire escape routes;
- external signs: identification of building, directional, information, flag poles;
- site security;
- car parking for public, disabled, visitors and staff: allow 20–30 m² per space.
- van and lorry parking for resident and/or touring companies

Consideration should be given to the visual effect of the external works during daylight hours, evening hours and when the building is not in use at night.

Form (Fig. 14.2)

The massing of alternative layouts, relating to site conditions and adjoining building or landscape, needs to consider:

- The dominance of the auditorium in the layout, as the focus of the circulation and support accommodation, but not necessarily the largest area, can be either expressed externally or suppressed within the body of the building.
- The problem of scale created by the large volumes of the auditorium and platform/stage, with the use of support accommodation to reduce the scale.
- The particular problem of the flytower, if included, which can be acknowledged as an essential feature and expressed architecturally, or the ancillary accommodation can be built up to disguise the flytower (Fig. 14.3).
- An overall thematic expression or distinct character to each functional area.
- The image: an appropriate image needs to be defined which communicates the style of the venue, and can be a civic edifice or a community-orientated building, formal or informal, traditional visual references or radical, emphasis on ritual or casual organization, elite expression or democratic, exclusive or open image, emphasis on public facade or overall sculptural composition.
- The method of ordering the building: geometric, organic expression, classicist approach, democratic expression with all the accommodation under a unifying roof form.
- Urban design context: isolated building, integrated into street frontage, within landscape setting, or related to a civic open space or atrium; building for the performing arts as generator of activity especially during evening hours; strategic view of public entrance and other architectural features, such as the flytower, within the urban context.

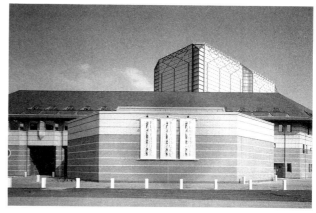

(a)

(b)

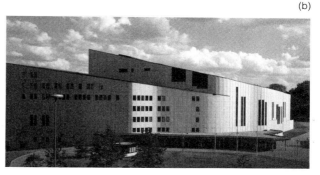

Fig. 14.3 *Flytower. (a) West Yorkshire Playhouse, Leeds: Flytower acknowledged as an essential feature seen as the visual pivot of the architectural composition and a decorative opportunity. (b) Opera House, Essen: Ancillary accommodation built up to disguise the bulk of the flytower: a common sloping roof allows the lower section over the public spaces and the higher over the tower and production spaces*

- Rural design context: heights of building in relation to trees, colour of external materials to complement or contrast with the landscape; as part of a landscape composition with the building as a visual focus.

Examples of massing are shown in Fig. 14.4.

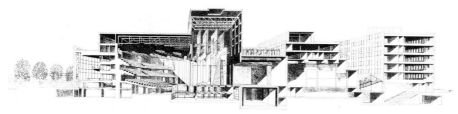

Fig. 14.2 *Three-dimensional organization. The section and perspective of the Opera House in Amsterdam shows the main functional areas and their organization: the public foyer and circulation levels relating to the auditorium levels, the auditorium including (in this example) two balconies, the ceiling zone over the auditorium including structure and services as well as acoustic treatment and performance lighting positions, the stage areas including the flytower and rear stage provision. The illustration also shows the building in its wider urban context with its link to the municipal offices, in this example*

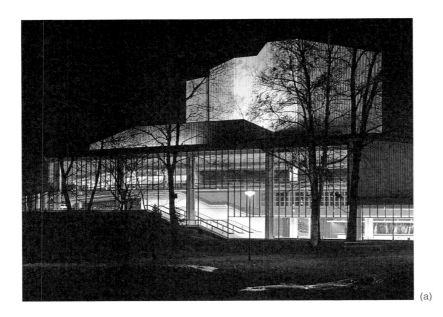

(a)

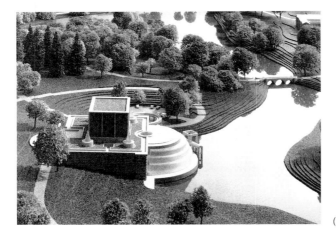

(b)

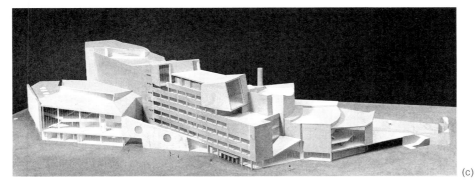

(c)

Fig. 14.4 *Massing. (a) Civic Theatre, Helsinki. Use of flytower to this theatre as a visual pivot, while the lower glazed foyer wraps around the auditorium, and allows views to, and from, the adjacent park. (Architects: Timo Penttila.) (b) Model of the proposed opera house at Compton Verney with a formal layout, emphasizing the central axis of the auditorium, stage and public spaces. The bulk of the rear stages and unloading and scene dock is visually lost with these facilities set within the hill behind. (Architects: Hans Larson.) (c) Model of the competition-winning scheme for a theatre in Mannheim. The sculptural form is located within the city square and is viewed from all sides. The orthogonal backbone of offices and flytower to the main auditorium contrasts with the organic spaces for the public to the two auditoria. (Architects: Hans Sharoun.)*

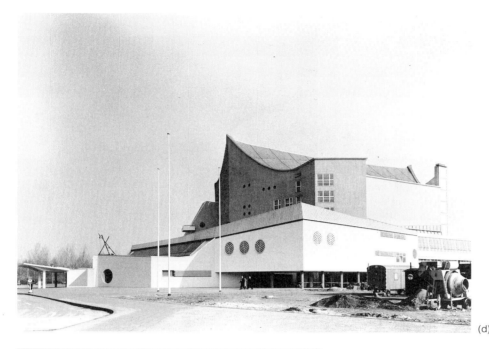

(d)

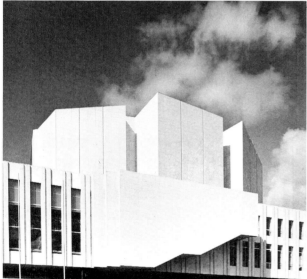

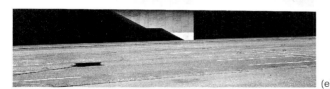

(e)

Fig. 14.4 continued *Massing. (d) Berlin Philharmonic. Three dimensional form, for a concert hall, expressing the organic nature of the layout, with the auditorium emerging from the lower large foyer spaces and ancillary accommodation. (Architects: Hans Sharoun.) (e) Finlandia, Helsinki, concert hall and conference centre. The sculptured auditorium form emerges from the lower foyer block. The staircase from the main foyer level to the balcony level is cantilevered from the main façade. (Architects: Alvar Aalto.)*

Approvals and legislation

Approvals affect all stages in design and building processes, and are concerned with public authorities applying appropriate legislation and regulations. The power and jurisdiction of these authorities vary from country to country. Extensive legislation controls new building work and adaptation of existing buildings, and requires discussion with, and formal application to, various public authorities. These include the bodies discussed in the following sections.

Planning application

An application for planning permission covers new development, change of use and extensions, including car-parking, disabled requirements, access, drainage and design policy. If an existing building is listed and subject to a conservation order, then consent to alter, convert and extend is also required.

Building regulations or codes

An application under building regulations covers mainly structure, construction, energy, fire, drainage and prevention of moisture penetration, as well as provision and access for disabled persons. Detailed drawings, specifications and structural calculations must be submitted and approval obtained before construction begins.

Reference is made, in Britain, to fire safety requirements to BS 5588 Part 6: 1991 'Fire Precautions in the design, construction and use of buildings, Code of Practice for places of assembly.'

Provision for disabled persons is similarly covered by BS 5180 1979 'Access for the Disabled to Buildings' and by BS 5588 Part 8: 1988 'Code of Practice for Means of Escape for Disabled People'.

BS 5588 refers to new buildings. Existing buildings are covered by the advisory document, the 'Home Office Manual: Guide to Fire Precautions in existing Places of Entertainment and Like Premises'.

Fire officer

The local fire authority requires to inspect and approve premises before issuing a fire certificate. Requirements may include maintenance of means of escape, staff numbers and training and fire drill.

Environmental Health Officer

The local Environmental Health Officer covers the health requirements of the bar and kitchen to the restaurant.

Local licensing court

Formal application is required, to show that local requirements for Places of Public Assembly and Licenced Areas are satisfied. The local licensing authority are able to produce their own requirements covering fire protection, building construction, equipment, safety and their maintenance.

Health and safety

Approval is required from the local Health and Safety Officer and Factory Inspector covering operational areas with technicians, as included in the Health and Safety at Work legislation.

The Health and Safety Executive has produced a *Guide to Health, Safety and Welfare at Pop Concerts and Similar Events*, covering mainly outdoor events and sections on crowd control, organization, stewarding and marquees as well as sound and noise.

Legal constraints

If the land and/or existing building is owned by others, they may impose conditions on the development and their approval will need to be obtained.

15

15 Time-scale

The realistic time-scale for the project requires to be considered, covering time for design, development and construction of the new or adapted building. The period varies according to the size and complexity of the project and may be weeks, months or years. There are several broad aspects which need to be examined and these are considered in the following sections.

Design, development and construction

The programme needs to acknowledge the time taken for each stage in the process, namely:

- client's proposal;
- feasibility;
- briefing process;
- design process;
- building process;
- hand-over;
- opening night.

Specific hurdles and key dates

Specific hurdles and key dates which may influence the programme, such as:

- external circumstances, such as the expiry of a lease on existing premises;
- dates for building commencement and completion, especially if the project is an adaptation of an existing building;
- planning permission, listed building consent, building regulations or codes approval and other permissions;
- financial implications: fund-raising programme, cash flow, income on investment versus interest paid on loan;
- time-scale of allied partners and their funding programme.

Client's decisions and procedure

Certain key decisions condition progress and are concerned with the ability to proceed to a following stage. These cover the decision to proceed from, as examples:

- client's proposal to feasibility study; feasibility study to detailed briefing; detailed briefing to scheme design;
- approval of scheme design;
- selection of contractor.

Decisions may require a formal and perhaps lengthy procedure involving various committees or alternatively a prompt decision may be reached quickly by a few with delegated responsibilities. Time for such decisions needs to be accommodated within the programme.

Existing buildings

For existing buildings for the performing arts which are being altered, then the period of time the building is closed may be critical and will require being reduced to a minimum to avoid loss of income and/or continuity of operation. For highly-restricted time periods and extensive adaptation then it may be necessary for prefabricated components to be prepared before closure.

Permanent or temporary building

The period of time the building is to function may vary and it could be a:

- permanent building;
- temporary building for a one-off event or restricted period of time, after which the building is removed;
- temporary conversion of an existing building;
- mobile building.

Staged development

A project may be designed to develop over time, i.e. the total complex consists of stages erected over varying periods of time, following, as examples, audience development programmes and cash-flow restrictions.

Other factors

Many factors can affect the time-scale of a project as it progresses, for example the consequence of seasons on building operations, the quality of work done, the availability of manpower and so on.

16

16 Financial appraisal

The financing of the project is often the most critical of the issues considered within the feasibility study. The client needs to identify the extent and sources of the capital costs, revenue costs and income, while the level of subsidy (if applicable) requires to be established and acknowledged. All estimates of costs need to allow for inflation across the design and development period of time.

Financial appraisal covers the following:

- cost estimates: identifying and estimating the capital cost, revenue costs and income;
- sources of capital funds;
- construction costs;
- cost planning;
- cash flow;
- financial viability.

Cost estimates

The cost estimates include the items discussed in the following three sections.

Capital expenditure

Capital expenditure refers to all the one-off costs required to achieve the building. For each of the proposed alternative layouts, the estimate of the capital expenditure should be established covering the following:

- Site purchase cost, including acquisition, site survey and soil investigation. The site may be leased at a nominal or market level.
- Demolition costs if the site contains existing buildings which have to be moved.
- Purchase costs of an existing building for conversion (if applicable), including fabric, structural and other surveys of the building.
- Construction costs, including allocation for fittings, furniture and specialist equipment as well as any infrastructure (roads, pedestrian routes, sewers, electricity cables and so on) and external works (parking, landscape, open spaces and so on).
- Associated design costs covering the work of the architect and other members of the design team as fees and expenses. Design fees are usually a percentage of the construction costs.
- Specialist advisors to the client such as solicitor, fund raiser, surveyor as fees and expenses. Such fees are usually calculated on an hourly charge or a lump sum.
- Client organization costs: project manager, fund raising, public relations, publicity and general administration of the project as well as travel and training costs, fees for planning and building control application and company registration.
- Bridging loan costs if necessary before funds are available.

Estimates of capital expenditure should be kept under review as the project progresses and at the completion of each stage in the design process the construction costs need to be checked against the initial estimates.

In addition funding, as a discrete sum, is required for the feasibility study.

Running costs

For each of the alternative layouts, the estimate of the running costs should be established. The client's policy on running costs – operational and maintenance requirements – should be considered at each stage of the design process. Not only will the running costs represent an increasing expense during the life of the completed building, but the success of a building design will probably be judged largely on the level of running costs with the lower cost being regarded as satisfactory. Costs cover:

- *Fixed costs*: Financing any loan, depreciation, rent, lease, local taxes, security, insurance and administrative overheads including staffing.
- *Semi-fixed costs*: Power, lighting, heating, ventilation, water rates, cleaning, maintenance of the building and services, redecoration and equipment replacement.
- *Production costs if a resident company*: Employment of performers, technical and company staff as well as publicity, marketing, materials and production of scenery, properties and costumes.

Careful planning can assist in reducing staff costs while a selection of materials and method of construction which require minimal or no maintenance will reduce the running costs. A trade-off will be necessary between increased capital expenditure and the cost of maintenance over the life span of the building. Similarly an increased capital expenditure can reduce the energy consumption costs over the life span.

Income

The prediction of income is important to the feasibility of the project, including the effect on the total capital sum. Certain sources of income may place conditions on the brief: sponsorship may necessitate entertaining facilities, while meeting rooms for hire may be included. Sources of income include the following:

- Admission charges. Income relates to audience capacity in the auditorium and the predicted number of people who will attend performance as a percentage of the audience capacity. Income also relates to the pricing of the admission tickets which may range form zero to the economic rate without subsidy. Pricing relates to the policy of the client's organization and is usually a balance between as much income from ticket sales as possible while not discouraging purchase by those in the catchment area.
- Sales: performance programme and advertising within, food and beverage, shops.

- Hire of facilities: art gallery, exhibition space, meeting room as well as the auditorium for conference and lectures.
- Hire of costumes and scenery: manufacture of costumes, properties and scenery for other companies.
- Franchise of bars and places to eat.
- Percentage of profit of touring performances initiated at the building and associated copyright.
- Hire by touring companies as lump sum or percentage of the profits.
- Annual grants from local, central government and regional arts boards, as well as other funding institutions.
- Sponsorship by individuals, companies, industry and institutions of productions or specific functions.
- Club membership subscription.

Sources of capital funds

A characteristic of the majority of buildings for the performing arts is the many sources of funds there may be for a single project, acquired from a broad base of contribution. Sources of funds may affect the phasing of the building programme or incorporation of special facilities. Sources include the following:

- One-off grants from local and central government, tourist authority, European Union, development corporation, regional arts boards and other similar organizations.
- Loans from local government, banks and financial institutions.
- Fund-raising activities from local businesses and industry, special events, individuals and charitable benefactors, including trusts and foundations.
- Sale of assets of existing building and land, if for example, a company owns its own facilities and is re-locating.
- Allocation within a large commercial project as part of a development brief, such as a lump sum contribution or part/total construction of the building by the developer.

The client should check the availability of funds and any constraints of time and conditions imposed by the funders. Experience from comparable client organizations and advisory bodies on fund raising should be sought.

Construction costs (Fig. 16.1)

Estimates of capital cost for the construction of a building are generally calculated by using a cost per square metre of floor area, based on an analysis of costs of the same, or similar, requirements in an actual construction of a particular building type. However buildings for the performing arts are not readily or usefully subject to a cost per square metre basis because there is a considerable variation between the auditorium costs and those of the ancillary accommodation.

The cost per seat, i.e. a multiplication of the number of seats in the auditorium by a cost index for one seat to give the overall cost of the building, does not recognize the variation of ancillary accommodation between, for example, a building hosting touring companies only and one with a resident company requiring production spaces.

One method is to recognize variation in construction, standards and finishes between different functional parts of the overall building: these cover the auditorium and platform/stage, other areas inside the building and external work and infrastructure.

The auditorium and platform/stage

These volumes will include large spans, possible complex geometry to the auditorium with air-conditioning, sound insulation and acoustic treatment. Stage and platform equipment and, if applicable, a flytower and its mechanism are items peculiar to the building type and their costs need to be established.

If the auditorium and platform/stage is an uncommitted space with raked seating and staging created within a simple shell for each production, then the shell with its services could be costed separately with the seating and staging occurring under specialist items or even running costs.

Multi-purpose auditoria will generate some mobile units: bleacher seating, rostra, air units and so on. These may be costed under specialist items.

The costing may be calculated on a cost per square metre basis, cost per seat or a combination, with specialist items as a separate heading. Application of a cost per seat will depend on the standard of comfort provided. Various categories can be identified ranging from a low level of space standard found in say a studio theatre with bench seating and minimum knee room (0.35 m^2) to luxurious level (0.90 m^2) with costs ranging from £40–200+.

Other areas

These include:

- public spaces;
- performance organization;
- performers' spaces;
- management spaces;
- storage;
- production spaces (if applicable).

Capital costs for construction can be based on the requirements identified during the development of the brief and include floor area required, the use to which each space is put, level of services (heating, ventilation, lighting, security, fire prevention) and the standard of finishes, fittings and equipment. For each of these main areas an estimate can be derived on a cost per square metre basis with information from comparable examples: the dressing and changing rooms for the performers may be comparable, in cost

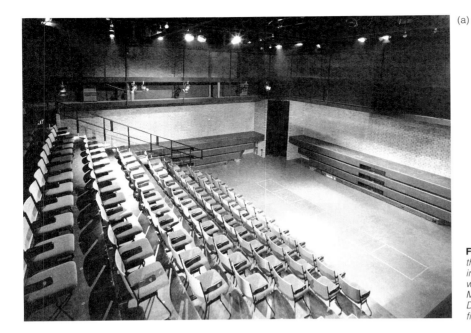

(a)

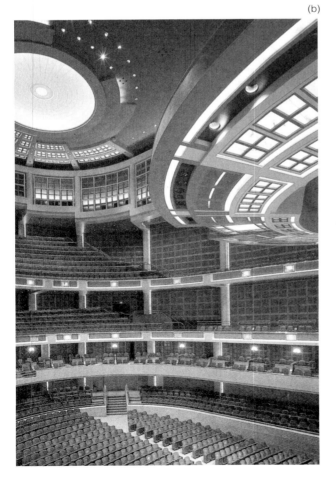

(b)

Fig. 16.1 *Expression. Expenditure on (a) the Cockpit Arts Centre, London – inexpensive, conspicuous thrift – contrasts with the concert hall interior of the (b) Morton H Meyerson Symphony Centre in Dallas, where brass, onyx and cherry wood finishes display a conscious quality*

terms, to domestic buildings, while the production workshops are similar to light industrial units.

External works and infrastructure

External works include all construction work beyond the building but within the site. Costs can be derived from comparable examples not necessarily associated with buildings for the performing arts.

A parallel calculation is the cost of the building in use covering maintenance, heating, lighting and ventilation: such costs relate to the capital expenditure on construction and quality of finishes, services installation and design details.

Cost planning

Once a realistic estimate is agreed a cost plan can be prepared. The plan allocates parts of the total cost to individual elements of the building: roof, external walls, wall finishes, heating installation and so on. It is a framework which can influence decision-making and can assist the detailed design and specification. Adjustments can be made through the design process but a cost plan allows a controlled approach whereby additional expenditure on one element is balanced by savings on others. The design team can therefore monitor the costing within these guidelines as part of the design process.

A further reason for the cost planning of a project is to ensure that the final cost of a building project does not exceed the client's original budget figure. The feasibility study should contain the cost limitations, set by the client, and a realistic estimate of the construction and other capital costs. A start should be made on analysing and controlling costs as early as possible within the briefing and design processes. This will avoid the costly and time-consuming changes that result when it is discovered that costs exceed the budget after a design has been prepared.

Cash flow

The ability to pay for the building and cover all costs is essential so that not only is there sufficient funding but also that there are sufficient funds available on a monthly basis to cover expenditure. The building project will last several years from clients' proposal to the completion of the construction and cash flow planning will be necessary so that available money matches expenditure. Grants may be given only after completion of a particular stage in the development and money may need to be borrowed, with subsequent charges, until the grants are handed over.

The major expenditure lies with the construction costs and the contracts payments usually stipulate on a monthly basis. The pattern of payment tends to follow a curve over the contract period i.e. the amount of the monthly payments start relatively low, increase during the middle period and then tail off towards the end.

The majority of the work of the design team occurs before the contract following the feasibility study, and payment tends to be made at the end of each stage of the design process. Feasibility is a minor expenditure in comparison to the building and design costs and may be subject to a separate funding arrangement.

Administrative costs are usually at a constant level through the whole of the project with certain peaks of expenditure due to publicity at completion of the various stages and opportunities within the building process.

Financial viability

There are two levels of financial viability involved in the costs associated with buildings for the performing arts: project cost–feasibility and cost–benefit analysis.

- *Project cost–feasibility* is concerned with the simple financial balance between capital costs, sources of funds, running costs and income generated. The calculations have to be seen against the financial objectives of either non-profit making with the necessity of subsidy and sponsorship, or the requirement to achieve a project.
- *Cost–benefit analysis* takes into account a wider perspective and is concerned with the identification of the economic (and other) benefits to the community or parent organization as a whole, especially to justify capital grants and income subsidy. These benefits may include:
  - employment of construction workers and professionals in the design and erection of the building, including suppliers of materials and components;
  - employment of management, technical and company staff and the performers in the building;
  - employment in service occupations associated with the functioning of the building including supply of materials, graphic design, production of posters and programmes and so on, as well as the specialist shops selling music scores, books, outfits and so on, established due to interest and participation in the performing arts generated by the proposal;
  - income generated throughout the area as a direct effect of visitor spending, especially where the building, among other possible attractions, is visited by tourists: also income is generated by visiting companies who stay in local hotels for the duration of a production;
  - building for the performing arts as a catalyst to attract new commercial and industrial development to an area.

In addition there are benefits which are less concerned with the local economy and include:

- improved image of, and prestige to, the area;
- social/educational/cultural benefits.

Cost–benefit analysis does not supersede project cost–feasibility but provides supplementary information to justify investment in the performing arts especially by the public sector.

Appendix 1: References and sources of information

General: buildings for the performing arts

Aloi, R. (1958) *Architecture per lo Spettacolo*, Hoepli, Milan

Armstrong, L. and Morgan, R. (1984) *Space for Dance: An Architectural Design Guide*, National Endowment for the Arts

Artaud, A. (1970) *The Theatre and its Double*, John Calder, London

Arts Council (1989) *An Urban Renaissance: sixteen case studies showing the role of the arts in urban regeneration*, Arts Council, London

Arts Council (1986) *Theatre is for all: Report of the Enquiry into Professional Theatre in England*, Arts Council, London

Baker, C. A. (1983) *Practical Law for Arts Administrators*, John Offord, London

Baur-Heinhold, M. (1967) *Baroque Theatre*, Thames and Hudson, London (first German edition, 1966)

Bay, H. (1974) *Stage Design*, Pitman, London

Bentham, F. (1970) *New Theatres in Britain*, Rank Strand, London (case studies from 1958)

Beranek, L. L. (1962) *Music, Acoustics and Architecture*, Wiley, New York (reprinted Krieger, Huntingdon, New York, 1979)

Bianchini, F. and Parkinson, M. (eds.) (1993) *Cultural Policy and Urban Regeneration*, Manchester University Press, Manchester

Billington, M. (1980) *Performing Arts: An Illustrated Guide*, MacDonald, London

Blundell-Jones, P. 'Beyond the Black Box', *Architectural Review*, July 1986, pp. 46–51

Brecht, B. (1973) *Brecht on Theatre – The Development of an Aesthetic*, Methuen, London and New York

Brook, P. (1968) *The Empty Space*, Penguin, Harmondsworth

Brook, P. 'L'Architecture d'Aujourd'hui' No. 152

Brown, C. P., Fleissig, W. B. and Morrish, W. R. (1984) *Building for the Arts*, Western States Arts Foundation, Sante Fe, New Mexico

Burris-Meyer, H. (1975) *Theatres and Auditoriums*, 2nd edition with new supplement (Burris-Meyer and Cole (eds.), Kriefer, R.E. New York, Huntingdon

Collins, V. (1984) *Recreation and the Law*, E. and F. N. Spon, London

Cope, E. (1976) *Performances: Dynamics of a Dance Group*, Lepus Books, London

Cotterell, L. E. (1984) *Performance*, John Offord, London (2nd edition)

Cremer, L. and Muller, H. A. (1982) *Principles and Applications of Room Acoustics*, 2 vols., Applied Science Publishers, London and New York (original German edition 1978).

Davies, A. (1987) *Other Theatres*, Macmillan, London

Department of the Environment *Action for Cities, Dormant Land: Wake it Up!*, leaflet, HMSO, London

Department of the Environment with URBED (1987) *Re-using Redundant Buildings: Good practice in urban regeneration*, Urban and Economic Development Ltd., London

Devlin, G. (1989) *Stepping Forward: Some suggestions for the development of dance in England during the 1990s*, Arts Council, London

Diggle, K. (1984) *Arts Marketing*, Rhinegold, London

England, A. (1990) *Theatre for the Young*, Macmillan, London

Foley, M. (1994) *Dance Spaces*, Arts Council, London

Forsyth, M. (1985) *Buildings for Music*, Cambridge University Press, Cambridge

Forsyth, M. (1987) *Auditoria: Design for the Performing Arts*, Batsford, London

Goodwin, J. (1989) *British Theatre Design*, Weidenfeld & Nicholson, London

Ham, R. with the Association of British Theatre Technicians (1987) *Theatres: Planning Guidance for Design and Adaptation*, Butterworth Architecture, Oxford

Hartnoll, P. (ed.) (1983) *Oxford Companion to the Theatre*, 4th edition, Oxford University Press, London

Hawkins, T. and Menear, P. *Stage Management and Theatre Administration*, A Phaidon Theatre Manual, Phaidon, Oxford

Health and Safety Commission/Home Office/The Scottish Office (1993) *Guide to the Health, Safety and Welfare at Pop Concerts and Similar Events*, HMSO, London

Holt, M. (1993) *Stage Design and Properties*, Phaidon, London

Hutchison, R. and Feist, A. (1991) *Amateur Arts in the UK*, Policy Studies Institute, London

Izenour, G. C. (1977) *Theatre Design*, McGraw-Hill, New York

Knappe, J. M. (1989) *The Magic of Opera*, Da Capo Press, New York

Lawson, F. (1988) *Restaurants, Clubs and Bars*, Butterworth Architecture, Oxford

Leacroft, R. (1973) *The Development of the English Playhouse*, Methuen, London and New York

Leacroft, R. and Leacroft, H. (1984) *Theatre and Playhouse*, Methuen, London

Lord, P. and Templeton, D. (1983) *Detailing for Acoustics*, Butterworth Architecture, Oxford

Lord, P. and Templeton, D. (1986) *The Architecture of Sound: planning and designing auditoria*, Butterworth Architecture, Oxford

Lounsberry, W. (1967) *Theatre Backstage*, University of Washington, Washington, DC

Macintosh, I., Sell, M. and Glasstone, V. (1982) *Curtains!!! or a New Life for Old Theatres*, John Offord, London

Mackenzie, R. K. (ed.) (1980) *Auditorium Acoustics*, Applied Science Publishers, London

Mackintosh, I. (1993) *Architecture, Actor and Audience*, Routledge, London

Marsh, C. (1989) *Planning Gain*, Planning Aid for London, London

Mulryne, R. and Shewing, M. (ed.) (1995) *Making Space for Theatre*, Mulryne and Shewing Ltd, Stratford-upon-Avon

Myerscough, J. (1988) *The Economic Importance of the Arts in Britain*, The Policy Studies Institute, London

Neufert, E. (ed.) (1980) *Architects' Data*, Granada Publishing Ltd, London and Halsted Press, New York

Nicholl, A. (1966) *The Development of the Theatre*, Harrap, London

Orrey, L. (1991) *A Concise History of Opera*, Thames & Hudson, London

Parker, W. (1968) *Scene Design and Stage Lighting*, Reinhart & Winston, New York

Parker, R. (ed.) (1994) *The Oxford Illustrated History of Opera*, Oxford University Press, Oxford

Pevsner, N. (1991) *A History of Building Types*, Thames & Hudson, London

Pilbrow, R. (1979) *Stage Lighting*, Cassell, London, 2nd edition

Pruen, J. and Paul, J. (1988) *Safety in the Built Environment*, Butterworth Architecture, London

Reid, F. (1982) *The Stage Lighting Handbook*, Adam and Charles Black, London, 2nd edition

Reid, F. (1978) *The Staging Handbook*, Pitman Publishing Ltd, London, and Theatre Arts Books, New York (reprinted Adam and Charles Black, 1983)

Reid, F. (1983) *Theatre Administration*, Adam and Charles Black, London

Reid, F. (1989) *Designing for the Theatre*, A & C Black, London

Rettinger, M. (1973) *Acoustic Design and Noise Control*, Chemical Publishing Company, New York

Rodgers, P. (1989) *The Work of Art: A Summary of the Economic Importance of the Arts in Britain*, Calouste Gulbenkian Foundation, Policy Studies Institute, London

Roose-Evans, J. (1984) *Experimental Theatre*, Routledge, London and New York

Schubert, H. (1971) *The Modern Theatre*, Pall Mall Press, London

Strong, J. (1990) *The Arts Council Guide to Building for the Arts*, Arts Council, London

Sweeting, E. (1969) *Theatre Administration*, Pitman, London

Tidworth, S. (1973) *Theatres, an Architectural and Cultural History*, Pall Mall Press, London

Warre, M. (1967) *Designing and Making Scenery*, Studio Vista, London

Wickham, G. (1985) *A History of the Theatre*, Phaidon, Oxford

de Zuvillaga, 'The Disintegration of Theatrical Space', *Architectural Association Quarterly*, Vol. 8, No. 4, 1976, pp. 24–31

Journals which are concerned with design and technology include:

ABTT Newsletter, Assocation of British Theatre Technicians, London
Actualité de la Scénographic, Paris
Acustics, Stuttgart
Applied Acoustics, Barking, Essex
Bauten der Kultur, Berlin (GDR)
Buhnentechnische Rundschau, Zurich
Cue, London
Journal of the Acoustical Society of America, New York
Journal of Japanese Institute for Theatre Technology, Tokyo
Journal of Sound and Vibration, London and New York
Sightline, Association of British Theatre Technicians, London
Theatre Crafts, Rodale Press Inc., Emmaus, USA
Theatre Design and Technology, Journal of the US Institute of Theatre Technology, New York

Magazines which illustrate buildings for the performing arts include:

A & U (Architecture & Urbanism), Tokyo
Architect (formerly *RIBA Journal*), London
Architects' Journal, London
Architectural Record, New York
Architectural Review, London
Architecture d'aujourd'hui, Paris
Architecture Today, London
Arkitektur DK, Copenhagen
Arkitectur, Stockholm
Baumeister, Munich
Building, London
Canadian Architect, Don Mills, Ontario
Casabella, Milan
Domus, Milan
Progressive Architecture, Stamford, CT
Werk, Bauen and Wohnen, Zurich

Provision for disabled persons

British Standards Institution (1979) 'Code of Practice for Access for the Disabled to Buildings: BS5819', BSI, Milton Keynes
Carnegie UK Trust (1988) *After Attenborough*, Carnegie UK Trust, Fife
Centre for Accessible Environments (1990) *Access Provision: Alterations and Extensions to Existing Public Buildings*, London
Centre on Environment for the Handicapped (1985) *Implementing Accessibility – Access Committee for England*, London
Department of Health and Social Security (1979) 'Can disabled people go where you go?', Silver Jubilee Committee on Improving Access for Disabled People, HMSO, London
Earnscliffe, J. (1992) *In Through the Front Door*, The Arts Council of Great Britain, London
Goldsmith, S. (1976) *Designing for the Disabled*, Royal Institute of British Architects, London, 3rd edition
Harkness, S. and Groom, J. N. (1976) *Building without Barriers for the Disabled*, Whitney, New York
London Boroughs Disability Resource Team (1988) *Towards Integration – The Participation of People with Disabilities in Planning*, London Strategic Policy Unit, London
Lord, G. (ed.) (1982) *The Arts and Disabilities. A Creative Response to Social Handicap*, Carnegie UK Trust, Fife

Morrison, E. (1991) *Equal Opportunities Policy and Practice – Disability*, Independent Theatre Council, London
Richards, A. (1988) 'Able to attend: a good practice guide on access to events for disabled people', National Council for Voluntary Organisations, London
Royal National Institute for the Deaf (1989) *Installation Guidelines for Induction Loops in Public Places*, RNID, London
Royal National Institute for the Deaf (1989) *A List of Audio Frequency Induction Loop Installers*, RNID, London
Thorpe, S. (1986) *Designing for People with Sensory Impairments*, Centre on Environment for the Handicapped, London
Thorpe, S. (1986) *Reading Plans – Layman's Guide to the Interpretation of Architects' Drawings*, Access Committee for England and Centre on Environment for the Handicapped, London

Fund raising

Blume, H. (1977) *Fundraising – A Comprehensive Handbook*, Routledge and Heagan Paul, London and New York
Doulton, A.M. (1994) *The Arts Funding Guide*, The Directory of Social Change, London (bi-annual publication)
Fitzherbert, L. and Forrester, S. (ed.) (1986) *A Guide to the Major Trusts*, The Directory of Social Change, London
Also
Bread and Circuses: information magazine on cultural developments in Europe. From IETM, 143 Boulevard Anspach, 1000 Brussels, Belgium
The Directory of Grant Making Trusts. Charities Aid Foundation, 48 Pembury Road, Tonbridge, Kent TN9 2JD

General references

Books

Bailey, S. (1990) *Offices*, Butterworth, Oxford
Bathurst, P. E. and Butler, D. A. (1980) *Building Cost Control Techniques*, (2nd edition), Heinemann, London
Beaven, L. and Dry, D. (1983) *The Architect's Job Book*, (4th edition), RIBA Publications, London
Cartlidge, D. P. and Mehrtens, E. N. (1982) *Practical Cost Planning*, Hutchison, London
Ferry, D. J. (1980) *Cost Planning of Buildings*, (4th edition revised by T. Brandon), Granada, London
Kemper, A. M. (1979) *Architectural Handbook: Environmental Analysis, Architectural Programming, Design and Technology, and Construction*, Wiley, New York
Lacey, R. E. (1978) *Climate and Building in Britain*, HMSO, London
Markus, T. A. and Morris, E. N. (1980) *Buildings, Climate and Energy*, Pitman, London
Palmer, M. A. (1981) *The Architect's Guide to Facility Programming*, American Institute of Architects, Washington
Preiser, W. (ed.) (1978) *Facility Programming: Methods and Applications*, Dowden, Hutchinson & Ross, Stroudsburg, PA
Speaight, A. and Stone, G. (1990) *AJ Legal Handbook*, (5th edition), Butterworth Architecture, Oxford
Tutt, P. and Adler, D. (eds.) (1979) *New Metric Handbook*, Butterworth Architecture
Underwood, G. (1984) *The Security of Buildings*, Butterworths, London
Vandenberg, M. and Elder, A. J. (eds.) (1974) *AJ Handbook of Building Enclosure*, The Architectural Press, London

Appendix 2: Main consultants and clients' advisors

Main consultants

Architects

The Royal Institute of British Architects (RIBA)
66 Portland Place, London W1N 4AD

The Royal Incorporation of Architects in Scotland (RIAS)
15 Rutland Square, Edinburgh EH1 2BE

The Royal Society of Ulster Architects (RSUA)
2 Mount Charles, Belfast BTZ 1NZ

The American Institute of Architects
1735 New York Avenue, NW, Washington DC 20006

The architect's role is to work with the client to establish what is needed in terms of spaces and facilities and to design a building which will fulfil these requirements, and additionally to administer a building contract fairly between contractor and client. The architect prepares the drawings and specification on which the contractor tenders and thereafter builds. The architect generally inspects the progress and quality of work.

The architect may be employed solely to assess the suitability of a site or building, or to prepare an outline design or feasibility study.

The three basic fee options are: percentage of the total construction cost; time charges; lump sum. The selection of the appropriate method will depend on various factors, including the service to be provided, the size and type of the project and negotiations between client and architect. The professional bodies will give advice on conditions of appointment and recommended fee scales.

Engineers

The Association of Consulting Engineers
1st Floor, Alliance House, 12 Caxton Street, London SW1H 0QL

The Institution of Civil Engineers (ICE)
1 Great George Street, London SW1P 3AA

The Institution of Structural Engineers (ISE)
11 Upper Belgrave Street, London SW1X 8BH

The Institute of Electrical Engineers
Savoy Place, London WC2R 0BL

The Institute of Mechanical Engineers
1 Birdcage Walk, Westminster, London SW1H 9JX

The American Institute of Consulting Engineers
345E, 47th Street, New York NY 10017

There are two main groups of engineers, civil and structural, and services engineers. From the first group it is usually structural engineers who form part of the design team, and assist with the design of the building sub-structure and superstructure. Services engineers are appointed to assist with the design of environmental control aspects, such as lighting, heating and air conditioning, and mechanical services. As these items can represent a high percentage of the total building costs, the appointment of the required consultants at an early stage for them to participate in the briefing process and feasibility studies is recommended. It is normal practice to make these appointments in consultation with the architect.

Advice should be sought from the Association of Consulting Engineers on the conditions of engagement for different types of appointment. They include recommended fee scales as guidelines to fee charging for the services of civil, structural, mechanical and electrical engineering work. Fees are charged either on a time basis, on a percentage of total cost of the building or as a lump sum.

Quantity surveyors

The Royal Institute of Chartered Surveyors (RICS)
12 Great George Street, Parliament Square, London SW1P 3AD

The Royal Institute of Chartered Surveyors in Scotland
7 Manor Place, Edinburgh EH3 7DN

Quantity surveyors work out the detailed construction cost of a building, from preliminary cost advice, estimates of alternative proposals and cost planning through to preparing bills of quantities, negotiating tenders, financial management and valuing work during construction, and the preparation of the final account. They form part of the design team and would normally be appointed in consultation with the architect.

Recommended fee scales are published by the RICS. The method of charging depends on the scale or complexity of the project, is on a time basis, on a percentage of the total building cost or as a lump sum.

Theatre consultants

Society of Theatre Consultants
47 Bermondsey Street, London SE1 3XT

Theatre consultants advise on management and feasibility studies, design briefs, general planning, auditorium studies and production requirements. Detailed technical advice covers the full equipment range from stage lighting and sound communications, stage machinery and flying systems. Theatre consultants are normally included in the design team for a performance related arts project.

Stage machinery consultants

Stage machinery consultants provide the same technical expertise as the theatre consultant, restricted to stage machinery, flying and other systems related to productions.

Acoustic engineers

Institute of Acoustics
PO Box 320, St Albans, Hertfordshire AL1 1PZ

Association of Noise Consultants
6 Trap Road, Gilden Morden, Royston, Hertfordshire SG8 0JE

Acoustic engineers advise on sound insulation, the design and installation of sound control systems, and how the shape, materials and internal surfaces of a building affect the quality and movement of sound. If an acoustician is to form part of the design team, their appointment is normally made in consultation with the architect.

Landscape consultants

The Landscape Institute
6/7 Barnard Mews, London SW11 1QU

The American Society of Landscape Architects
4401 Connecticut Avenue NW, Washington DC 20008-2302

The landscape consultant can appraise the site conditions, provide site survey information, prepare sketch plans through to contract drawings and specification to obtain tenders, administer the contract and check the work executed. The professional bodies can provide information and methods of fee charging.

Clients' advisors

Accountants

Institute of Chartered Accountants in England and Wales
Chartered Accountants Hall, 2 Moorgate Place, London EC2P 2BJ

Institute of Chartered Accountants in Scotland
27 Queen Street, Edinburgh EH2 1LA

Accountants can advise on cash flow projections, loan facilities, and detailed financial information required for loans and grants.

Building surveyors

The Royal Institution of Chartered Surveyors (RICS)
12 Great George Street, Parliament Square, London SW1P 3AD

The Royal Institute of Chartered Surveyors in Scotland
7 Manor Place, Edinburgh EH3 7DN

A building surveyor can provide a consultancy or an advisory service on a diagnosis of building defects and resultant remedial work, planned maintenance and structural surveys. The institute will give advice on the type of work and recommended fee scales.

Clerk of works

The Institute of Clerk of Works of Great Britain
41 The Mall, Ealing, London W5 3TJ

The clerk of works inspects the building work on site on behalf of the employer under the directions of the architect. If the client organization does not employ a clerk of works as part of their permanent staff, consultation on selection should be made with the architect and the clerk of works' appointment initiated prior to the tendering stage of the project.
     The institute will advise on appointments and conditions of contract.

Disabled persons consultants

Centre for Accessible Environments
60 Gainsford Street, London SE1 2NY

This organization provides an architectural advisory service, which consists of a register of architects who have expertise in provision for the disabled for different building types.

Fund-raising consultants

Institute of Charity Fundraising Managers
208/210 Market Towers, 1 Nine Elms Lane, London SW8 5NQ

The fund raisers advice on current practice, legislation on sponsorship and charitable giving, sources of finance and planning and overseeing a fund-raising campaign.

Graphic designers and interior designers

The Chartered Society of Designers
29 Bedford Square, London WC1B 3EG

International Interior Designers Association
341 Merchandise Mart
Chicago, IL 60654

Graphic and interior designers generally provide similar design and technical services to those of an architect but restricted to exhibitions and interiors. A design consultant may also be commissioned in an advisory capacity or for particular services.

Insurance advisers

British Insurance and Investment Brokers Association
BIIBA House, 14 Bevis Marks, London EC3A 7NT

Insurance advisers deal with aspects of insurance cover during the building process and after occupation.

Land surveyors

The Royal Institution of Chartered Surveyors (RICS)
12 Great George Street, Parliament Square, London SW1P 3AD

The Royal Institution of Chartered Surveyors in Scotland
7 Manor Place, Edinburgh EH3 7DN

Land surveyors cover surveys of property boundaries, sites, buildings, setting out of buildings, aerial photography and photogrammetry.

Lighting designers

The International Association of Lighting Designers (IALD)
1 Bovingdon Green, Bovingdon, Hertfordshire HP3 0LD

The International Association of Lighting Designers (IALD)
18 East 16 Street, Suite 208, New York, NY 10003–3193

This association provides lists of members who specialize in lighting design, normally working in close association with the architect in the project.

Management consultants

Institute of Management Consultants
5th Floor, 32–33 Hatton Gardens, London EC1N 8DL

Institute of Leisure and Amenity Management (ILAM)
Lower Basildon, Reading, Berkshire RG8 9NE

A management consultant can advise on the structure of the organization, programme planning, staffing structures and facility requirements.

Planning consultants

Royal Town Planning Institute
26 Portland Place, London W1N 4BE

Royal Town Planning Institute
15 Rutland Square, Edinburgh EH1 2BE

A planning consultant can be appointed where issues of planning law require specialist advice.

Public relations consultants

Public Relations Consultants Association
Willow House, Willow Place, Victoria, London SW1P 1JH

Public relations consultants undertake research to determine if support exists for a project, advise on how this support can be activated, establish links with the press and media, and help with the design and presentation of material and other aspects of a publicity campaign.

Security consultants

British Security Industry Association
Security House, Barbourne Road, Worcester WR1 1RS

Security consultants can advise on guard and patrol, security systems, CCTV, safe and lock and security equipment.

Solicitors

The Law Society
113 Chancery Lane, London WC2A 1PL

The Law Society of Scotland
26 Drumsheugh Gardens, Edinburgh EH3 7YR

A solicitor advises on matters which have legal connotations, such as entering into any form of contract, setting up a company or registering as a charity.

Valuers

Incorporated Society of Valuers and Auctioneers,
3 Cadogan Gate, London SW1X 0AS

Valuers can advise on the market value of a site or property. They are often qualified surveyors, working in a firm of estate agents, valuers and surveyors.

Advisory organizations

The main advisory organizations covering the performing arts are:

Association of British Theatre Technicians (ABTT)
47 Bermondsey Street, London Se1 3XT

The United States Institute of Theatre Technology (USITT)
1501 Broadway, New York, NY 10036, USA

Other organizations:

Arts Council of England
14 Great Peter Street, London SW19 3NQ

Arts Development Association (ADA)
The Arts Centre, Vane Terrace, Darlington, County Durham DL3 7AX

Association of Community Technical Aid Centres Ltd.
Royal Institution, Colquitt Street, Liverpool L1 4DE

Centre on Environment for the Handicapped
35 Great Smith Street, London SW19 3B

Business in the Community
227a City Road, London EC1V 1LX

Charities Aid Foundation
48 Pembury Road, Tonbridge, Kent TN9 2JD

Charity Commission
St Alban's House, 57–60 Haymarket, London SW1

Crafts Council
1 Oxendon Street, London SW1E 5EH

European Union (EU)
European Social Fund Unit, Department of Employment, 11 Belgrave Street, London SW1V 1RB

Independent Theatres Council,
4 Baden Place, Crosby Row, London SE1 1YN

National Council for Voluntary Organisations
26 Bedford Square, London WC1B 3HU

Scottish Arts Council,
12 Manor Place, Edinburgh EH3 7DD

Theatrical Management Association,
Bedford Chambers, The Piazza, Covent Garden, London WC2 HQ

Theatres Trust,
10 St Martins Court, London WC12 4AJ

Welsh Arts Council,
Holst House, Museum Place, Cardiff CF1 3NX

Index

Aalto, Alvar, 134, 209
Aartelo and Piironen, 46
Abbey Theatre, Dublin
    view of public face, and canopy, 160
access, 98 *see also* circulation;
        entrances; foyers; wheelchairs
    box offices, 188
    for deliveries, 185, 195
    for disabled persons, 115, 120, 188,
        189, 201
    and location of supplementary
        facilities, 186, 187, 188
    performance lighting, 182–183
    staff restrooms, 189
acoustic performance, 112–113
acoustic strategy, 203–204
acoustics, 36–37 *see also*
        amplification; recording studios;
        sound control rooms
    for auditoria, design considerations,
        111–112
    classical music, 103–104
    computer-aided design, 113
    insulation and noise, 114
    model simulation, 112
    physical adjustment, 112–114
    and seating, 115
    and site surveys, 98
adaptation, 83, 102 *see also*
        conversion
    and building surveys, 99
    examples of, 36, 45, 64–65, 107–108
    multi-purpose formats, 108
advisory organisations, 223
air-conditioning, 129–130, 205
Alhambra, Bradford
    emphasized proscenium opening,
        142
amateur companies, 173
amphitheatres, 64–65, 110
amplification, 11, 104, 109, 114, 131
    sound mixing, 183
Amsterdam Opera House
    foyer design and layout, 165
Appleton Partnership, 43, 135, 152,
    163
approvals and legislation, 209
arenas, 23, 24, 35–36
art works, 206 *see also* exhibitions
Arthur Erickson/Mathers and Haldenby
    Associated Architects, 133
arts workshops or centres, 24, 49–51
Arup Associates, 65, 136
Atelier One, 63
audience surveys *see* surveys
audiences, 84
    actual and potential, 92–93, 94
    assessment of demand, 92–94
    attendance phases, 14
    characteristics, 14, 93
    trends, 14–15
auditorium character
    examples of, 133–137
    explanation of, 132–133
auditorium design, 84, 102–133,
        134–137 *see also* multi-purpose
        formats; open stage formats;
        proscenium formats

acoustics, 111–114
adaptation, 123–124
air-conditioning, heating and
    ventilation, 129–130
attendants, 123
aural and visual limitations, 109
broadcasting requirements, 123
cabaret layout, 129
ceiling zone, 132
circulation, 120–122
definitions and checklist, 102
escape, means of, 120
fire protection, 131
latecomers, 123
levels, 110–111
lighting, 130–131
promenade performance, 129
seating capacity, 132
seating layout, 114–120
sightlines, 124–128
sound equipment, 131
sound insulation and noise control,
    114
standing, 129
structure, 131–132
wheelchair location, 122–123
auditorium forms, 104, 105

balconies, 110–111
    sightlines, 126, 127, 128
balcony handrails, 111,112
ballet *see* dance
Barbican Theatre, London
    view of balconies and side slips, 110
Barton Hall, Horndean Community
    School, Hampshire
    external and internal views, plan and
        traverse section, 52
Bastille Opera House, Paris
    sketch of public face, and arch, 160
Bayreuth, Germany, 9
Berlin City Council, 27
Berlin Philharmonic
    foyer design and layout, 164
    interior view, auditorium, 134
    massing, 209
    orchestra stage, 138
    seating, 117
    view of public face, and canopy, 160
Berlin Philharmonic Orchestra, 27
Birmingham Arena
    internal views and plan, 35–36
Birmingham City Council, 35
Birmingham Symphony Hall
    interior view, auditorium, rectangular
        box, 133
    orchestra stage, 138
box offices, 161, 187–188
    plan and section, 189
boxes, 110–111
brief writers, 86–87
briefing process, 85–87 *see also*
        feasibility studies
    identification of user's requirements,
        86–87
briefs *see* briefing process
broadcasting and recording, 131
Broadgate, London

external view, open space, 65
building codes *see* building regulations
building design considerations,
        200–210
    checklist, 200
    relationships between functions, 200,
        201, 202
building maintenance, 88, 190
building process, 88
building regulations, 209–210
building surveys *see* surveys
building types, 22–25 *see under*
        specific category
    checklist, 22
    locational hierarchy, 22–25
buildings in use *see* building
    maintenance
buildings, existing, 96, 99, 212
buildings, temporary, 63–64, 212

canopies, 59, 159, 160–161
capital funds, sources, 215
catering, 192 *see also* refreshments
ceiling zone, 132
Center Stage, Baltimore
    interior view, 90 degree fan and
        shallow balcony, 136
Centre Pompidou, 36
Chaix, Philippe and Jean-Paul Morel,
    34
Chamber Music Hall, Berlin
    external and interior views, and long
        section, 27–28
chamber music, 27–28
changing rooms, 171–174
    associated areas, 175–176
    dance, 172
    location and access, 176
    multi-auditoria centres, 173
    musicals, 173
    opera, 171–172
    orchestral and choral, 171
    pop/rock and jazz, 171
    requirements, 173
choral music, 8
    changing rooms, 172
    company organization, 191
    performers' spaces, relationship
        between, 179
    proscenium formats, 102–104
    sightlines, 124, 125, 128
    venues, 26–27
    visual limitations, 109
Christchurch Town Hall, Sussex
    interior view, auditorium, 134
circulation
    auditorium access, 165–167
    and design considerations, 201–203
    routes, 162–167
    vertical, 166, 167
    within auditorium, 120–122
City of Edinburgh District Council, 49
Civic Theatre, Helsinki
    massing, 208
    stage layout, 140
    view of public face, and canopy, 160
cleaning, 190, 205

Clickhinin Leisure Centre, Shetland
Islands
exterior and interior views, and plan,
53–54
client partnerships, 72
client types and roles *see also* clients,
in design and development
process
commercial sector, 18–19, 72, 73
community organizations, 19, 72
educational institutions, 18, 72
local government, 18, 72, 73
private trusts/independent
organizations, 19, 73
voluntary sector, 19, 72
client's proposals
associated activities, 82
development options, 82–83
formulation of ideas and outline of
requirements, 80
objectives checklists, 81–82
reason for building, 80–81
scope, 82
clients' advisors, 222–223 *see also*
clients, in design and development
process
clients, in design and development
process *see also* briefing process;
feasibility studies
advisors, 75, 222–223
decision-making, 212
checklist, 72–73
structure, 73
development committee, 72
initiating, 72
organization, 74
project management, 75
cloakrooms, 161–162
Cockpit Arts Centre, London
expenditure on, 216
combined music, drama and other
functions, 51–52, 136
commissioning, 88
communications, 205
community schools, 24, 52
Compton Verney
massing, 208
Concert Bowl, Kenwood House,
London
general view, 59
concert halls, 23, 26–27, 46, 48
auditorium and platform/stage
formats, 102–103
conference facilities, 26, 35, 43, 46, 52
constraints on development, 98
construction of a new building *see* new
build
construction works, 88
consultants, 78, 86, 87, 222–223 *see
also* briefing process; design
process
contemporary dance *see* dance
contractors, 88
contracts, 88
control rooms *see* lighting control
rooms; sound control rooms;
television and radio transmission
control rooms

conversion, building, 83
examples of, 47, 49, 60, 136, 137
cost plans, 216–217
costs *see also* feasibility studies
and cash flow, 217
capital expenditure, 214
construction, 215–216
financial viability
cost-benefit analysis, 217
project cost-feasibility, 217
income, 214–215
justification of support, 5
planning, 216–217
running, 214
costumes, 185
preparation sequence, 197
courtyard theatre, 110
example of, 48–49
Courtyard Theatre, West Yorkshire
Playhouse, Leeds *see* West
Yorkshire Playhouse, Leeds
crèches, 161
crowd control, 129
Cunningham, Merce, 10

dance, 9–10
changing rooms, 172
company organization, 191
dressing rooms, 172
noise rating, 114
orchestra pit, 145
performers' spaces, relationship
between, 179
proscenium formats, 104
sightlines, 124
stage layout, 140, 141
venues, 29–31, 41–42, 45, 49–51
visual limitations, 109
dates, key, 212
deaf aids, 131
demand studies, 92–93 *see also*
feasibility studies
demolition of old buildings, 96
Denys Lasdun and Partners, 31, 135
derelict sites, 35, 57
Derngate, Northampton
view of main entrance, and plan,
51–52
design and development *see also*
client's proposals; clients, in
design and development;
feasibility studies; briefing
process; building types
definition and context, vii
issues, 70
process, 70
stages in, 80–88, 212
design process
stages in, 87
traditional and alternative methods,
88
development options, 82–83
development policy, 97
dimmer rooms, 182
disabled persons *see also* access;
wheelchairs
consultants, 222
deaf aids, 131

exit routes, 120
external access, 201
gangways, 115
special needs, 158
district centres, 24
functional linkages with other
activities, 96–97
Dixon, Jeremy, 164
drama, 11–12 *see also* theatre
dressing rooms, 173
noise rating, 114
orchestra, 146
performers' spaces, relationship
between, 179
proscenium formats, 104–105
sightlines, 124, 127
stage layout, 140, 141
venues, 23, 24, 31–34, 38–52,
56–58,152,155
dressing rooms, 171–174
associated areas, 175–176
dance, 172
drama, 173
location and access, 176
multi-auditoria centres, 173
musicals, 172
opera, 172
pop/rock, jazz, 171
requirements, 174–175

Edinburgh Theatre Workshop, 49
external view, plan and section,
50–51
electronic music, 198
end stage *see* open stage formats
energy efficiency *see* energy strategy
energy strategy, 204
entrances, 159–162, 162, 163–164
entry points, 120–122
environmental health officers, 210
Epidaurus, Greece, 110
escape, means of, 120, 203 *see also*
exits
gangways, 120–121
travel distance, 120
Euripides, 11
exhibitions, 168–169
exits, 120
experimental music workshops, 36–37
external works *see* landscape and
siting proposals; massing

Faulkener-Brown, Hendy, Watkinson,
Stonor, 53
feasibility studies, 70, 74 *see also*
assessment of demand; audiences
and brief, 85
consideration of local conditions,
83–84
progress of, 84–85
specific areas of study, 84
Festival Theatre, Adelaide
view of stepped and raked boxes,
111
Festival Theatre, Edinburgh
view of public face, 159
financial appraisal, 214–217 *see also*
feasibility studies

finishes and components, 206
Finland National Opera Company, 28
Finlandia, Helsinki
    massing, 209
fire officers, 210
fire protection, 131, 204
Fisher, Mark, 150
flexibility of use, 27, 47–48, 51–55, 62,
    136, 152–156
    multi-use stage, 150–151
floors, flat, 151–152
flytowers, 104, 105, 140, 144–145, 146,
    151, 207
food services see refreshments
form see massing
format selection, 12
foyers, 161, 162–164, 165, 166
Frazer, Vivian, 38
free-standing rigid pneumatic
    structures, 62
functional linkages see site location
fund raising, 74–75, 84, 85 see also
    capital funds, sources; feasibility
    studies
    consultants, 222

gangways, 115, 120–121
    sightlines, 127
Garsington Manor
    view of canopy, isometric and long
        section, 63–64
general policy see provision, pattern of
Georgian Theatre, Richmond,
    Yorkshire, 110
Gibberd Hedes Minns, 36
Gilbert and Sullivan, 10
Glasgow City Council, 27
Globe Theatre, 12
Glyndebourne Opera House, Sussex
    interior view, auditorium, horse-shoe
        form, 135
Graham, Martha, 10
green rooms, 175
Groves-Raines, Nicholas, 39
Guide to Health, Safety and Welfare at
    Pop Concerts and Similar Events,
    210

Hampshire County Council, Architects
    Department, 52
hand over and opening night, 88
handrails, 120–121
Hardy Holyman Pfeiffer Associates,
    137
Harland and Wolff Shipyard, Glasgow
    view of stage, plan and traverse
        section, 107–108
health and safety, 210
Health and Safety Executive, 210
hearing aids see deaf aids
heating and ventilation, 129–130, 205
Hertzberger, Herman, 134
historic building use, 24, 64–65
historic forms, 106
HOK Sports Facilities Group, 35
Holzbauer, Wilhelm and Cees Dam,
    135
Howell Killick Partridge and Amis, 57

Humphries, Mark, 60
Hurd Rolland, 137
Hyuamaki Karhunen Parkkinen, 28

informal external spaces, 23, 24, 65
Institute for Research and Co-
    ordination in Acoustics and Music
    (IRCAM), Paris, 36
    general view and long section, 37
integrated design, 26
invitation of tenders, 87
IRCAM see Institute for Research and
    Co-ordination in Acoustics and
    Music

Jackson's Lane Community Centre
    Association, 47
Jacksons Lane Community Centre,
    London
    general and interior views, and plan,
        47–48
James R. Grieves Associates, 136
James Stirling Michael Wilford and
    Associates, 41, 136
jazz clubs, 60–61
jazz, 10–11
    changing rooms, 171
    loudspeakers, 131
    performers' spaces, relationship
        between, 178
    proscenium formats, 104–105
    sightlines, 127
    stage design, 149–150
    venues, 26–27, 48, 60–61
    visual limitations, 109
John Dangerfield Associates, 62

key dates see dates, key
King's Theatre, Glasgow
    interior view, side boxes, 111
Kirklees Metropolitan Council, Design
    Practice, 137

landscape and siting proposals,
    206–207
Larson, Hans, 208
Law and Dunbar Nasmith Partnership,
    56
Lawrence Bately Theatre, Huddersfield
    interior view, auditorium, conversion,
        137
legal constraints, 210
Levitt Bernstein Associates, 48
licensed bars, 168
licensing court, local, 210
lighting
    artificial, 205
    auditorium, 130–131
    dimmers, 182
    equipment
        repair and maintenance, 185
        storage, 185
    exhibitions, 168
    follow spots, 182–183
    installation, 205
    natural, 205
    performance, 130
lighting control rooms, 181–182

Lincoln Centre, New York, 97
local licensing court see licensing
    court, local
London County Council, 164
loudspeakers, 131
Lyttleton Theatre, Royal National
    Theatre, London
    See Royal National Theatre, London

make-up rooms, 176
Maltings Concert Hall, Snape
    interior view, auditorium, conversion,
        136
management policy, 158, 167, 187
management role, 123
management structure, of buildings,
    73–74 see also client types and
    roles; clients, in design and
    development process
    staff categories, 73
management style, 73
managerial spaces, 186–190
    relationship between activities, 189
market surveys see surveys
Martin, Sir Leslie
    with RMJM, 26
    with William Nimmo & Partners, 43
massing, 207–209
Matcham, Frank, 33
meeting rooms, 169
metropolitan centres, 23
    functional linkages with other
        activities, 96
Michael Hopkins and Partners, 135
Milton Keynes Bowl, Milton Keynes
    general view, and plan, 58–59
Milton Keynes Development
    Corporation, 54, 58
Monteverdi, Claudio, 9
Morton H. Meyerson Symphony Centre,
    Dallas
    expenditure on, 216
    foyer design and layout, 165
Mozart, Wolfgang Amadeus, 9
multi-auditoria complexes, 203
multi-form multi-function theatre, 51–52
multi-purpose formats, 106–108, 152–
    156 see also open stage formats;
    proscenium formats
    seating adaptation, 123–124
multi-purpose halls, 24, 25, 53–54
multi-use, 24, 25, 26–27, 35–36, 41–42,
    45–54
Music Centre, Vredenburg, Utrecht
    foyer design and layout, 166
    interior view, auditorium, square
        plan, 134
musical instruments see also piano
    store
    storage and delivery, 185
musicals, 10
    changing rooms, 173
    company organization, 191
    dressing rooms, 172
    noise rating, 114
    orchestra pit, 145
    performers' spaces, relationship
        between, 179

musicals (*Cont'd*)
proscenium formats, 104
sightlines, 124
stage layout, 141
venues, 45

National Jazz Centre, London
plans and general section, 60
National Theatre Company, 57
neighbourhood centres, 24
functional linkages with other
activities, 96–97
Netherlands Dance Company, 29
Netherlands Dance Theatre, The
Hague, Netherlands, 29
general and interior views, plan and
long section, 29–31
New Bubble Theatre Project, London
layout and long section, 62
new build, 83, 87, 96 *see also* design
process
Newcastle City Council, 45
Noise Rating (NR), 114
non-performance activities *see* box
offices; creches; exhibitions;
meetings rooms; refreshments;
shops; toilets

observation rooms, 184
offices, 180–181 *see also* box offices
administrative, 186–187
child supevisor's, 176
company management, 176
production, 194
touring companies, 176
Old Vic, London
external and internal views, and
plan, 33–34
Olivier Theatre *see* Royal National
Theatre, London
OMA, 29
open stage formats, 12, 102, 104,
105–106
drama, 105
end stage, 104, 105, 146, 154, 156
fan-shaped, 106, 146, 147
opera, dance and musicals, 104
performers' vomitory, 122
pop/rock and jazz, 105
theatre-in-the-round, 55, 106,
147–149, 155
thrust stage, 106, 146–147, 156
traverse stage, 106
open-air auditoria, 23, 24, 58–59
opening night *see* hand over and
opening night
opening of a building *see* hand over
and opening night
Opera House, Amsterdam
form, three-dimensional organization,
207
interior view, auditorium, wide fan,
135
Opera House, Essen
flytower, 207
interior view, auditorium, eccentric
fan proscenium format, 134
stage layout, 140

Opera House, Helsinki, Finland, 28
general view, interior of horse-shoe
auditorium, and plan, 28–29
opera houses, 23, 28–29
opera, 8–9
changing rooms, 171–172
company organization, 191
dressing rooms, 172
noise rating, 114
orchestra pit, 145
performers' spaces, relationship
between, 179
proscenium formats, 104
sightlines, 124
stage layout, 140, 141
venues, 28–29, 41–42, 45, 46, 63
visual limitations, 109
orchestra pit, 145–146
orchestral, 8
changing rooms, 171
company organization, 191
noise rating, 114
performers' spaces, relationship
between, 177
proscenium formats, 102–104
sightlines, 124, 127, 128
stage layout, 141
venues, 26–27, 46–47, 48, 59
visual limitations, 109
organisation, performance *see*
performance organization
outdoor areas, 98
ownership
community organization, 47
educational institution, 41, 43
limited company, 29
local government, 27, 35, 45, 49, 51,
52, 53
national company, 28, 62
private, 63
trust, 31, 39, 43, 48, 54, 56

paint frames, 195
parking, 97–98, 159, 185
partnerships *see* client partnerships
pattern of provision *see* provision,
pattern of
pattern of use, 81, 190 *see also*
demand studies
Pentagram Design, 62
Penttila, Timo, 208
Percy Thomas Partnership, 133
performance areas, 105, 141
performance lighting *see* lighting
performance organization, 176–186,
187, 188
opera, musical dance and drama
supplementary facilities, 180
location and access, 186
supplementary functions, 178–180
orchestral and choral music
supplementary facilities, 177–178
location and access, 186,187
supplementary functions, 177
pop/rock, jazz
supplementary facilites, 180
location and access, 186, 188
performers' spaces, 170–176

associated areas, 175–176
functional relationships
classical music, 177
jazz, 178
musicians, 180
opera, dance, musicals, drama,
179
pop/rock music, 178
performing arts
definition of, 5
Performing Arts Centre, Cornell
University, Ithaca, New York
general and interior views, plan and
perspective, 41–42
rehearsal studio, 193
Peter Moro Partnership, 135, 153, 162
physical therapy rooms, 176
Piano and Rogers, 36
piano store, 185 *see also* musical
instruments
pilot schemes testing demand, 94
Pink Floyd concert tour
temporary stage, 150
Pitlochry Festival Theatre, Pitlochry
general and interior views, plan and
long section, 56–57
Places of Public Assembly and
Licenced Areas, 210
planning applications, 209
plant rooms, 206
platform *see* stage
plumbing and drainage requirements,
205
policy, open, 158
political support, 5–6, 75, 82, 84
pop/rock, 11
changing rooms, 171
company organization, 191
loudspeakers, 131
performers' spaces, relationship
between, 178
proscenium formats, 104–105
sightlines, 125, 127
stage design, 149, 150
standing, 129
venues, 26–27, 34–36, 45
video screens, 150
visual limitations, 109
power points, 205
production information, 87
production spaces, 190–198
trial assembly area, 195
production, types of *see* under specific
category of performing art
project management, 75
properties store rooms, 184–185 *see
also* storage
proposals *see* client's proposals
proscenium formats, 12, 102–108 *see
also* flytowers; multi-purpose
formats
drama, 104–105
with flytower, 140–141
without flytower, 146
fore-stages, 150–151
horizontal sightlines, 128
jazz/pop/rock, 104–195
opera, dance and musicals, 104

orchestral and choral classical music, 102–104
seating, 118–119
small-scale productions, 104
proscenium openings, 141
provision, pattern of, 5–6, 22–23, 186
see also financial appraisal
and politics, 5–6
policy, general and public, 5–6
public funding, 5–6
public policy see provision, pattern of
public spaces, 158–170
outdoor areas, 169–170
type and numbers of users, 158
purpose-built, 27, 28, 29–31, 34–35, 36–37
single direction relationships, 102

Quarry Theatre, West Yorkshire Playhouse, Leeds see West Yorkshire Playhouse, Leeds
Queens Hall, Edinburgh
interior view, auditorium, conversion, 137
quick-change areas/rooms, 184

ramps, 115, 120 see also disabled users
recital rooms, 23, 24, 27–28, 46
for jazz, 104
recording studios, 184
facilities, 197–198
relationship between functions, 198
rectangular box, 102–103
refreshments, 167–168 see also catering
refuse, 184
regional centres, 23–24
functional linkages with other activities, 96–97
rehearsal spaces, 192–194
Renton Howard Wood Levin, 33, 45, 51
resident companies, 18, 73, 94
resorts, 24 see also rural resorts
Richard Hamblett Associates, 49
RMJM, 26
role of management see management role
Rolling Stones tour 1994
temporary stage, 150
Ronnie Scott's Jazz Club, Birmingham, 60
plan, general view and section, 61
rostra, 123–124
Roy Thomson Hall, Toronto
foyer design and layout, 166
interior view, auditorium, elliptical form with two balconies, 133
Royal Festival Hall, London, 111
interior view, side boxes, 111
sketch of canopy, 161
staircase access, 164
Royal Glasgow Concert Hall, 26
external and interior views, plan and long section, 26–27
sub-platform store, 140
view of public face, canopy, 159

Royal National Eisteddfod Mobile Theatre of Wales
external view, 62
Royal National Theatre, London, 31
foyer design and layout, 165
general and interior views, plan and long section 31–33
Lyttleton Theatre
eroded proscenium opening, 142
interior view, proscenium theatre, 135
stage layout, 141
Olivier Theatre, 110, 117
seating, 117
Royal Opera House, London, 73
drawing of public circulation showing two entrances, 164
Royal Scottish Academy of Music and Drama, Glasgow
general view, and plan, 42–43
Royal Theatre, Northampton, 51 see also Derngate, Northampton
rural resorts, 24, 25, 56–57

safety see also health and safety
first aid room, 162
legislation, for standing, 129
safety curtains, 143
Sandy Brown Associates, 60
model simulation, acoustic characteristcs, 112
scenery, 144, 184 see also flytowers; properties store rooms; workshops
scenic projectors, 183
Scharoun, Hans, 134, 163, 208, 209
and Edgar Wisniewski, 27
scheme design, 87
school of music and drama, 42–43
seating
adaptation, 123–124
bleacher, 55, 123
density, 117, 120
fixed, 116
gangways, 115
geometry, 115, 117–119
layout design and dimensions, 114–115
loose, 116
raked, 123–124
and sightlines, 125–127
rows, 115, 117
temporary, 123–124
types, 116–117
and wheelchair locations, 122–123
seating capacity, 110, 114, 115, 117–120 see also
and car parking, 97
by category of building, 132
financial appraisal
maximum and actual, 132
security, 190, 204
consultants, 223
services, integration and distribution, 206
Shakespearean histories, 11
shops, 161
sightlines, 110–111
horizontal (seated audience), 128

stage (platform) height, 138, 140
standing, 129
vertical (seated audience), 124–128
wheelchair users, 122–123
signage, 206
Silva Hall, Hult Centre for the Performing Arts, Eugene Oregon
interior view, auditorium, proscenium form, two balconies, 137
site
acquisition, 75, 98–99
characteristics, 98
checklist, 96–99
conditions, 98
costs, 99
location
development policy, 97
functional linkages, 96–97
site surveys see surveys
sites, single, 97
sound control rooms, 123, 183
sound effects and music see recording studios
sound equipment, 131, 185, 197
sound locks, 197, 203
soundproofing
lighting control room window, 181
television and radio transmission and recording, 183
South Bank Centre, London, 97
sports facilities, 35, 36, 51, 53
Staatgallerie Theatre, Stuttgart
interior views rectangular box, 136
vertical circulation, 166
staffing arrangements see management structure of buildings
stage
access, performers' and scenery, 143
basement, 143
floor, 143–142
fore, 150–151
layouts, 139
with flytower, 140
without flytower, 146
multi-use, 150–151
raised, 151–152
side and rear, 143
temporary, 150
stage design, 133, 138–156 see also main entries open stage formats; proscenium formats
checklist, 102
combination with flat floor, 151–152
jazz music, 149
multi-use stage, 150–151
open stage formats, 146–149
orchestral and choral music, 138–140
pop/rock music, 149, 150
proscenium formats, 140–146
stage door
location and access, 176
stage management, 176–181
stage managers
performance control, 184
Stantonbury Campus Theatre, Milton Keynes

Stantonbury Campus Theatre (*Cont'd*)
  interior view, and plan, rectangular
    box, 54–55
Stockholm Folk Opera, 9
storage, 190
  costumes, 185
  gallery, 168
  lighting equipment, 185
  musical instruments, 185
  piano, 185
  production materials, 195
  properties, 184–185
  scenery, 184
  sound equipment, 185
structure, 206
  auditorium, 131–132
  stage and flytower, 144–145
structures, pre-fabricated, 34–35
structures, temporary, 59, 150
Studio Theatre, Hong Kong Centre for
    the Performing Arts, 153
  stage plans, 156
Studio Theatre, Theatre Royal, Bristol
  interior view, auditorium, 136
surveys
  audience, 92–93
  building, 99
  site, 98–99
Sydney Theatre Company, Walsh Bay,
    Sydney
  interior view, auditorium, plan and
    cross section, 38–39

Tampere Hall, Finland, 46
  external and interior views, plan and
    long section, 46–47
television and radio transmission
    control rooms, 183–184
television cameras, 123
testing of design criteria *see*
    commissioning theatre
  amateur, 24
  commercial, 23, 33–34
  community, 24, 47–49, 54–55
  dance, 23, 29–31
  drama, 11–12, 23–24, 31–34, 38–52,
    56–58, 152–153, 154–155
  mobile, 25, 62
  small- and medium-scale drama, 23,
    24, 38–40, 136, 152–156
  specialist, 57–58
  touring, 24, 26, 29, 35, 43, 45–46,
    48, 51–52
theatre consultants, 78
theatre restoration, 33–34, 45

Theatre Royal, Newcastle, 45
  exterior view, plan and long section,
    45
Theatre Royal, Plymouth
  interior view, auditorium, proscenium
    with two balconies, 136
  public entrance and foyer,
    circulation, 162
  stage layout, 141
Theatre, Mannheim
  massing, 208
  public entrance, 163
Theatre-in-Education programme, 43
theatre-in-the-round *see* open stage
    formats
Tim Ronalds Architects, 47
time-scale, 212
toilets, 162
  staff restrooms, 189
touring companies, 18, 73, 86, 94
  changing and dressing rooms, 171
  location and access for costumes
    and instruments, 186
  offices, 176
  productions, provision for, 192
  relationship between functions, 201
  stage layout, 141
touring music and drama, 24, 45–47,
    51
town centres, 24
  functional linkages with other
    activities, 96–97
transport *see also* parking
  patterns, 93
  production requirements, 198
traverse stage *see* open stage formats
Traverse Theatre, Edinburgh
  exterior and interior views, seating
    layout and section, 39–40
trusts
  ownership, 31, 39, 43, 48, 54, 56
  running of facility, 49
Tyrone Guthrie Theatre, Minneapolis
  seating, 117
  stage layout, thrust stage, 147

university provision, 41–42
urban design context, 207
urban revitalization *see* development
    policy
user requirements *see* briefing process

ventilation *see* heating and ventilation
Verona Amphitheatre, Italy
  general views, 64–65

video screens, 150

Wagner, Wilhelm Richard, 9
wardrobe, 196–197 *see also* costumes
  relationship between activities, 196
Warren and Mahoney, 134
Wembley Arena, London
  interior view and plan, 36
West Yorkshire Playhouse, Leeds, 43
  Courtyard Theatre, 152
    interior view, 153
    plan and section, end stage
      layout, 154
    plan and section, theatre-in-the-
      round, 155
  flytower, 207
  foyer design and layout, 165
  Quarry Theatre
    interior view, auditorium and
      projection view, 44
    interior view, auditorium, 90
      degree fan, 135
    stage layout, 90 degree fan, 147
  rehearsal room, 193
  scenery workshop, 194
  view of public entrance, 43, 163
  view of public face, 160
  wardrobe, 197
wheelchairs, 115, 120, 181 *see also*
    access; disabled users
  access to box offices, 188, 189
  dimensions, 122
  location within the seating, 122–123
wig store and hairdresser's room, 176
Wilde Theatre, Bracknell
  external and interior views, plan and
    long section, 48–49
William Nimmo & Parnters, 43
Williams, Sir Owen, 36
workshops, 194–196
  relationship between activities, 196
  sequence of operations, 195–196

Year of Culture, 1990, 27
Young Vic, London, Young People's
    Theatre Complex
  general and interior views, plan and
    long section, 57–58
youth productions, 57–58 *see also*
    pop/rock

Zenith 2, Montpellier
  external and interior views, plan and
    cross section, 34–35